Yoga Myths Debunked

✔ **Yoga is only for double-jointed people.**

Yoga is for everyone and can be tailored to your individual needs. It doesn't require you to turn into a pretzel.

✔ **Yoga is only for Asian people.**

Yoga originated in the East (India to be precise), but it is universally applicable. Besides, many of its practices have been modified to suit contemporary Western needs and tastes.

✔ **Yoga is just a bunch of mindless exercises.**

The popular image of Yoga as gymnastics is wrong. The physical exercises form only a part of its comprehensive approach. What's more, the exercises are far from mindless but instead call for focus and mindfulness.

✔ **Yoga is only for weaklings.**

Yoga favors a gentle approach, but its advanced exercises certainly call for strength and stamina. Many athletes use Yoga to complement their other forms of exercise.

✔ **You can't gain muscle strength through Yoga.**

Yoga has a whole range of exercises that help strengthen your chest, back, stomach, arm, and leg muscles. Take a look at advanced practitioners; their muscular strength and development may surprise you!

✔ **You need a guru to do Yoga.**

If you couldn't try out some basic Yoga exercises by yourself, we wouldn't have written *Yoga For Dummies.* Consulting with a Yoga teacher or instructor can be helpful, but a guru is only necessary when you want to engage in Yoga as a full-fledged spiritual practice.

✔ **Yoga requires you to believe in all kinds of strange ideas.**

Yoga is based on universal principles shared by many other systems that have a holistic orientation to life. The fundamental approach of Yoga is to test the principles it is based on and find out for yourself whether they work for you. The philosophical ideas of Yoga have been formulated over many millennia of experimentation. You either find them useful or you don't, but no belief in bizarre ideas is necessary.

✔ **People over 50 can't learn Yoga.**

Yoga is for people of all ages. Some people start in their 70s and 80s. It is never too late — or early — to start practicing Yoga.

✔ **Yoga can only offer a handful of exercises.**

Yoga has a vast repertoire of exercises, and Yoga teachers are constantly adding new variations on these exercises to refine the system and make it suitable for the widest range of people possible. In addition to improving your flexibility, Yoga can help you combat stress and keep you generally fit. It even has great restorative power and, because of this, is recommended by knowledgeable physicians around the world.

✔ **You can practice Yoga once a month and achieve good results.**

As with any other exercise system, you only get out of Yoga what you put into it. Regular daily Yoga practice gives the best results. But in Yoga, a little effort goes a long way.

Yoga For Dummies®

Cheat Sheet

Keys to a Successful Yoga Practice

✔ **Be clear about your goals.**

Decide what you want to accomplish (flexibility, fitness, better health, and/or inner peace, for example).

✔ **Make a realistic commitment.**

In light of your goals, use the advice given in this book to design your own program.

✔ **Get your physician's approval.**

If you have a health challenge or are pregnant, be sure to consult a physician before embarking on a Yoga exercise program. Consult a physician who is basically sympathetic to exercise and is reasonably familiar with Yoga so that you can be sure you're getting the best — and most relevant — advice.

✔ **Enjoy gentle Yoga.**

You don't need to be competitive with yourself or anyone else. Allow Yoga to gently unfold the potential of your body and your mind. Don't overdo exercising. Keep the enjoyment factor high.

✔ **Keep a practice journal.**

Chronicle your experience with Yoga, and periodically read through your journal to see the progress you have made. Progress is the best motivator.

✔ **Create a support system for yourself.**

You can always find strength in numbers. Find other people who enjoy Yoga so that you can motivate and inspire each other. If you prefer to practice on your own at home, you may still want to consider participating in a Yoga class occasionally, if only to get feedback or find encouragement.

✔ **Vary your program periodically.**

Even the best program can get boring. Prevent your enthusiasm from flagging by changing your exercise routine occasionally.

✔ **Educate yourself.**

Continue to educate yourself about Yoga. Education helps to make your Yoga practice more meaningful. Many good books and magazines are available on the subject. Take the time to read and study. You'll be pleasantly surprised about the depth you can discover in Yoga.

✔ **Be a Yoga enthusiast, but not a bore.**

By all means, be enthusiastic about your Yoga practice, but know that not everyone shares your enthusiasm, including the dearest members of your family. Yoga's positive effect on your body and mind is the best advertising, so let those effects speak for themselves rather than annoying your family and friends with constant talk of Yoga.

✔ **Focus on a personal ideal.**

We all need ideals. You don't need to worship a hero, but being able to look up to someone who, in your eyes, has succeeded and whom you find inspiring is always a good idea. Keep your ideal or ideals always vivid in your mind.

For Dummies: Bestselling Book Series for Beginners

Praise for Yoga For Dummies

"No one in our culture knows the ins-and-outs of Yoga better than Dr. Georg Feuerstein. He is the leading authority on Yoga today. Yoga can be transformative. To learn how, read this book."
— Larry Dossey, M.D., author of *Be Careful What You Pray For, Prayer is Good Medicine*, and executive editor of *Alternative Therapies in Health and Medicine*

"Larry Payne is a gifted Yoga teacher. His 'User-Friendly Yoga' program is now offered for the first time at the UCLA Medical School. I am very impressed by *Yoga For Dummies*. It is a tremendous service for Yoga enthusiasts and health professionals alike."
— Richard Usatine, M.D., Associate Professor of Family Medicine and Assistant Dean, UCLA School of Medicine

"*Yoga For Dummies* is destined to reach and benefit many people who have wanted a reliable introduction. Dr. Feuerstein, author of 30 books, writes beautifully and meaningfully. He is the perfect person to introduce readers to the Yoga path for health and well-being."
— Eleanor Criswell, Ed.D., Professor of Psychology, Director of the Novato Institute for Somatic Research and Training, and author of *How Yoga Works*

"Larry Payne is a gifted teacher. His *User-Friendly Yoga* was my reintroduction to Yoga, and has been very valuable."
— Michael Keaton, actor

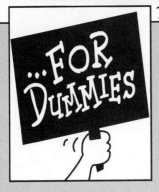
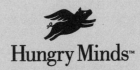

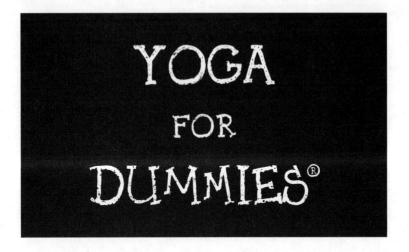

YOGA FOR DUMMIES®

by Georg Feuerstein, Ph.D.
& Larry Payne, Ph.D.

Foreword by Lilias Folan

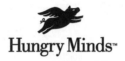

Hungry Minds™

Best-Selling Books • Digital Downloads • e-Books • Answer Networks • e-Newsletters • Branded Web Sites • e-Learning

New York, NY ◆ Cleveland, OH ◆ Indianapolis, IN

Yoga For Dummies®

Published by
Hungry Minds, Inc.
909 Third Avenue
New York, NY 10022
www.hungryminds.com
www.dummies.com

Library of Congress Catalog Card No.: 99-60532

ISBN: 0-7645-5117-5

Printed in the United States of America

10

1B/QR/RR/QR/IN

Distributed in the United States by Hungry Minds, Inc.

Distributed by CDG Books Canada Inc. for Canada; by Transworld Publishers Limited in the United Kingdom; by IDG Norge Books for Norway; by IDG Sweden Books for Sweden; by IDG Books Australia Publishing Corporation Pty. Ltd. for Australia and New Zealand; by TransQuest Publishers Pte Ltd. for Singapore, Malaysia, Thailand, Indonesia, and Hong Kong; by Gotop Information Inc. for Taiwan; by ICG Muse, Inc. for Japan; by Intersoft for South Africa; by Eyrolles for France; by International Thomson Publishing for Germany, Austria and Switzerland; by Distribuidora Cuspide for Argentina; by LR International for Brazil; by Galileo Libros for Chile; by Ediciones ZETA S.C.R. Ltda. for Peru; by WS Computer Publishing Corporation, Inc., for the Philippines; by Contemporanea de Ediciones for Venezuela; by Express Computer Distributors for the Caribbean and West Indies; by Micronesia Media Distributor, Inc. for Micronesia; by Chips Computadoras S.A. de C.V. for Mexico; by Editorial Norma de Panama S.A. for Panama; by American Bookshops for Finland.

For general information on Hungry Minds' products and services please contact our Customer Care Department within the U.S. at 800-762-2974, outside the U.S. at 317-572-3993 or fax 317-572-4002.

For sales inquiries and reseller information, including discounts, premium and bulk quantity sales, and foreign-language translations, please contact our Customer Care Department at 800-434-3422, fax 317-572-4002, or write to Hungry Minds, Inc., Attn: Customer Care Department, 10475 Crosspoint Boulevard, Indianapolis, IN 46256.

For information on licensing foreign or domestic rights, please contact our Sub-Rights Customer Care Department at 212-884-5000.

For information on using Hungry Minds' products and services in the classroom or for ordering examination copies, please contact our Educational Sales Department at 800-434-2086 or fax 317-572-4005.

Please contact our Public Relations Department at 212-884-5163 for press review copies or 212-884-5000 for author interviews and other publicity information or fax 212-884-5400.

For authorization to photocopy items for corporate, personal, or educational use, please contact Copyright Clearance Center, 222 Rosewood Drive, Danvers, MA 01923, or fax 978-750-4470.

Hungry Minds™ is a trademark of Hungry Minds, Inc.

About the Authors

Photo by: Kathleen Sohn Foster

Georg Feuerstein, Ph.D., has been studying and practicing Yoga since his early teens. He is internationally respected for his contribution to Yoga research and the history of consciousness and has been featured in many national magazines both in the United States and abroad. He has authored over 30 books, including *The Yoga Tradition, The Shambhala Encyclopedia of Yoga, Tantra: The Path of Ecstasy,* and *Lucid Waking.* In the early '70s, he taught Hatha Yoga (physical exercises) to the British women's Olympic ski team for one season, but his main focus is on Jnana Yoga (the path of wisdom) and Raja Yoga (the royal path of meditation).

Georg is founder-director of the Yoga Research Center in Northern California, a coeditor of *Yoga World,* a patron of the British Wheel of Yoga, a fellow of the Indian Academy of Yoga, a contributing editor of *Yoga Journal* and *Intuition* magazine, and he also serves on the advisory board of the Integral Health Network. His Web site is located at www.yogaresearchcenter.org.

Photo by: Richard Kephart

Larry Payne, Ph.D., is an internationally prominent Yoga teacher and workshop leader. He used Yoga to overcome his own serious back problems which he developed during his previous career as an advertising sales executive. Larry regards his own early injuries from numerous competitive sports, his experience in a high-stress profession, and a previously inflexible body as invaluable preparation for helping others.

In Los Angeles, Larry is the founder of the corporate Yoga program at the J. Paul Getty Museum, cofounder of the Yoga program at the UCLA School of Medicine, and he also has founded similar programs for Rancho La Puerta Fitness Spa, The Ritz Carlton and Lowes Hotels, and numerous corporations. Larry is chairman of the International Association of Yoga Therapists and has received Outstanding Achievement Awards for Yoga in Europe, South America, and the United States. Larry has appeared on national television, syndicated radio and has been featured in numerous international magazines, as well as *The New York Times* and the *Los Angeles Times.* He is featured in the video and audio programs "User Friendly Yoga" and "User Friendly Back Yoga." His Web site is located at www.samata.com.

Authors' Acknowledgments

Joint Acknowledgments

We would jointly and warmly like to thank the staff of Hungry Minds, especially Tami Booth (for signing us up and keeping us going, and for superbly combining intelligent efficiency with gracefulness), Jennifer Ehrlich (for cheerfully shepherding the book through the whole editorial process), Kelly Ewing (for getting us started), Tammy Castleman, Linda Stark, and Wendy Hatch (each for her considerable copyediting skills and good humor), Carol Susan Roth (our dynamic agent for her constant encouragement and for unfailingly championing our cause), Richard Rosen (for benefiting our book with his expert technical review), and Blaine Michioka (our photographer extraordinaire who shot all the photos in this volume). Our gratitude and appreciation also extend to our featured models Margarite Baca (Yoga teacher and writer), Christopher Beaumont (screen writer for television), Arleen Bocatija (police officer), Helga Anne Desmet (esthetician trainer and beauty consultant), Colette Foster Groves, M.D. (dermatologist), Lisa Galizia (nutritionist and Yoga teacher), Wah (singer, songwriter, and performer), as well as our Malibu Yoga students in the group photograph — Bob Allen, Chris Briscoe, Zorica Denton, Cheryl Dinow, Paul Eckstein, Ingrid Kelsey, Pam Miller — all for happily and patiently modeling the postures for this book. Last but not least, we would like to cordially thank Lilias Folan for her gracious foreword and also for inspiring American Yoga for so many years.

Additional Acknowledgments from Georg

I would especially like to thank Larry for a beautiful friendship that has sprung from the challenges of coauthoring this work, and as always my wife, Trisha, for happily helping out in so many ways.

Additional Acknowledgments from Larry

Since this is my first major book, I have more people to thank than my dear friend Georg, who wrote his first book at age 19 and hasn't stopped since. First, I would like to thank my immediate family who have always been my greatest supporters. My mother Dolly; brothers Harold, Chris, and James; sister Lisa; nieces Natale and Maria; my 95-year-young grandmother Clara; uncle Sonny and father Harry, who is smiling down from somewhere up above. Next, I would like to acknowledge the teaching I have received in India, in particular the privilege of studying with Yoga master T.K.V. Desikachar, my main inspiration. I also would like to acknowledge my gratitude to A.G. Mohan and his wife Indra; Evarts Loomis, M.D., for inspiring me to change my life all those many years ago; my first Yoga teachers Ragavand Dass, Renee Taylor, and David Luna; Bill Grant and Teri Daniels for dragging me to my first classes; Richard Miller, Ph.D., who has been and always will be a teacher of mine; Chris Fletcher, my invaluable personal assistant; my writing coach Richard Rosen; my personal health professional support team, Clare and Kathy McDermott, An Than, Ph.D., Professor Sasi, Steve Ostrow, J.D., Rick Morris, D.C., Bruce Parker, D.C., Ron Lawrence, M.D., Jesse Hanley, M.D., Steve Paredes, D.C., Sherry Brourman, P.T., Val Gross, Benjamin Shield, C.R., Marvin Worchell, D.D.S., David Freeman, Ditta Smolka, and Tara Kamath. In addition, I would like to thank Lilias Folan for her inspiration and for recommending me for this assignment, and finally Georg Feuerstein for being a true friend with a big heart, a mentor, and an example of what Yoga is all about.

Publisher's Acknowledgments

We're proud of this book; please register your comments through our Online Registration Form located at www.dummies.com.

Some of the people who helped bring this book to market include the following:

Acquisitions and Editorial

Senior Project Editor: Jennifer Ehrlich

Executive Editor: Tammerly Booth

Copy Editors: Tamara Castleman, Linda S. Stark

Technical Editor: Charles Richard Rosen

Editorial Manager: Mary C. Corder

Editorial Assistant: Alison Walthall

Special Help

Kelly Ewing, Wendy Hatch, Elizabeth Netedu Kuball, David Mehring

Production

Project Coordinator: Regina Snyder

Layout and Graphics: Daniel Alexander, J. Tyler Connor, Angela F. Hunckler, Todd Klemme, Jane E. Martin, Anna Rohrer, Brent Savage, Rashell Smith, Kate Snell, Michael A. Sullivan, Brian Torwelle

Special Photography: Blaine Michioka/ Rainbow Photography

Proofreaders: Christine Berman, Kelli Botta, Brian Massey, Arielle Carole Mennelle, Rebecca Senninger, Ethel M. Winslow, Janet M. Withers

Indexer: Liz Cunningham

Hungry Minds Consumer Reference Group

Business: Kathleen A. Welton, Vice President and Publisher; Kevin Thornton, Acquisitions Manager

Cooking/Gardening: Jennifer Feldman, Associate Vice President and Publisher

Education/Reference: Diane Graves Steele, Vice President and Publisher

Lifestyles/Pets: Kathleen Nebenhaus, Vice President and Publisher; Tracy Boggier, Managing Editor

Travel: Michael Spring, Vice President and Publisher; Suzanne Jannetta, Editorial Director; Brice Gosnell, Publishing Director

Hungry Minds Consumer Editorial Services: Kathleen Nebenhaus, Vice President and Publisher; Kristin A. Cocks, Editorial Director; Cindy Kitchel, Editorial Director

Hungry Minds Consumer Production: Debbie Stailey, Production Director

Contents at a Glance

Cartoons at a Glance

By Rich Tennant

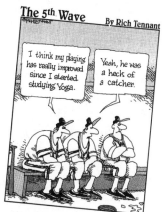

page 333

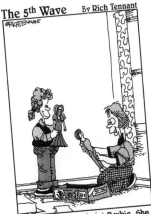

"...and this one's Yogini Barbie. She doesn't come with a lot of stuff, but you can bend her into 13 different positions without anything breaking."

page 229

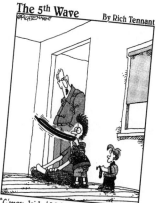

"C'mon kids! We've asked you not to do that when your Mom's doing her deep breathing exercises."

page 41

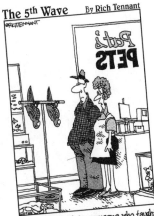

"They belonged to someone who taught Yoga, and aside from hanging upside down from time to time, they're very quiet and well behaved."

page 261

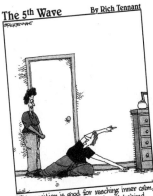

"This position is good for reaching inner calm, mental clarity, and things that roll behind the refrigerator."

page 87

page 9

Cartoon Information:
Fax: 978-546-7747
E-Mail: richtennant@the5thwave.com
World Wide Web: www.the5thwave.com

Table of Contents

· ·

Foreword

1 must admit to feeling shocked when I first heard Yoga was about to join the well-known *...For Dummies* series. Dummies indeed! All my concerns dissolved, however, when I learned that my two highly respected colleagues Georg Feuerstein, Ph.D., and Larry Payne, Ph.D., were going to coauthor this book. I knew then that all beginning Yoga students were in very good hands.

Like two separate eyes seeing as one, Georg and Larry bring a unique understanding and experience to a subject that can be remote and difficult. They have taken the care to honor Yoga's ancient past and our contemporary needs.

I first met Georg when I was teaching at a *Yoga Journal* conference. During a break, I wandered through the busy booths that were selling Yoga props, books, and tapes. I felt drawn to a quiet little cubicle displaying large photos of some of the great Yoga saints and sages. Stillness and joy seemed to roll out from each image like waves. I sat down, closed my eyes, and breathed in the sweet energy of this little oasis. I was to find out later that it was the booth of the Yoga Research Center, founded and directed by Georg.

Larry Payne, director of the Samata Yoga Center in Los Angeles, is a long-time soul friend and Yoga companion. I have spent many happy times being the student in the back row of his dynamic Yoga classes. He brings to this book his many years of experience and study. His user-friendly, warm, and caring approach to Yoga and life is contagious.

I know that these two great teachers will bring to both the beginner and the more experienced practitioner inspiration and encouragement. Every page in this book contains easy practical tools and tips needed to accompany you on your journey toward health, greater happiness, and joy of living.

Lilias Folan

TSI Yoga, P.O. Box 43101, Cincinnati, OH 45203

Lilias Folan is described by *Yoga Journal* as "one of the luminaries of American Yoga." Since 1972, she has hosted and co-produced the nationally syndicated PBS series *Lilias!* She is an author and popular speaker, and conducts Yoga and meditation seminars and conferences worldwide. Her audio and video tapes include *Lilias! Silver Yoga Series, Lilias! Yoga Workout Series* (2 volumes), and *The Inner Smile.* Her workshop schedule can be found at www.liliasyoga.com.

Introduction

● ●

More than six million Americans practice Yoga of one kind or another, and more or less regularly. Many more millions of Yoga practitioners live in other parts of the world. They aren't all dummies, and neither are you, really. The fact that you are reading *Yoga For Dummies* proves that curiosity is alive and kicking in you and that you are willing to learn. In our definition, a dummy is not someone who is abysmally ignorant and stupid, but someone who knows that he or she doesn't know something and actively seeks to fill this gap with the best knowledge available. Someone like you.

Yoga originated 5,000 or so years ago somewhere in India. It only reached the shores of Europe and America a hundred years ago. But the modern Yoga boom didn't start until the 1960s, largely thanks to Richard Hittleman's extraordinarily successful TV series. This was followed in the 1970s by Lilias Folan's TV series (still showing in parts of the country). This was also the time when TM (Transcendental Meditation) — a form of Yoga — became hugely popular largely because of the Beatles. It attracted hundreds of thousands who were in search of stress reduction and a more meaningful life.

More recently, celebrities like Jane Fonda, Madonna, Michelle Pfeiffer, Michael Keaton, and Kareem Abdul Jabar have put Yoga on the map for the wider public. Hollywood, ever quick to catch on, promptly created a successful TV show — *Dharma and Greg* — in which the lead character, Dharma, is a delightfully quirky Yoga instructor. So you are in illustrious company.

About This Book

Perhaps *Yoga For Dummies* is the first book on Yoga you have ever held in your hands. In this case, you are starting at the right place. More likely, however, you have leafed through quite a few other books (there is definitely no shortage of publications dealing with Yoga exercises). Not all of those publications are either sound or helpful. Why, then, should you take this book seriously? We have a two-part answer for you.

First, the information you will find in *Yoga For Dummies* is based on our extensive study and practice of Yoga. Between us, we have 55 years of experience with Yoga. One author (Georg Feuerstein) is internationally recognized as a leading expert on the Yoga tradition and has authored many seminal works on it (see the resources at the end of this book). The other author (Larry Payne) has a thriving practice as a Yoga teacher in Los Angeles, where he teaches and responds to his clients' specific health challenges, notably back problems, and is featured in popular Yoga and back videos. In this book, we have merged our respective areas of expertise to create a reliable and user-friendly introductory book that can also serve you as a beginner's reference work on an ongoing basis.

Second, we are both dedicated to motivating you to practice this system, which we have seen work minor and major miracles. We have committed our lives to making Yoga available to anyone who cares about the health and wholeness of their body and mind. In short, you are in the best of hands.

Yoga For Dummies guides you slowly, step by step, into the treasure house of Yoga. And it is a fabulous treasure house! You will find out how to unlock your body's extraordinary potential and enlist your mind to do so, and in the process strengthen your mind as well. Remember the old Latin saying, *Mens sana in corpore sane.* A sound mind in a sound body. We show you how to improve or regain the health and wholeness of your body and mind.

Whether you are interested in becoming more flexible, fitter, less stressed out, or more peaceful and joyful, this book contains all the good counsel and practical exercises to start you in the right direction. Our presentation is based on the rich heritage of Yoga, which is the oldest system of total well-being in the world.

Thus, *Yoga For Dummies* contains enough information to be useful also to those who have taken the first few steps into the world of Yoga and want to know about coming attractions. Above all, we have endeavored to make this book relevant to busy people like yourself. And if, after reading this guide, you become more serious about studying and practicing Yoga, consider taking a Yoga class with a qualified instructor. This book is a great guide, but nothing compares to hands-on teaching.

Yoga is not a fad. It has been around in this country for over a hundred years and has a history of approximately five millennia. It is clearly here to stay. Yoga has brought health and peace of mind to millions of people. It can do the same for you.

Conventions Used in This Book

The focus of this book is on Hatha (pronounced *haht-ha*) Yoga, which is that branch of Yoga that works primarily with the body through postures, breathing exercises, and other similar techniques. Our overall orientation, however, is more comprehensive, and we include enough material about the other branches of Yoga to give you a basic understanding of them.

When necessary, we provide helpful photos or illustrations to help you better understand the exercises or postures. Because breathing is an important part of yogic exercises, many of the photos or illustrations include the word *Inhale* or *Exhale* (with an arrow) to help you breathe properly. This means that, for example, if an illustration shows a right-pointing arrow with the word *Exhale* next to it, you know that you are to exhale as you move to the next posture depicted to the right. You get the idea.

For your safety, when practicing the exercises be sure to read all the instructions. Don't just glance at the illustrations and think you can leap right in. Although the illustrations are very helpful tools, they don't give you the whole story needed to practice safe and effective Yoga.

What You're Not to Read

We must admit that we hope you read every word in this book at some point in your yogic journey. We also confess that there are a few tidbits of information that we included just to get your mind going and make you think. While these tidbits are interesting and important in their own right, they're not essential to your practice of the various postures. We've clearly marked this text with the Technical Stuff icon. Feel free to skip 'em, but plan to go back and read them at some point. You'll be glad you did!

Foolish Assumptions

We're not here to judge, but we have made some general assumptions about you, the reader. First, we assume that you are interested in reaping some benefits from practicing Yoga. Second, we assume that you don't have much (if any) experience with Yoga. Finally, we assume that you are curious and willing to find out more. That's it. Nothing fancy. If you fall into this category, then *Yoga For Dummies* is for you!

How This Book Is Organized

This book is organized according to the characteristic design of all ...*For Dummies* books. It answers all the important questions you need to know for a successful practice of Yoga. Here are some of the questions for which you will find optimal answers:

- How much time do I need to dedicate to Yoga for it to be useful to me?
- Am I too old to practice Yoga?
- Does an illness or disability prevent me from practicing Yoga?
- Can I discover Yoga from a book or do I need to find a teacher?
- Is it better to practice Yoga in a private session or in a class?
- How long does it take before I see results, and what kind of results will I see?
- Do I need to believe any weird ideas to practice Yoga? (A preview answer: No!)
- Is it true that Yoga is a spiritual teaching?
- What are the best exercises to practice?
- When should I practice Yoga?
- Does Yoga have anything to say about diet?
- What about Yoga for the whole family?
- Is Yoga deadly serious or will it be enjoyable?

Yoga For Dummies is conveniently divided into six parts. Here is what you will encounter in them:

Part I: Off to a Good Start with Yoga

This opening part sets the stage for the discussions and practices that follow. In Chapter 1, we explain what Yoga is and clear up some widespread misunderstandings about it. We also introduce the five basic approaches to and twelve principal branches of Yoga and review how these relate to your health and happiness. This will help you to ask yourself the right sort of questions to discover the most appropriate orientation and style for yourself. In Chapter 2, we provide you with down-to-earth practical advice on getting started with your own Yoga practice, showing you how you can make it both safe and effective. In particular, we answer all your questions about participating in a class or practicing on your own.

Part II: Getting in Shape for Yoga

With this part, we jump straight into Yoga practice. In Chapter 3, we cover everything you need to do to prepare for a Yoga session, including cultivating the right state of mind, for the mind is a key ingredient in all forms of Yoga. Chapter 4 introduces the art of relaxation, which is fundamental to a successful Yoga practice. In Chapter 5, we explain the importance of correct breathing both during the execution of the Yoga postures and as a discipline in its own right.

Part III: Postures for Health Maintenance and Restoration

In this third part, which is the backbone of our book, we guide you systematically into the practice of simple but potent Yoga postures. We start out, in Chapter 6, by giving you the key formula for a well-rounded practice. It is important to pay close attention to preparation (warm-up) and the sequencing of postures to gain maximum benefit and avoid injury. In Chapters 7 to 14, you successively discover sitting postures, standing postures, balancing exercises, special practices for your abdominals, inversions, bends, and twists, as well as the popular dynamic movement called the "Sun Prayer." In Chapter 15, we offer you several recommended routines, which can help you get started right away. For your convenience, we have put together an 8-week program as well as short routines for those busy days when you have only 5 to 15 minutes of leisure time.

Part IV: Creative Yoga

This part is all about making your Yoga sessions creative, enjoyable, efficient, and safe. In Chapter 16, we give you a classic formula that will allow you to design your own exercise routines, depending on the available amount of time (from 5 to 60 minutes) and your specific needs and goals. We also cover the advantages and disadvantages of practicing singly, with a partner, and in groups, or with and without props. In case you think you are too busy to practice, we give you well-tested suggestions for overcoming this ever-popular obstacle. Chapter 17 reviews available props — such as walls, chairs, inversion benches, straps, blocks, and so on — for facilitating your practice of postures.

Part V: Yoga as a Lifestyle

When adopted as a lifestyle, Yoga extends over the entire day. In this part, we explain how this can be done and why it makes sense. As we show in Chapter 18, Yoga has much to say about positive mental attitudes toward work, leisure, diet, family, and other people. Chapter 19 outlines Yoga's good advice about how to make sex regenerative and a means of increasing happiness. In Chapter 20, we introduce you to the art of meditation. If the postures are the backbone, meditation is the heart of Yoga. Regular meditation puts you in touch with the joy and peace that is your mind's natural condition. It enables you to become a happier and freer person. Freedom is the ultimate goal of traditional Yoga. Chapter 21 deals with special situations, notably Yoga for people suffering from back problems and women during pregnancy, menstruation, and menopause. Chapter 21 also includes our thoughts on how you can adapt Yoga for children, who are a "special situation" all their own. They can be taught simple, fun exercises to practice along with you or by themselves. Many children respond very well to Yoga.

Part VI: The Part of Tens

All ...*For Dummies* books have a Part of Tens section, which is a kind of capstone. Here we give you top-ten lists that provide you with useful and practical information. Thus in Chapter 22, we give you important hints on a successful and enjoyable Yoga practice with a focus on relaxation, and in Chapter 23, tell you the best places to visit if you are interested in learning Yoga from a competent teacher and/or in a group setting. Finally, in Chapter 24, we list ten principal and many secondary good reasons for practicing Yoga — if you still need them after reading our book and applying its techniques.

We encourage you to explore Yoga further, and so in the appendix at the end of the book we give you the necessary resources to do just that. We cover prominent organizations, list some of the best books, audiotapes, and videos on the various aspects of Yoga, and also share with you our favorite Yoga sites on the World Wide Web.

Icons Used in This Book

Throughout this book you'll notice little pictures in the margins. We call them *icons*. You can use these icons in a couple of different ways:

  ✔ **As helpful "flags" to use as you read.** For example, if you decide to read an entire chapter from beginning to end, the icons serve as signposts along the way and tell you how to use the information you've just encountered.

✔ **As a tour guide to help you find your way through the book.** For example, if you've become familiar with Yoga and just want to find the exercises, flip through the book looking for the Exercise icon.

Following is the list of icons used in this book:

This icon points you toward helpful information that can make your yogic journey a little smoother. Be sure to read these morsels!

This icon flags danger ahead. Be sure to check out the information marked by this icon; you'll be glad you did!

This icon marks nerdy technical stuff that's interesting to know, but probably not necessary to your understanding of Yoga. Read this and impress your friends at your next dinner party.

The paragraphs sitting next to this baby are pretty noteworthy. You may want to jot them down somewhere or circle them in the book.

Sometimes the terms used in association with Yoga can be fairly jargony and strange-sounding to most people. This icon flags such words so you can pay special attention to them. If you're not careful, you may start sounding like a pro!

This icon leads you to the various routines, exercises, and postures scattered throughout the book. If it's exercises you want, keep your eyes peeled for this icon.

This icon sits next to text that cuts through the myth and mystery to expose the truth about Yoga. This is interesting stuff!

Look for this icon to find out some personal experiences we've encountered during our 55 combined years in the world of Yoga. You'll laugh, you'll cry, and you may even learn something!

Where to Go from Here

Yoga For Dummies is designed to be both an *introduction* and a *beginner's reference work*. You can read the chapters one after the other and practice along with us, or you can dip into the book here and there reading up on the things that are of immediate interest to you, such as how to find the right kind of style or Yoga class for your needs, or what helpful props you can use to make your practice easier.

If you are a newcomer to Yoga, we recommend that you spend some time with the table of contents. You may even want to leaf through this book to get a general sense of how we have structured and approached the material.

If you are not new to Yoga and simply want a refresher course, *Yoga For Dummies* can also be used as a reliable guide in answering your questions. Just flip to the index to find the information you need or check out the appendix, which refers you to a variety of sources of information on specific topics relating to Yoga.

What are you waiting for? Dig in!

Part I
Off to a Good Start with Yoga

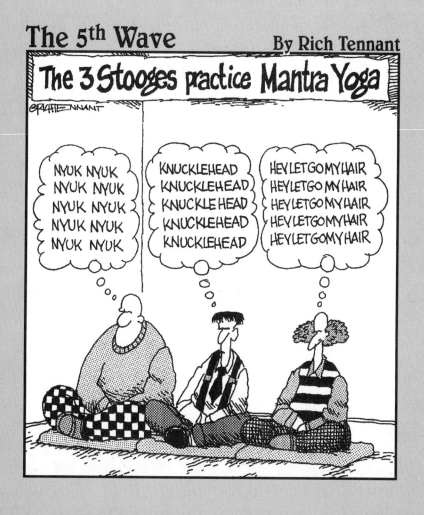

In this part . . .

Yoga is very comprehensive and includes a great
variety of approaches. Before you go off hiking in the
countryside, you need to take a quick look at the map
or risk getting lost. Before you start experimenting with
Yoga, it helps to know what it is and how it works. That's
how you can guarantee that your practice of Yoga will be
both enjoyable and safe.

In the two chapters of this first part, we give you a road
map that allows you to take the first step and the next in
what will be an exciting and rewarding journey of discovery for you.

Chapter 1

Yoga 101: What You Need to Know

· ·

In This Chapter

▶ Debunking myths about Yoga

▶ Deciphering the word *Yoga*

▶ Exploring the eight main branches of Yoga

▶ Understanding the five basic approaches to Yoga

▶ Defining popular styles of Hatha Yoga

▶ Taking control of your life with Yoga

· ·

Two or three decades ago, some people still occasionally confused *Yoga* with *yogurt*. Today, Yoga is a household word.

The fact that just about everyone has heard the word *Yoga*, however, doesn't mean that everyone knows exactly what it means. Many misconceptions still exist, even among those who practice Yoga. In this chapter, we clear up the confusion and explain what Yoga really is and how it relates to your health and happiness. We also help you see that Yoga, with its many different branches and approaches, really does offer something for everyone.

Whatever your age, weight, flexibility, or beliefs may be, you can practice and benefit from Yoga. Although it originated in India, Yoga is for all of humanity.

Headed to the capital

In English, you customarily write *yoga* in lower-case letters. However, throughout this book, we write the word with an initial capital letter — *Yoga* — to emphasize that Yoga is a self-contained system or tradition, like Zen, Taoism, or Hinduism. The adjective form of *Yoga* is *yogic*, which you encounter frequently in this book.

Understanding the True Character of Yoga

Whenever you're told Yoga is *just* this or *just* that, your nonsense alert should kick into action. Yoga is too comprehensive to reduce to any one thing. Yoga is like a skyscraper with many floors and numerous rooms at each level. Here's what Yoga is not:

- ✔ Yoga is not *just* gymnastics.
- ✔ Yoga is not *just* fitness training.
- ✔ Yoga is not *just* a way to control your weight.
- ✔ Yoga is not *just* a technique for stress reduction.
- ✔ Yoga is not *just* meditation.
- ✔ Yoga is not *just* the "huffing and puffing" of proper breath control.
- ✔ Yoga is not *just* a way to improve and maintain your health.
- ✔ Yoga is not *just* a spiritual tradition from India.

To put it simply, Yoga is all these things — the catch is that it's also a great deal more. (You would expect as much from a tradition that's been around for 5,000 years.) Yoga includes physical exercises that look like gymnastics — some of which have even been incorporated into Western gymnastics. These exercises help you become or stay fit and trim, control your weight, and reduce your stress level. Yoga also offers a whole range of meditation practices, including breathing techniques that exercise your lungs and calm your nervous system or charge your brain and the rest of your body with delicious energy.

Moreover, you can use Yoga as an efficient system of health care, one that has proven its usefulness both in restoring and maintaining health. Yoga continues to gain acceptance within the medical establishment. More and more physicians are recommending Yoga to their patients not only for stress reduction but also as a safe and sane method of exercise, as well as physical therapy (notably, for the back and knees).

But Yoga is more than even a system of preventative or restorative health care. Yoga looks at health from a broad, holistic perspective that's only now being rediscovered by avant-garde medicine. This perspective appreciates the enormous influence of the mind — your psychological attitudes — on physical health.

Finding meaning: The word Yoga

The word *Yoga* comes from the ancient *Sanskrit* language spoken by the traditional religious elite of India, the *brahmins*. Yoga means "union" or "integration" and "discipline," so the system of Yoga is called a *unitive* or *integrating discipline*. Yoga seeks unity at various levels. First, Yoga seeks to unite your body and mind. All too often, people separate their minds from their bodies. Some people are chronically "out of the body." They can't feel their feet or the ground beneath them, as if they hover like ghosts just above their bodies. They're unable to cope with the ordinary pressures of daily life and collapse under stress. Often, they're confused and don't understand their own emotions. They're afraid of life and easily hurt.

Many people suffer from slighter forms of this syndrome, which can make facing life squarely and mindfully a difficult task. Because they are not fully "in" the body, they tend to also be somewhat disconnected from the world around them. This causes them to daydream and avoid, rather than face, life's challenges. Through Yoga, they can reconnect their mind and emotions to the body, enabling them to live life more fully and with enjoyment.

A second problem that Yoga tackles is the split between the rational mind and the emotions. All too often, people bottle up their emotions and don't express their real feelings, choosing instead to rationalize these feelings away. If done chronically, this avoidance can become a serious health hazard. Sometimes people aren't even aware that they're suppressing their feelings — especially anger. Then anger or frustration consumes them from the inside out.

Here's how Yoga can help you with your personal growth:

- Yoga can put you in touch with your real feelings and balance your emotional life.

- Yoga can help you become less fragmented inwardly and more whole and real. In other words, it can help you understand and accept yourself and feel comfortable with who you are. You won't have to "fake it" or reduce your life to constant role-playing.

- Yoga can greatly improve your "hook-up" to other people. That is, you become more able to empathize and communicate with others.

Yoga is a powerful means of psychological integration. It makes you aware that you're part of a larger whole, not merely an island unto yourself. Humans can't thrive in isolation. Even the most independent individual is greatly indebted to others. Once your mind and body are happily reunited, this union with others comes about naturally. The moral principles of Yoga are all embracing, encouraging you to seek kinship with everyone and everything. We say more about this in Chapter 18.

Finding yourself: Are you a yogi (or yogini)?

Someone who's dedicated to the discipline of balancing mind and body through Yoga is traditionally called a *yogi* (if male) or a *yogini* (if female). In this book, we use both terms at random. Alternatively, we also use the English term *Yoga practitioner*.

A yogi or yogini who has really mastered Yoga is called a *Yoga master* or an *adept*. If such an adept also teaches (and not all of them do), he or she traditionally is called a *guru*. The Sanskrit word *guru* means literally "weighty one." According to traditional esoteric sources, the syllable *gu* signifies spiritual darkness and *ru* signifies the act of removing. Thus a *guru* is a teacher who leads the student from darkness to light.

Very few Westerners have achieved complete mastery of Yoga, mainly because Yoga is still a relatively young movement in the West. However, at the level at which Yoga is generally taught outside its Indian homeland, many competent Yoga teachers or instructors can lend a helping hand to beginners. In this book, we hope to do just that for you.

Considering Your Options: The Eight Main Branches of Yoga

When you take a bird's-eye view of the Yoga tradition, you see a dozen major strands of development, each with its own subdivisions. Picture Yoga as a giant tree with eight branches — each branch has its own unique character, but each is also part of the same tree. With so many different paths, you're sure to find one that's right for your personality, lifestyle, and goals. In this book we focus on Hatha Yoga, the most popular branch of Yoga, but we avoid the common mistake of reducing it to mere physical fitness training. Thus, we also talk about meditation and the spiritual aspects of Yoga.

Here are the eight principal branches of Yoga, arranged alphabetically:

- ✔ **Bhakti Yoga:** the Yoga of devotion
- ✔ **Guru Yoga:** the Yoga of dedication to a Yoga master
- ✔ **Hatha Yoga:** the Yoga of physical discipline
- ✔ **Jnana Yoga:** the Yoga of wisdom
- ✔ **Karma Yoga:** the Yoga of self-transcending action

- ✓ **Mantra Yoga:** the Yoga of potent sound
- ✓ **Raja Yoga:** the Royal Yoga
- ✓ **Tantra Yoga (including Kundalini Yoga):** the Yoga of continuity

These eight branches are described in the following paragraphs.

Bhakti Yoga: The Yoga of devotion

Bhakti Yoga (pronounced *bhuk-tee*) practitioners believe that a supreme being transcends their lives, and they feel moved to connect or even completely merge with that supreme being through acts of devotion. Bhakti Yoga includes such practices as making flower offerings, singing hymns of praise, and thinking about the divine being.

Guru Yoga: The Yoga of dedication to a master

In Guru Yoga (pronounced *goo-roo*), one's teacher is the main focus of spiritual practice. Such a teacher is expected to be enlightened or at least close to being enlightened (see Chapter 20 for more about enlightenment). In Guru Yoga, you're asked to honor and meditate on your guru until you merge with him or her. Because the guru is thought to be one with the ultimate reality, this merger is believed to duplicate his or her spiritual realization in you.

Feeling enlightened

To get a sense of the nature of enlightenment, sit in a warm room as still as possible, with your hands in your lap. Now sense your skin all over, which is your body's boundary separating you from the air surrounding you. As you become more aware of your body's sensations, pay special attention to the connection between your skin and the air. After a while, you'll realize that there is really no sharp boundary between your skin and the "outside" air. In your imagination, you can extend yourself further and further beyond your skin into the surrounding space. Where do you end, and where does the space begin? This experience can give you a sense of the all-comprising expansiveness of enlightenment, which knows no boundaries.

Hatha Yoga: The Yoga of physical discipline

All branches of Yoga seek to achieve the same final goal, enlightenment (see Chapter 20), but Hatha Yoga (pronounced *haht-ha*) approaches this goal through the body rather than through the mind or through the emotions. Hatha Yoga practitioners believe that unless the body is properly purified and prepared, the higher stages of concentration, meditation, and ecstasy are virtually impossible to achieve — such an attempt would be like trying to climb Mt. Everest without the necessary gear. Much of this book focuses on this branch of Yoga.

The body is a precious possession. Yoga asks you to take proper care of it, so that you can enjoy not only health but also longevity and, ultimately, enlightenment.

Jnana Yoga: The Yoga of wisdom

Jnana Yoga (pronounced *gyah-nah*) teaches the ideal of *nondualism* — that reality is singular and your perception of countless distinct phenomena is a basic misconception. What about the chair or sofa that you're sitting on? Isn't that real? What about the light that strikes your retina? Isn't that real? Jnana Yoga masters answer these questions by saying that all these things are real at your present level of consciousness, but they aren't ultimately real as separate or distinct things. Upon enlightenment, everything melts into one, and you become one with the immortal spirit.

Good karma, bad karma, no karma

The Sanskrit term *karma* means literally "action." It stands for activity in general but also for the "invisible action" of destiny. According to Yoga, every action of body, speech, and mind produces visible and also hidden consequences. Sometimes the hidden consequences — destiny — are far more significant than the obvious repercussions. Don't think of karma as blind destiny. You are always free to make choices. The purpose of Karma Yoga is to regulate how you act in the world so that you cease to be bound by karma. The practitioners of Karma Yoga seek to not only prevent bad (black) karma but also go beyond good (white) karma to no karma at all. According to this Yoga branch, all karma binds you to the state of unenlightenment. This state is undesirable because in it, you are neither free nor blissful.

The sacred syllable OM

The best known traditional mantra, used by Hindus and Buddhists alike, is the sacred syllable *om* (pronounced *ohmmm*. It's said to be the symbol of the absolute reality, the Self or spirit. It's composed of the letters *a, u, m,* and the nasal humming of the letter *m*. A corresponds to the waking state; *u* corresponds to the dream state; *m* corresponds to the state of deep sleep; and the nasal humming sound represents the ultimate reality. We introduce several other traditional mantras in Chapter 20 in our coverage of meditation.

Karma Yoga: The Yoga of self-transcending action

Karma Yoga (pronounced *kahr-mah*) seeks to influence destiny positively. This path's most important principle is to act unselfishly, without attachment, and with integrity. Karma Yoga practitioners believe that all actions — whether bodily, vocal, or mental — have far-reaching consequences for which we must assume full responsibility.

Mantra Yoga: The Yoga of potent sound

Mantra Yoga (pronounced *mahn-trah*) makes use of sound to harmonize the body and focus the mind. It works with *mantras,* which can be a syllable, word, or phrase. Traditionally, practitioners receive a *mantra* from their teacher in the context of a formal initiation. They are asked to repeat it as often as possible and to keep it secret. Many Western teachers feel that initiation is not necessary and that any sound will do. You can even pick a word from the dictionary — such as *love, peace,* or *happiness.*

Raja Yoga: The Royal Yoga

Raja Yoga (pronounced *rah-jah*) means literally "Royal Yoga" and is also known as *Classical Yoga.*

When you mingle with Yoga students long enough, you can expect to hear them refer to the *eightfold path,* as codified in the *Yoga-Sutra* of Patanjali. This is the standard work of Raja Yoga. Another name for this yogic tradition is *ashtanga-yoga* (pronounced *ahsh-tahng-gah),* the "eight-limbed Yoga" — from *ashta* ("eight") and *anga* ("limb"). The eight limbs of this prominent approach, which are designed to lead to enlightenment, or liberation, are as follows:

- ✔ *Yama* (pronounced *yah-mah*): Moral discipline, consisting of the practices of nonharming, truthfulness, nonstealing, chastity, and greedlessness (for an explanation of these five virtues, see Chapter 18).

- ✔ *Niyama* (pronounced *nee-yah-mah*): Self-restraint, consisting of the five practices of purity, contentment, austerity, self-study, and devotion to a higher principle.

- ✔ *Asana* (pronounced *ah-sah-nah*): Posture, which serves two basic purposes — meditation and health.

- ✔ *Pranayama* (pronounced *prah-nah-yah-mah*): Breath control, which raises and balances your psychosomatic energy, thus boosting your health and mental concentration.

- ✔ *Pratyahara* (pronounced *prah-tyah-hah-rah*): Sensory inhibition, which internalizes your consciousness to prepare the mind for the various stages of meditation.

- ✔ *Dharana* (pronounced *dhah-rah-nah*): Concentration, or extended mental focusing, which is fundamental to yogic meditation.

- ✔ *Dhyana* (pronounced *dhee-yah-nah*): Meditation, the principal practice of higher Yoga (this practice and the next are explained in Chapter 20).

- ✔ *Samadhi* (pronounced *sah-mah-dhee*): Ecstasy, or the experience of unitive consciousness in which you become inwardly one with the object of your contemplation.

Tantra Yoga: The Yoga of continuity

Tantra Yoga (pronounced *tahn-trah*) is the most complex and most widely misunderstood branch of Yoga. In the West and in India, Tantra Yoga is often confused with "spiritualized" sex. While sexual rituals are used in some schools of Tantra Yoga, this isn't a regular practice in the majority of schools. Tantra Yoga is actually a strict spiritual discipline involving fairly complex rituals and detailed visualizations of deities. These deities are either visions of the divine or the equivalent of Christianity's angels and are invoked to aid the yogic process of contemplation.

Another name for Tantra Yoga is Kundalini Yoga (pronounced *koon-dah-lee-nee*). The latter name, which means "she who is coiled," hints at the secret "serpent power" that Tantra Yoga seeks to activate: the latent spiritual energy stored in the human body. If you are curious about this aspect of Yoga, you may want to read the autobiographical account by Gopi Krishna (see the appendix in the back of this book).

Uncovering Where You Fit In: The Three Primary Qualities

After you review the various branches of Yoga and diverse styles of Yoga, one question may remain: How do you want to proceed? To help you in your consideration, we introduce the traditional model of the three primary qualities (called *gunas* in Sanskrit). According to Yoga, everything that exists (other than the ultimate superconscious reality itself) is composed of three basic constituents. These are named *sattva, rajas,* and *tamas,* respectively.

- ✔ *Sattva* is the principle of lucidity.
- ✔ *Rajas* is the principle of dynamism.
- ✔ *Tamas* is the principle of inertia.

These three principles or forces exist in an infinite number of combinations both in the material and the mental realm. Some things are more *tamasic,* others more *rajasic,* and a few more *sattvic.*

The purpose of Yoga is to increase the principle of lucidity in all your actions, thoughts, and feelings. We call this process *sattvification.* While you are alive, you can never be completely sattvic, but you can certainly train your mind to overcome the limitations of *tamas* and *rajas.* When your mind is freed from the negative influence of *tamas* and *rajas,* it is like a highly polished mirror that faithfully reflects the light of the spirit, or higher consciousness.

Finding Your Niche: Five Basic Approaches to Yoga

Since the late nineteenth century when Yoga was introduced to the Western hemisphere from its Indian homeland, it has undergone various adaptations. Today, Yoga is practiced in five major ways:

- ✔ As a method for physical fitness and health maintenance
- ✔ As a sport
- ✔ As body-oriented therapy
- ✔ As a comprehensive lifestyle
- ✔ As a spiritual discipline

We take a look at these five basic approaches in the upcoming sections.

Yoga as fitness training

The first approach, Yoga as fitness training, is the most popular way that Westerners practice Yoga. It's also the most radical revamping of traditional Yoga. More precisely, it's a revision of traditional *Hatha Yoga* (see Chapter 2 for more about Hatha Yoga). Yoga as fitness training is concerned primarily with the physical body — its flexibility, resilience, and strength. This is how most newcomers to Yoga encounter this great tradition. Fitness training is certainly a useful gateway into Yoga, but later on, some people discover that Hatha Yoga also includes moral and spiritual practices that are designed to lead to enlightenment. From the earliest times, Yoga masters have emphasized the need for a healthy body. But they've also always pointed beyond the body to the mind and other important aspects of being.

Yoga as a sport

This second approach, Yoga as a sport, is especially prominent in some Latin American countries but is widely controversial. Its practitioners, many of whom are excellent athletes, master hundreds of extremely difficult Yoga postures to perfection and demonstrate their skills and beautiful physiques in international competitions. But this new sport, which also can be regarded as an art form, has drawn much criticism from the ranks of more traditional Yoga practitioners. They feel that competition has no place in Yoga. Yet this athletic orientation has done much to put Yoga on the map in some parts of the world. We see nothing wrong with good-natured Yoga competitions as long as self-centered competitiveness is held in check.

Yoga as therapy

The third approach, Yoga as therapy, applies yogic techniques to restore health or full physical and mental functioning. In recent years, some Western Yoga teachers have begun to use yogic practices for therapeutic purposes. Although the idea behind Yoga therapy is very old, its name is fairly new. Yoga therapy is, in fact, a whole new professional discipline, calling for far greater training and skill on the part of the teacher than is the case with ordinary Yoga. Commonly, Yoga is intended for those who don't suffer from disabilities or ailments requiring remedial action and special attention. Yoga therapy, on the other hand, addresses these special needs. For example, Yoga therapy may be able to help you find relief from certain ailments such as chronic back pain, asthma, rheumatism, and many others. Chapter 21 shows you some basic yogic techniques for back pain, a widespread problem in Western society.

Seeing the potency of Yoga therapy, several insurance companies now offer coverage for it as a part of their alternative therapies programs. Other insurance companies will no doubt follow suit before long. See the appendix for the address of the International Association of Yoga Therapists.

Yoga as a lifestyle

The fourth approach, Yoga as a lifestyle, enters the proper domain of Yoga. Yoga once or twice a week for an hour or so is certainly better than no Yoga at all. And Yoga can be enormously beneficial even when practiced only as fitness training. But you unlock the real potency of Yoga when you adopt it as a lifestyle. This means *living* Yoga; practicing Yoga every day, whether it's physical exercises or meditation. Above all, it means applying the wisdom of Yoga to everyday life and to live lucidly, that is, with awareness. Yoga has much to say about what and how you should eat, how you should sleep, how you should work, how you should relate to others, and so on. It offers a total system of conscious and skillful living.

Don't think that you have to be a yogic superstar to practice lifestyle Yoga. You can begin today. Just make a few simple adjustments in your daily schedule and keep your goals vividly in front of you. Whenever you are ready, make further positive changes — one step at a time.

Yoga as a spiritual discipline

Lifestyle Yoga is concerned with healthy, wholesome, functional, and benevolent living. Yoga as a spiritual discipline, the fifth and final approach, is concerned with all that *plus* the traditional ideal of *enlightenment* — that is, discovering your spiritual nature. (We discuss the journey to enlightenment in Chapter 20.)

The word *spiritual* has been abused a lot lately, so we need to explain how it's used here. *Spiritual* relates to *spirit* — your ultimate nature. In Yoga, it is called the *atman* (pronounced *aht-mahn*) or *purusha (poo-roo-shah)*.

According to Yoga philosophy, the *spirit* is one and the same for everyone. It's formless, immortal, superconscious, and unimaginably blissful. It is one and the same in all beings and things. It is transcendental because it exists beyond the limited body and mind. You discover the spirit in the moment of your enlightenment.

What all approaches to Yoga have in common

The five approaches to Yoga share at least two *fundamental practices:* the cultivation of awareness and relaxation.

✔ *Awareness* is the peculiarly human ability to pay close attention to some-thing, to be consciously present, to be mindful. Yoga is attention training.

To see what we mean, try this exercise: Pay attention to your right hand for the next 60 seconds. That is, feel your right hand and do nothing else. Chances are, your mind is drifting off after only a few seconds. Yoga consists in reining in your attention whenever it strays.

✔ *Relaxation* is the conscious release of unnecessary and therefore unwholesome tension in the body.

Both awareness and relaxation go hand in hand in Yoga. Without bringing awareness and relaxation to Yoga, the exercises would be merely exercises — not *yogic* exercises.

Conscious breathing is often added to awareness and relaxation as a third foundational practice. Normally, breathing happens automatically. In Yoga, awareness is brought to this act, which then makes it into a powerful tool for training the body and the mind. We say much more about these aspects of Yoga in Chapter 5.

Getting the Scoop on the Prominent Styles of Hatha Yoga

In its voyage from antiquity to modernity, Hatha Yoga has undergone many transformations. The most significant adaptations were made during the past several decades, particularly to serve the needs of Western students. Of the many styles of Hatha Yoga available today, the following are the best known:

Viniyoga (pronounced *vee-nee yoh-gah*) is the approach developed by Shri Krishnamacharya and continued by his son T. K. V. Desikachar, whose school is located in Madras, India. As the teacher of well-known Yoga masters B. K. S. Iyengar, K. Pattabhi Jois, and Indra Devi, Shri Krishnamacharya can be said to have launched a veritable Hatha Yoga renaissance in modern times, which is still sweeping the world. Viniyoga works with what is called "sequential process," or *vinyasa krama* (*vee-nyah-sah krah-mah*). The emphasis is not on achieving an external ideal form but on practicing a posture according to one's individual needs and capacity. Regulated breathing is an important aspect of Viniyoga, and the breath is carefully coordinated with the postural movements.

B. K. S. Iyengar, the brother-in-law of Shri Krishnamacharya and uncle of T.K.V. Desikachar, created Iyengar Yoga, which is the most widely recognized approach to Hatha Yoga. This style is characterized by precision performance and the aid of various props, such as cushions, benches, wood blocks, straps, and even sand bags. Iyengar has trained thousands of teachers, many of whom are in the United States. His Ramamani Iyengar Memorial Yoga Institute, founded in 1974 and dedicated to his late wife Ramamani, is located in Pune, India.

Ashtanga Yoga originated with K. Pattabhi Jois, who was born in 1916 but who has a suitably modern outlook to draw eager Western students to his Ashtanga Yoga Institute located in Mysore, India. He was a principal disciple of Shri Krishnamacharya who, apparently, instructed him to teach the sequences known as Ashtanga, or Power Yoga. This is by far the most athletic style of Hatha Yoga. Ashtanga Yoga differs from Patanjali's eightfold path, though it is theoretically grounded in it.

Kripalu Yoga, inspired by Kripalvananda and developed by his disciple Yogi Amrit Desai, is a three-stage Yoga tailored for the needs of Western students. In the first stage, postural alignment and coordination of breath and movement are emphasized, and the postures are held for a short duration only. In the second stage, meditation is included into the practice and postures are held for prolonged periods. In the final stage, the practice of postures becomes a spontaneous "meditation in motion." See Chapter 23 for more information about the Kripalu Yoga Center in Massachusetts.

Integral Yoga was developed by Swami Satchidananda, a student of the famous Swami Sivananda of Rishikesh, India. Swami Satchidananda made his debut at the Woodstock festival in 1969, where he taught the Baby Boomers to chant *om,* and over the years has attracted thousands of students. As the name suggests, this style aims to integrate the various aspects of the body-mind through a combination of postures, breathing techniques, deep relaxation, and meditation. Function is given preeminence over form. See Chapter 23 for more information about the Satchidanana Ashram in Virginia.

Sivananda Yoga is the creation of the late Swami Vishnudevananda, also a disciple of Swami Sivananda, who established his Sivananda Yoga Vedanta Center in Montreal in 1959. He has trained over 6,000 teachers, and there are numerous Sivananda centers around the world. This style includes a series of 12 postures, the Sun Salutation sequence, breathing exercises, relaxation, and *mantra* chanting. See Chapter 23 for more information about the Sivananda Yoga Vedanta Center in New York.

Ananda Yoga is anchored in the teachings of Paramahansa Yogananda and was developed by Swami Kriyananda, one of his disciples. This is a gentle style designed to prepare the student for meditation, and its distinguishing features are the affirmations associated with postures. This Yoga style includes Yogananda's unique energization exercises, first developed in 1917, which involve consciously directing the body's energy (life force) to different organs and limbs. See Chapter 23 for more information about Ananda in California.

Bikram Yoga is the style taught by Bikram Choudhury. Bikram Choudhury, who achieved fame as the teacher of Hollywood stars, teaches at the Yoga College of India in Bombay, Beverly Hills, and other locations around the world, including San Francisco and Tokyo. This approach is fairly vigorous and requires a certain fitness level for participation.

Kundalini Yoga is not only an independent approach of Yoga but also the name of a style of Hatha Yoga, originated by the Sikh master Yogi Bhajan. Its purpose is to awaken the serpent power *(kundalini)* by means of postures, breath control, chanting, and meditation. Yogi Bhajan, who came to the United States in 1969, is the founder and spiritual head of the Healthy, Happy, Holy Organization (3HO), which has headquarters in Los Angeles and numerous branches around the world.

Hidden Language Yoga was developed by the late Swami Sivananda Radha, a German-born female student of Swami Sivananda. This style seeks to promote not only physical well-being but also self-understanding by exploring the symbolism inherent in the postures. Hidden Language Yoga is taught by the teachers of Yasodhara Ashram in British Columbia.

Somatic Yoga is the creation of Eleanor Criswell, Ed.D., a professor of psychology at Sonoma State University in California who has taught Yoga since the early 1960s. She is managing editor of *Somatics* magazine, which was launched by her late husband, Thomas Hanna, inventor of Somatics. Somatic Yoga is an integrated approach to the harmonious development of body and mind, based both on traditional yogic principles and modern psychophysiological research. This gentle approach emphasizes visualization, very slow movement into and out of postures, conscious breathing, mindfulness, and frequent relaxation between postures. For more about Eleanor Criswell's book, see this book's appendix.

You also may hear or see a mention of other Yoga styles, including Tri Yoga (developed by Kali Ray), White Lotus Yoga (developed by Ganga White and Tracey Rich; see the appendix), Jivamukti (developed by Sharon Gannon and David Life), and Ishta Yoga (developed by Mani Finger and made popular in the United States by his son Alan).

Empowering Yourself with Yoga

Outside agents like physicians, therapists, or remedies can help us through major crises, but we ourselves are primarily responsible for our own health and happiness. Especially the source of lasting happiness lies within us. Yoga reminds us of this truth and helps us mobilize the inner strength to live responsibly and wisely.

Maintaining health and happiness

What is health? Most people answer this question by saying that health is the opposite of illness. But health is *more* than the absence of disease. It's a positive state of being. Health is wholeness. To be healthy means not only to possess a well-functioning body and a sane mind but also to vibrate with life, to be vitally connected with one's social and physical environment. To be healthy also means to be happy.

Finding out what being healthy really means

Because life is constant movement, you shouldn't expect health to be static. Perfect health is a mirage. In the course of your life, you can expect inevitable fluctuations in your state of health — even cutting your finger with a knife temporarily upsets the balance. Your body reacts to the cut by mobilizing all the necessary biochemical forces to heal itself. Regular Yoga practice can create optimal conditions for self-healing. You achieve a baseline of health, with an improved immune system that enables you to stay healthy longer and heal faster.

Healing rather than curing

Yoga is about healing rather than curing. Like a really good physician, Yoga takes deeper causes into account. These causes, more often than not, are to be found in the mind, in the way you live. That's why Yoga masters recommend self-understanding.

Taking an active role in your own health

Most people tend to be passive in health matters. They wait until something goes wrong, and then they rely on a pill or a physician to fix the problem. Yoga encourages you to take the initiative in preventing illness and restoring or maintaining your health. Taking control of your health has nothing to do with self-doctoring (which can be dangerous); it's simply a matter of taking responsibility for your health. A good physician will tell you that healing is greatly facilitated when the patient actively participates in the process. For example, you may take various kinds of medication to deal with a gastric ulcer, but unless you learn to eat well, sleep adequately, avoid stress, and take life more easy, you're bound to have a recurrence before long. You must change your lifestyle.

Following your bliss

Yoga suggests that the best possible meaning you can find for yourself springs from the well of joy deep within you. That joy or bliss is the very nature of the spirit, or transcendental Self (refer to "Yoga as a spiritual discipline," earlier in this chapter). Joy is like a 3-D lens that captures life's bright colors and motivates you to embrace life in all of its countless forms. Yoga points the way to happiness, health, and life-embracing meaning.

Something for nothing?

The computer industry has coined thousands of new terms. One is particularly relevant to Yoga practice: *gigo,* which means "garbage in, garbage out." It captures a simple truth: The quality of a cause determines the quality of the effect. In other words:

- Don't expect health from junk food.
- Don't expect happiness from miserable attitudes.
- Don't expect good results from shoddy Yoga practice.

- Don't expect something from nothing.

Yoga is a powerful tool, but you must learn to use it properly. You can buy the latest super-duper computer, but if you only know how to use it as a typewriter, that's all it is. You get out of Yoga what you put into it.

Keep an open mind. Allow yourself to be surprised by Yoga's comprehensiveness. Don't settle for *just* this or that. Even after decades of Yoga practice and study, we're still discovering new things about Yoga.

Realizing Your Human Potential with Yoga

Don't put a ceiling on your own potential and growth! In 1865, Richard Webster ran one mile in 4:36.5. In 1993, Noureddine Morceli took only 3:44.39 to do the same. At the first Olympic Games in Athens in 1896, Ellery Clark reached 5 feet 11.25 inches in the running high jump event. A century later, at the Olympic Games in Atlanta, Georgia, Charles Austin improved the record to 7 feet 10 inches. The story is similar for other sports.

You may never be a world-class athlete. You (and we) are, however, *in principle* capable of anything that great Yoga masters can do. We all share the same human potential. Whether you actualize it depends largely on how determined you are and whether you find the right method for tapping into your own inner strength and wisdom.

Yoga makes good use of the mind, which is an incredible resource. Don't ask us to define what the mind is. We'd have to answer in the words of a comedian and say, "It doesn't matter." (When asked what matter is, the same comedian replied, "Never mind.") When speaking about the mind, we usually mean the mental attitudes that shape your behavior.

The power of Yoga

One of Yoga Master Sri Chinmoy's students, Ashrita Furman, holds the *Guinness Book of World Records* record for the most world records. In early 1997, 39-year-old Ed Kelley, another student of Sri Chinmoy, completed a 3,100-mile ultramarathon in 47 days, 15 hours, 19 minutes, and 56 seconds. You can't do this sort of thing without the cooperation of the mind. And the mind has been the playground of the masters of Yoga throughout the ages.

At the Menninger Foundation in Topeka, Kansas, in 1970, the late Swami Rama demonstrated that he could mentally control the functioning of his heart muscle. He also conclusively showed that he'd achieved extensive control over his brain waves. At will, he generated theta waves, which usually appear only in deep, dreamless sleep, and yet he could remember what had transpired in the lab more completely and clearly than the experimenters and technicians themselves. Similar accomplishments have been demonstrated by other Yoga masters to the amazement of the physicians and psychologists studying them.

Although Yoga is mind training, it isn't *just* mind training. It includes the physical body, which Yoga views as a great treasure. Having a body provides you with valuable experiences and lessons, and the body is the foundation on which you build your entire life. Yoga asks you to take proper care of your body through reasonable diet and physical exercise, as well as appropriate rest and sleep. At the same time, Yoga tells you that you're not *just* the body but also the mind, and not *just* the mind but also a greater "something" beyond body and mind — what we call the *spirit*.

Balancing Your Life with Yoga

Hindu tradition explains Yoga as the discipline of balance. This is another way of expressing the ideal of unity through Yoga. Everything in you must harmonize to function optimally. A disharmonious mind is disturbing in itself, but sooner or later, it also causes physical problems. An imbalanced body can easily warp your emotions and thought processes. If your relationships with others are strained, you cause distress not only for them but for yourself as well. And when your relationship to your physical environment is disharmonious, well, you trigger serious repercussions for everyone.

A beautiful and simple Yoga exercise called "The Tree" (described in Chapter 9) is meant to improve your sense of balance and promote your inner stillness. Even when conditions force a tree to grow askew, it always balances itself out by growing a branch in the opposite direction in which it's forced to lean. In this posture, you stand still like a tree, perfectly balanced.

Yoga helps you apply this principle to your life. Whenever life's demands and challenges force you to bend to one side, your inner strength and peace of mind serve as counterweights. Rising above all adversity, you can never be uprooted.

Chapter 2

Ready, Set, Yoga!

. . . .

In This Chapter

▶ Making up your mind

▶ Finding the right Yoga style, class, and teacher for yourself

▶ Preparing for a Yoga session

. . . .

This chapter gives you everything you need to begin your Yoga practice. Before you start, pause, take a deep breath, exhale slowly, and then ask yourself: What do I want from my Yoga experience? You may find your own answer by taking a few moments to ponder the following questions:

✔ Do I simply want to try Hatha Yoga because it's a trendy thing to do?

✔ Am I hoping to find a way to decompress (clear the mind and alleviate stress)?

✔ Is physical fitness my main interest?

✔ Do I simply want to have a more flexible body?

✔ Does meditation intrigue me?

✔ Do the spiritual aspects of Yoga interest me?

✔ Do I have health concerns, such as lower back problems or hypertension that I expect Yoga to help handle?

After you're clear about your motivation and expectations, don't just think it — *ink it*. Write down your goals so that you can really focus on your specific needs. For example, you may want to be able to cope with stress better. This is your *goal*. In order to achieve it, you have to take your particular situation into account. If you are a super-busy mom and have only half an hour of slack time at night during the week and perhaps a full hour on Sundays, you obviously have to keep your Yoga program very simple. This is your *need*.

No excuses, please

Most people are aware of how fast time flies in the 24 hours they're given each day. Yet if you look more closely at how you spend your days, you may find that not everything you do is necessary, and that in idle moments, you may miss the opportunity to recharge yourself or tap into your inner well of joy. But if you've picked up this book and are reading these lines, chances are you have *enough* time to practice Yoga regularly.

For those who think they're not capable of practicing Hatha Yoga because it requires too much flexibility or it's otherwise too demanding physically, turn your attention to this truth: You can be as stiff as a board and still benefit from Yoga! The whole point of the yogic postures is to help you become more flexible, whatever your starting point. Don't gauge yourself by the photos you may see in some Yoga books. They usually show advanced practitioners at their best. This book focuses on the needs of beginners. After you take the first few steps, the next big leap may not seem quite so challenging.

Make sure that you are physically ready before you begin this new venture with Yoga or any fitness activity. Consult with your doctor, especially if you have an existing health challenge. Even if your medical history includes experience with hypertension, heart problems, arthritis, or chronic back pain, you can benefit from Yoga. In more severe cases, you may want to work closely with a competent Yoga therapist to create just the right routines and to monitor your progress.

"Class Is in Session"

So, you're sure that you want to take the Yoga plunge. What's your safest bet? To put it plainly, set your sights on a suitable Yoga class or teacher instead of sailing away as a strict do-it-yourselfer. Although you can explore some basic practices by reading about them (this book makes sure of that!), a full-fledged, safe Yoga routine really requires proper instruction from a qualified teacher. After a few classes and the benefit of an instructor's expert advice, you can certainly continue practicing and exploring Yoga on your own (see the section "Skipping Class" later in this chapter). In that case, you may still want to check in with a teacher every so often, just to make sure that you haven't acquired any bad habits in executing the various postures and other practices. By the way, many Yoga schools offer introductory courses (four to six weeks), so you won't have to jump into the deep end.

Which way do I go?

If you live in a big city, you're bound to have several choices for group classes, but if you live in a small town you may have to be more resourceful. Here are some suggestions for finding the Yoga class that's right for you:

- ✔ Tell your friends that you want to join a Yoga class; some of them may start raving about their classes or teachers.

- ✔ Consult the resource guide in this book's appendix.

- ✔ Look at bulletin boards in health food stores and adult education centers.

- ✔ Check online resources (see the appendix at the end of this book).

- ✔ Look into possibilities at your local health club (but before joining a Yoga session, make sure that the teacher is really qualified: how much training has he or she had and is a certificate hanging on the office walls).

- ✔ Ask your local librarian.

- ✔ Head toward the back of the local Yellow Pages to check out listings under Yoga Instruction.

We think that visiting a few places and teachers is important before committing to a course or a series of classes. Some Yoga schools give out the telephone numbers of their teachers, and you may want to have a phone conversation before making a special trip to the school. When you visit a Yoga center or classroom, pay attention to your intuitive feelings about the place. Consider how the staff treats you and how you respond to the people attending class. Stroll around the facility and feel its overall "energy." First impressions are often (although not always) accurate.

Bring a written checklist to your class visit. Don't feel embarrassed about being thorough. If you don't want to be so obvious, memorize the points that you want to check out. Here are some ideas for your list:

- ✔ How do I feel about the building or classroom's atmosphere? Some teachers will let you quietly look in on a class; others find this too distracting for their students. What is my gut response to the teacher?

- ✔ Do I want a male or female teacher? Does it matter?

- ✔ What are the teacher's credentials?

- ✔ Does the teacher or school have a good reputation?

- ✔ How do I respond to other students?

✔ Do the programs suit my needs?

✔ How big are the classes, and can I still get proper, individual attention from the teacher?

✔ Would I be happy coming here regularly?

✔ Can I afford the classes?

If you are a beginner, look for a beginner's course. You're likely to feel more comfortable in a group that's starting at the same skill level instead of being surrounded by advanced practitioners who can perform difficult postures easily and elegantly. Whatever the skill level of a class, there's no need to feel self-conscious. None of the advanced students will stare at you to see whether the new kid in class is any good. You might get a few encouraging smiles, though.

Beginner classes are sometimes advertised as *Easy Does It Yoga* or *Gentle Yoga.*

As a beginner, be leery of mixed-level classes that lump together Yoga freshmen with postgraduates. Your teacher won't be able to give you the attention you deserve to ensure your safety. We recommend that you stay away from overly large classes (more than 20 students) for the same reason, at least until you feel more comfortable with the practice. Many of the more experienced teachers, however, are quite popular, and their classes tend to be large. You have to decide what is most important to you.

When checking out a Yoga center, don't hesitate to quiz the instructor or other staff members about any concerns. In particular, find out what *style* of Hatha Yoga they are offering. Some styles — notably the Ashtanga, or *Power Yoga* — demand athletic fitness. Others embody a more relaxed approach. In this book, we favor the latter. However, we can readily appreciate that some vigorous people may feel attracted to and benefit from yogic routines that are the equivalent of a workout and that call for strength, endurance, high flexibility, and a drench of perspiration.

If you're not familiar with the style of a particular school, don't hesitate to ask for an explanation (check out our explanation of styles in Chapter 1). Yoga practitioners are usually pretty friendly folk, eager to answer your questions and put your mind at ease. If they aren't, put a mark in the appropriate box in your mental checklist. Remember that even nice people, including Yoga practitioners, can have occasional off-days. But if you don't feel welcome and comfortable on your first visit, you probably won't receive better treatment later on.

TIP

Backyard studios and home classes

Throughout the world, many Yoga teachers hold sessions in their homes or in backyard studios. Don't let this practice turn you off — you may find a great opportunity. Some of the most dedicated Yoga teachers work this way because they want to avoid commercialism and the details of administering a full-scale center. Backyard studios often offer a great sense of community, and you can also expect lots of valuable, personal attention from the teacher because the groups tend to be smaller than those in larger centers.

Public or private?

Decide whether you want to learn Hatha Yoga in a group or from a private instructor. In practice, most people start with a group class because of the cost and the boost in motivation that comes from practicing with other people. If you can afford private lessons, however, even a few sessions can be extremely beneficial. Importantly, if you have a serious health challenge, you need to work privately with a Yoga therapist (see the appendix for a list of organizations specializing in Yoga therapy). Here is a sampling of the advantages of private lessons:

- ✔ You get personalized attention.
- ✔ You have the opportunity to interact more with the teacher during class.
- ✔ Your routines can vary more, with proper supervision.
- ✔ You can work more intensively with those exercises that are more challenging for you.
- ✔ If you're shy or easily distracted, you won't have to worry about the company of other people.

Here are a few advantages of group practice:

- ✔ You experience the support of the group.
- ✔ Your motivation is strengthened by seeing others succeed.
- ✔ You can make good, like-minded friends.
- ✔ Group sessions are easy on your pocketbook.

What to wear, what to wear?

Yoga practitioners wear a wide variety of exercise clothing. Practically speaking, what people wear depends on the difficulty level of the class and the temperature of the room. Of course, there's also the matter of personal expression. A handful of eccentric groups practice in the nude, which really isn't a good idea because it's bound to distract some folks. Besides, it's easy to catch a chill. Even when you practice on your own, you need to cover your lower trunk to protect your kidneys and abdomen.

Women often wear leotards, sweats, shorts, and tops. Men usually wear shorts, sweats, T-shirts, and tank tops.

The key is to wear clean, comfortable, and decent clothes that you can move and breathe in. If you want to be fashionable, you can now readily obtain Yoga clothing through mail-order catalogs (see the appendix).

If you are practicing outdoors or in a poorly heated room, you may want to layer your clothing so that you can peel off a layer when you are getting too warm from your Yoga practice. Also, extra clothing can come in handy when you get to the relaxation or meditation part of the class.

What do I pack in my Yoga suitcase?

Before attending a class, find out what kind of floor you'll be practicing on. If the floor is carpeted, then a towel or a sticky mat will suffice (we describe sticky mats and similar useful items in Chapter 17). A hardwood floor may require more padding, especially if your knees are sensitive. In that case, bring along a thick Yoga mat or a rug remnant that is a little longer then your height and a little wider then your shoulders. If you have a tendency to get cold, bring a blanket to cover yourself during final relaxation. A folded blanket is also helpful if you need a pad under your head when you're lying down. As your teacher becomes familiar with your unique needs, he or she may suggest some other personalized props for you to bring to class. As we discuss in Chapter 1, some Yoga styles — notably Iyengar Yoga — work more with props than others. Following are some things you may want to bring to class with you:

✔ Your own Yoga mat or rug

✔ A towel

✔ A blanket

✔ Extra clothing to layer on if the room is too cool or to take off if you're too warm

✔ Bottled water (to balance your electrolytes after the session)

✔ Enthusiasm, motivation, and good humor

If you're serious about your Yoga practice (and if you're concerned about hygiene), we recommend that you invest in your own personal mat and other equipment. Although many Yoga centers furnish this stuff, consider bringing your own. If you ever have to pick from the bottom of the bin after yet another sweaty class, you will know what we mean.

Paying the price: How much should Yoga cost?

In general, group Yoga classes are pretty affordable. The cheapest classes are usually available at adult education centers and community and senior centers. YMCA and YWCA classes also tend to be reasonably priced, or your health club may even include free Yoga classes as part of a fitness package. Most regular Yoga centers in metropolitan areas, however, charge on average $10 to 15 per class. A one-time drop-in fee (for those who haven't committed to taking more than one class) is usually a couple of dollars higher. Some schools offer the first class free, and others charge as much as $25.

You can do your own pricing research by phone, fax, and computer. More and more Yoga sites advertise on the Internet (see the appendix). They usually don't mention fees, but they do provide you with an e-mail address or a phone number. When you're considering a commitment to a Yoga center, check into the larger packages — they're often a good investment. Obviously, private lessons are quite a bit more expensive than group classes and range from $50 to $150.

Occasionally, some would-be students think that Yoga instruction should be free. Much as we hate to admit it, though, Yoga teachers need to eat and pay the bills, too. Unfortunately, some teachers do exploit their popularity and charge exorbitant amounts for their classes. Whenever you smell commercialism, you can be fairly sure your nose isn't deceiving you. If you're uncomfortable with the price you're quoted for Yoga classes, just search out a more reasonable offer.

How long will a Yoga class be?

The length of a group Yoga class varies from 50 to 90 minutes. Health clubs, fitness spas, and corporate classes are normally 50 to 60 minutes long, while beginning classes at Yoga centers usually last from 75 to 90 minutes long. A private Yoga lesson customarily lasts one hour.

Going co-ed

All Yoga classes that we're familiar with welcome both genders, with an average of seven women to three men enrolled in any session. Some of the more physically demanding styles of Hatha Yoga, however, attract an even number of athletic men and women.

What makes a good teacher?

A good Yoga teacher should be an example of what Yoga is all about: a balanced person who is not only skillful in the postures, but also courteous and thoughtful toward others and adaptive and attentive to your individual needs. Check out the teacher's credentials to be sure that he or she has been properly trained or is certified in one of the established traditions. Consult Chapter 23 and the appendix for our recommendations on some of the well-established larger Yoga organizations.

We caution you to steer clear of teachers who have taken only a few workshops on Yoga or received their diplomas in a three-day course. They may be excellent aerobics instructors or fitness trainers who know nothing about Yoga. Also avoid the drill sergeant type or anyone who makes you feel intimidated about your level of skill in performing the postures. By the way, under no circumstances allow your instructor to push or coerce you into a posture that doesn't feel right or that causes you pain.

Putting safety first

The most important factor for determining the safety of a Yoga class is your personal attitude. If you participate with the understanding that you are not competing against the other students or the teacher and that you also must not inflict pain upon yourself, you can enjoy a safe Yoga practice. The popular maxim "No pain, no gain" doesn't apply to Yoga. On the contrary: *There is no gain with negative pain* — to coin a phrase.

By *negative pain,* we mean discomfort that causes you distress or increases the likelihood of injury. Of course, if you haven't exercised for a while, you can expect to encounter your body's resistance at the beginning. You may even feel a little sore the next day, which just reflects your body's adjustment to the new adventure. The key to avoiding injury is to proceed gently. It's better to err on the side of gentleness than to face torn ligaments. A good teacher always reminds you to ease into the postures and work creatively with your body's physical resistance. Nonharming is an important moral virtue in Yoga — and observation toward all beings includes yourself!

If you have any physical limitations (recent surgeries, knee, neck, or back problems, and so on), be sure to inform the center and the teacher beforehand. In a classroom setting, instructors have to split their attention among several students; your up-front communication can help prevent personal injury.

Paging Miss Manners

Think of your Yoga class as a theater of expression and enlightenment. Now, imagine your enjoyment of the Yoga experience if one or more of your senses is distracted by the sight, sound, or smell of something that you find mildly offensive or — on the higher end of unpleasant — downright disgusting.

In all social settings, common courtesy calls for sensitivity to others; those same rules of responsible conduct apply to your participation in Yoga group sessions. So, sift through all the good manners you've accumulated from a lifetime of human interaction, and pack them as required equipment for your next trip to class. Before you go, check your bags for these etiquette essentials:

✔ Show up on time; don't wander into class "fashionably" late.

✔ If you show up early and students from the class before are still relaxing or meditating, respect their quiet time.

✔ Leave your shoes, chewing gum, cell phones, beepers, and crummy attitudes outside the classroom.

✔ Avoid smoking cigarettes or drinking alcohol before class.

✔ Bathe and take a restroom break before your Yoga session.

✔ Keep classroom conversation to a minimum — some people arrive early to meditate or to just sit quietly.

✔ Be sure to take your socks off if you practice on a slippery surface (just don't leave them near your neighbor's face). If you're self-conscious about your feet ("those ugly things"), remember that their 26 bones do a great job at propping up your body all day long — besides, everyone else is far too busy to focus on your feet.

✔ Avoid excessive, clanky jewelry.

✔ Be sure that your, um, private parts are appropriately covered if you choose to wear loose-fitting shorts or super-tight outfits.

✔ Don't wear heavy perfume or cologne.

✔ Cut back on your garlic consumption on the day that you go to class.

✔ Sit near the door or window if you require a lot of air.

✔ Sit close to the instructor if you have hearing difficulties; many teachers speak softly to generate the right mood.

✔ If you have used any props in class, put them away neatly.

✔ Pay your teacher on time, without having to be reminded.

Skipping Class

Traditionally, Yoga is passed down from teacher to student. However, a few accomplished yogis and yoginis are self-taught. These independent spirits set a precedent for those who enjoy exploring new territory on their own. If you live in an isolated area and don't have easy access to a Yoga instructor or class, don't be disheartened. You still have several choices that can help you begin your yogic journey (and in the appendix we provide you with a fairly extensive list of resources). Here's an abbreviated version:

✔ Audiocassettes

✔ Books

✔ Magazines

✔ Newsletters

✔ Newspapers

✔ Television

✔ Videos

Because Yoga is a motor skill, most people without access to a teacher rely on a video for instruction. If you opt for this particular approach, we recommend that you learn a routine and then begin listening only to the instructor's voice rather than focusing on the screen. Yoga emphasizes more inner work than outer activity; watching a video interferes with this process. Listening to a disembodied voice works better. According to Yoga, the eye is an active and even aggressive sense, whereas the ear is a more passive receptor. That's why audiotapes also can work well, provided they're accompanied by informative illustrations.

We prefer a good Yoga book over magazine or newspaper articles, simply because the creation of a book usually requires more in-depth, detailed consideration of subject matter and presentation. Look for our book recommendations in the appendix. But don't discount the value of a newsletter from a backyard Yoga studio. The publication can be a real find if it comes from a legitimate source. You'll undoubtedly come across some interesting and informative newsletters as your circle of Yoga friends widens.

The difficulty with self-tutoring at the beginning is that you may have trouble judging "good form" from "bad form." It takes time to understand how your body responds to the challenge of a posture and determine the proper correction for your body's own optimal form. Some people use a mirror to check the postures, but that only tells one side of the story and, more importantly, it externalizes the whole process too much.

Become comfortable with checking from the inside, through inwardly *feeling* your body. Until you are proficient at doing so, seek out a competent instructor if at all possible. He or she sees you objectively — from all sides — and can thus give you valuable feedback about your body's specific resistances and requirements.

Being a Committed Yogi or Yogini

The traditional practice time for Yoga is 24 hours a day (see Chapter 18). But even full-fledged yogis and yoginis don't perform postures and other similar exercises for more than a few hours daily. (Of course, some of them don't practice any physical exercises at all, but pursue meditation exclusively.) Some people can carve out a regular Yoga practice time in their daily schedules. Many others, however, find this commitment completely impractical. Yet you can still benefit by attending classes *twice a week*. Even attending a group session *once a week* may introduce a little balance into a hectic lifestyle. There also are many opportunities during the day to work in a few Yoga postures or breathing exercises — during car rides or coffee breaks, or while going shopping.

How much time you allocate to your postural practice depends entirely on your goals and lifestyle. Inevitably, the busier you are with work, chores around the house, and social life, the less time you have available for Yoga. Consider starting with twice a week for a minimum of 15 minutes and see if you can build to 30 minutes as a realistic goal in the first 3 months. If you are able to dedicate more time to Yoga, then try to practice *daily*. But set a realistic goal for yourself so that you don't stress-out about Yoga or give up on it before you're able to enjoy its benefits. Also, remember that even if you don't have much time during the week, what you learn from each session can be applied anytime and anywhere!

The amount of time that you dedicate to Yoga is a personal choice — no need to feel guilty about your decision. Guilt is counterproductive and has no place in Yoga practice.

Making Time for Yoga

For centuries, the traditional time for Yoga practice has been sunrise and sunset, which are thought to be especially auspicious. These days, busy lifestyles can toss out lots of obstacles to your best intentions: Be pragmatic and arrange your Yoga practice at your convenience. Just keep in mind that statistically, you have a 30 percent greater chance of accomplishing a fitness goal if you practice in the morning. More important than holding tight to a preset time is just making sure that you work Yoga into your schedule *somewhere* — and sticking with it.

Practicing at roughly the same time during the day can help you create a positive habit, which may make it easier to maintain your routine.

Eating before Yoga Practice

Whether you're taking a Yoga class or practicing on your own, the guidelines for eating before Yoga practice are similar to the advice given for most physical activities. With even the lightest meal, such as fruit or juice, allow at least one hour before class. For larger meals with vegetables and grains, allow two hours and for heavy meals with meat, three to four hours. Eating right after class is okay; you may notice that this snack or meal turns into a pleasant social event with classmates. (If the socializing aspect sounds like fun, remember that you're not likely to enjoy the same opportunities with private lessons.)

Keeping a Yoga Diary

Keeping a regular journal is a good way to chronicle your growth with Yoga. Beyond just writing down your physical experiences with Yoga, you can record your insights and ideas, as well as your dreams (both the ones visiting you during sleep and the ones you create with your conscious mind). Prolonged regular practice can definitely change you — not just your body but also your inner and outer life. Your journal may add to your overall understanding about Yoga while enhancing your self-understanding. Some people's journal entries are elaborate and analytical, others consist of a few catch phrases. Some folks enjoy exercising their poetic imagination as expression of their experiences with Yoga.

Part II

Getting in Shape for Yoga

The 5th Wave   By Rich Tennant

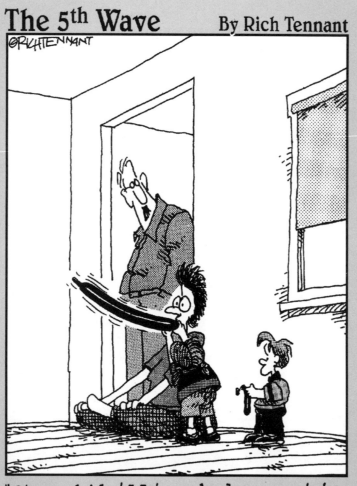

"C'mon kids! We've asked you not to do that when your Mom's doing her deep breathing exercises."

In this part . . .

1f you arrived here by skipping the first two chapters, well, you can still fill in some of the missing information by reading the three chapters of the present part. (But, please, do read the chapters in Part I — and carefully too — because they provide you with vital practical knowledge about Yoga.)

In this part, we provide you with guidelines for proper preparation to make your practice safe. Then we introduce you to the two pillars of good Hatha Yoga practice: relaxation and conscious breathing.

Chapter 3

Prep Before Pep

. . . .

In This Chapter

▶ Approaching Yoga with a healthy attitude

▶ Leaving the competition behind

▶ Translating your own mind-body language

▶ Doing it your way without regret

. . . .

In Yoga, *what* you do and *how* you do it are equally important — and both mind and body contribute to your actions. Yoga respects the fact that you are not merely a physical body but a psychophysical *body-mind*. Full mental participation in even the simplest of physical exercise enables you to tap into your deeper potential as a human being.

This chapter is about the right attitude toward practice, especially the yogic postures, which is the best preparation for success in Yoga. Among other things, we examine the spirit of competitiveness, which has no place in Yoga. We encourage you to find your own pace, without pushing yourself and risking injury. We also express the importance of function over form, proposing that you modify the "ideal form" of an exercise to suit your specific needs.

Yoga is not a military drill but a creative endeavor that asks you to call on the formidable powers of your own mind as you explore and enjoy yogic possibilities.

Cultivating the Right Attitude

Your attitudes reveal a lot about you and your social background. Attitudes are enduring tendencies in your mind, which show themselves not only in your speech but also in your behavior. Yoga encourages you to examine all your basic attitudes to life to discover which ones are wrong and dysfunctional so that you can replace them with better, more appropriate attitudes.

One of the attitudes worth cultivating is balance in everything.

A balanced attitude in this context means that you're willing to build up your Yoga practice step by step instead of expecting instant perfection. It also means not basing your practice on wrong assumptions, including the mistaken notion that Yoga is about tying yourself in knots. On the contrary, Yoga tries to loosen all our bodily, emotional, and intellectual knots.

Pretzels are not us!

Many people are turned off when they see publications featuring photographs of adept practitioners in advanced postures, with their limbs tied into knots.

Those publications sometimes neglect to tell you that most of the yogis and yoginis in the photographs have practiced Yoga several hours a day for many years to achieve their level of skill. Trust us! You don't have to be a pretzel to experience the undeniable benefits of Yoga. You derive no additional therapeutic benefit, for example, from bending backward until your toes touch your ears or raising one leg like a flagpole straight above your head while standing upright.

In Yoga sports — one of five orientations mentioned in Chapter 1 — more than 2,000 postures are possible. Many of these call for such great strength and flexibility that only a top gymnast can perform them flawlessly. The postures certainly look beautiful and intriguing when mastered, but their health benefits are the same as the 20 or so fundamental postures that make up most practitioners' daily routines. So, unless you aim to participate in Yoga competitions, you won't have to worry about all those glamorous-looking postures you may find in some books and magazines or on colorful posters. Most of these postures are new inventions, whereas Yoga masters have been content for centuries with just a handful of practices that have stood the test of time.

What's in a number?

The traditional Sanskrit texts of Hatha Yoga state that 8,400,000 postures exist, which correspond to as many species of living creatures. Of these, it is said, only 84 are useful to humans and 32 are especially important.

The number 84 has symbolic value and is the product of 12 × 7. The number 12 represents the fullness of a chronological cycle (as in the 12 months of the year, or the 12 signs of the zodiac). The number 7 stands for structural fullness (as in the 7 energy centers or *cakras* of the human body — see Chapter 20).

Practice at your own pace

People who are natural pretzels are typically double-jointed. If you're not inherently noodle-like, you can expect to have to practice regularly to increase your body's flexibility and muscular strength. We advocate a graduated approach. In Chapters 6-15, you can find all the preparatory and intermediary steps that lead up to the final forms for the various postures. The late Yoga master T. Krishnamacharya of Madras, India, who is the source of most of the best-known orientations of modern Hatha Yoga, expressed the importance of tailoring Yoga instruction to the needs of each individual. He recommended that Yoga teachers take a student's age, physical ability, emotional state, and occupation into account — we agree completely. So, our best advice to you is basic and simple: Proceed gently, but steadfastly.

If you like to learn Yoga from books, choose them carefully. Especially look closely at whether the exercise descriptions include all the stages of developing comfort with a particular posture. To ask a middle-aged newcomer to Yoga to imitate the final form of many of the postures without providing suitable transitions and adaptations is a prescription for disaster. For instance, in almost every book on Hatha Yoga — except ours — you will see the headstand featured quite prominently. This posture has become something of a symbol for Yoga in the West. Headstands are powerful postures, to be sure, but they also count among the more advanced practices. Because this beginner's book emphasizes exercises that are both feasible and safe, we have chosen not to include the headstand. We say more about this in Chapter 11, which introduces safe inversion practices. Instead, we give you several adaptations that are easier to perform and have no risk attached to them.

Send the scorekeeper home

Americans often grow up in a highly competitive environment. From childhood on, we are encouraged to do more, push harder, and secure success. In sports like football, basketball, and soccer, young players are indoctrinated with the spirit of competitiveness. Although competition has its place in society, elbowing one's way to victory can be harmful to oneself and others. And this type of competitive behavior has no place in the practice of Yoga.

Many years ago, a middle-aged man came to one of our classes. He was a friendly enough fellow, but extremely competitive and hard on himself. He announced right away that he was intent on mastering the lotus posture within a few weeks and pushed himself during our classes. We cautioned him repeatedly to proceed more slowly. After only a few visits, he failed to show up and never returned. Later we learned from a mutual friend that he had asked his wife to sit on his legs to force them into the lotus posture. Her weight had seriously injured both knees!

Yoga is about peace, tranquillity, and harmony — the exact opposite of the competitive mindset. Yoga doesn't require you to fight against anyone, least of all yourself, or to achieve some goal by force. On the contrary, you are invited to be kind to yourself and others and, above all, to collaborate with rather than coerce your body or do battle with your mind. Yoga is gentle. In its gentleness, however, it is extremely powerful.

No pain, no gain — NOT!

The idea of "no pain, no gain" — a completely mistaken notion — often reinforces competitiveness. Yoga does not ask you to be a masochist. Pain and discomfort are part of life, but this realization doesn't require you to invite them. On the contrary, the goal of Yoga is to overcome all suffering. Therefore never flog your body, always only coax it gently. Our motto is: *No gain from pain.*

Picture yourself in the posture

We encourage you to use visualization in the execution of postures. For example, before you do the cobra, shoulder stand, or triangle, take ten seconds or so to visualize yourself moving into the final posture. Make your visualization as vivid as possible. Enlist the powers of your mind!

Enjoying a Safe and Sound Yoga Practice

As you travel through yogic postures, you begin to build awareness of the communications taking place between your body and mind. Do you feel peacefully removed from the raging storm of life around you, comfortable and confident with your strength, motion, and steadiness? Or are you painfully in tune with the passage of time, sensing a physical awkwardness or strain in your movements? Listening to your own rhythms — and acknowledging their importance — can help make your Yoga experience an expression of peace, calm, and security. And that positive message is what Yoga practice is all about.

Making sense of the perfect posture myth

Some modern schools of Hatha Yoga claim that they teach "perfect" postures that you can slip into as easily as a tailor-made suit. But how can a perfect posture exist when we are all different? Should a 15-year-old athlete perform a posture or an entire postural routine following the same guidelines that apply to a 60-year-old retiree? Surely not. Besides, these schools disagree among themselves about what constitutes a perfect posture. So, to spell it out, the perfect posture is perfectly mythical.

Posture, as explained by the great Yoga master Patanjali 2,000 years ago, has only two requirements: A posture should be *steady* and *comfortable*. What could be more plain and simple? Although Patanjali was thinking primarily, perhaps even exclusively, in terms of meditation postures, his formula applies to all postures equally.

- ✔ **Steady posture:** A steady posture is a posture that's held stable for a certain period of time. The key isn't freezing all movement, though. Your posture becomes steady when your mind is steady. As long as your thoughts run wild and your negative emotions are not held in check, your body also remains unsteady. As you become more skilled in self-observation, you begin to notice the ever-revolving carousel of your mind and become sensitive to the tension in your body. That tension is what Yoga means by "unsteadiness."

- ✔ **Comfortable posture:** A posture is comfortable when it is enjoyable and enlivening rather than boring and burdensome. A comfortable posture increases the principle of clarity — *sattva* — in you (see Chapter 1). But please don't confuse comfort with slouching. *Sattva* and joy are intimately connected. The more *sattva* is present in your body-mind, the more relaxed and happy you will be.

Listening to your body

No one knows your body like you do. The more you practice Yoga, the better you can become at determining your limitations with each posture: Each posture presents its own unique challenge. Ideally, you want to feel encouraged to explore and expand your physical and emotional boundaries without risking strain or injury to yourself.

Some teachers speak of practicing at the *edge*. The edge is the point of intensity where a posture challenges you but does not cause you pain or unusual discomfort. The idea is to gradually — very slowly and carefully — push that edge farther back and open up new territory. To be able to practice at the edge, you must cultivate self-observation and pay attention to the feedback from your body.

Each Yoga session is an exercise in self-observation without being judgmental. Listen to what your body is telling you through its ongoing communications. Signals constantly travel from your muscles, tendons, ligaments, bones, and skin to your brain. Train yourself to become aware of them. You want to be in dialogue with your body instead of indulging in a monologue that focuses on your own mind without awareness of your body. Pay particular attention to signals coming from the neck, lower back, jaw muscles, abdomen, and any known problem areas of your body (such as a "difficult" knee or a "chronic" shoulder muscle).

To gauge the intensity of a difficult Yoga posture, use a scale from 1 to 10, with 10 being at the threshold of pain. Imagine a flashing red light and an alarm bell going off after you pass level 8. Notice the signals and heed them. Especially watch your breath. If your breathing becomes labored, it's usually a good indication that, figuratively speaking, you are going over the edge. You are the world's foremost expert on what your body is trying to tell you.

Beginners commonly experience trembling when holding certain Yoga postures. Normally, the involuntary motion is noticeable in the legs or arms and is nothing to worry about, as long as you aren't straining. The tremors are simply a sign that your muscles are working in response to a new demand. Instead of focusing on the feeling that you've become a wobbly bowl of jelly, make your breath a little longer if you can and allow your attention to go deeper within. If the trembling starts to go off the Richter scale, then you need to either ease up a little or end the posture altogether.

Moving slowly but surely

All postural movements are intended for slow performance. Unfortunately, most of the time, we're on automatic. Our movements tend to be unconscious, too fast, and not particularly graceful. We stumble, bump into things, and are generally unaware of our bodies. The yogic postures oblige you to adopt a different attitude. Among the advantages of slow motion are:

✔ You enhance your awareness, which enables you to *listen* to what your body is telling you and to practice at the *edge* (see the earlier section, "Listening to your body").

✔ You lower the risk of straining or spraining muscles, tearing ligaments, or overtaxing your heart. In other words, your practice becomes much safer.

✔ You experience relaxation more quickly.

✔ You don't get out of breath, and your breathing overall is improved.

✔ You enable more muscle groups come into action to share the workload.

For the best results, practice your postures at a slow, steady pace while calmly focusing on your breath and the postural movement (see Chapter 5). Resist the temptation to speed up, but instead savor each posture. Remember to relax and be present here and now. If your breathing becomes a little bit labored or you begin to feel fatigued, just rest until you're ready to go on.

If you find yourself rushing through your program, pause and ask yourself why you're in a hurry. If you have an actual reason, such as an imminent appointment, your best bet is to crop your program by focusing on fewer exercises. Or, if you cannot shake the feeling of being pressured by time, you may want to postpone your Yoga session altogether and practice conscious breathing (see Chapter 5) while you go about your other business.

However, if you're rushing through your program because you're feeling bored or distracted for some other reason, pause and remind yourself why you're practicing Yoga in the first place. Renew your motivation by telling yourself that you have plenty of time to complete your session; you have no earthly reason to be in any hurry. Boredom is a sign that you are detached from your own bodily experience and are not living in the present moment. Resume your Yoga practice as a full participant in the process. If you need more than a mental reminder, use one of the relaxation techniques that we describe in Chapter 4 to slow yourself down. As we explain in Chapter 5, full yogic breathing in one of the resting postures also has a wonderful calming effect.

Practicing function over form with Forgiving Limbs

In Yoga, as in life, function is more important than form. Beginners, in particular, need to adapt postures to enjoy the function and benefits of a given posture early in their practice experiences.

We call one very useful adaptive device *Forgiving Limbs*. With Forgiving Limbs, you give yourself permission to slightly bend your legs and arms instead of keeping them fully extended. You don't need to feel like a wimp if you're kind to your body in order to help you achieve the function of a posture. Although bent arms and legs don't look flashy, they enable you to move your spine more easily, which is the focus of many postures and the key to a healthy spine. For example, the primary mechanical function of a standing forward bend is to stretch your lower back. If you have a good back, take a moment to see what we mean in this adapted posture that's safe for beginners:

1. **Stand up straight and *without forcing anything* bend forward and try to place your head on your knees with the palms of your hands on the floor (see Figure 3-1a).**

   Very few men or women can actually do this, especially beginners.

2. **Now stand up again, separate your feet to hip width, and bend forward, allowing your legs to bend until you can place your hands on the floor and almost touch your head to your knees (see Figure 3-1b).**

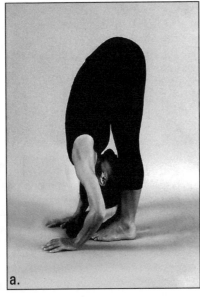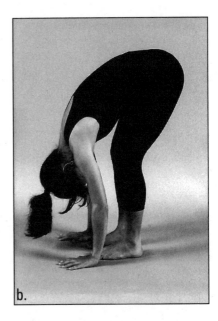

Figure 3-1:
Classic
form (a) and
modified
form with
"Forgiving
Limbs" (b).

a.   b.

As you become more flexible — and you will! — gradually straighten your legs until you can come closer to the ideal posture. A common lower back injury occurs when weekend warriors, inspired by young nubile instructors, try to do the seated version of the straight-legged forward bend and push too far.

Bending your legs and arms to achieve the intended function of a posture is perfectly all right; especially for beginners, bending is safer than attempting to achieve the final form.

Approaching exercise with open eyes

Many Yoga conferences entertain the question of whether you should keep your eyes open or closed during Yoga practice. In a nutshell, if you're comfortable with your eyes closed, then we recommend you close them. You may feel more focused and able to hear your body's signals. However, standing and balancing postures require you to keep your eyes open.

With a little practice, you can stay focused even with your eyes open. In general, Yoga favors an open-eyed approach to life's challenges. The yogis and yoginis like to know what's in front of them, and therefore many seasoned practitioners also execute the postures with open eyes. Seasoned meditators, by the way, can enter into deep meditation without shutting their eyes, though don't be surprised if they have a blank look; they have effectively withdrawn their awareness from external reality and are happily conscious at a different level. You can expect to experience something of this attitude as you master the various postures and breathing exercises.

Chapter 4

Relaxed Like a Noodle: The Fine Art of Letting Go of Stress

• •

In This Chapter

▶ Understanding the nature of stress

▶ Dealing with stress

▶ Relaxing the body

▶ Acquiring a calm mind

• •

*L*ife in general — not merely modern life — is inherently stressful. Even an inanimate object, such as a rock, experiences an element of stress. Not all stress is bad for you, however. The question is whether that stress is helping you or killing you.

Psychologists distinguish between *distress* and *eustress* (good stress). Yoga can help you minimize distress and maximize good, life-enhancing stress. For example, a creative challenge that stimulates your imagination and fires your enthusiasm, but that doesn't cause you anxiety or lost sleep, is a positive event. Even a joyous celebration is, strictly speaking, stressful; but the celebration's not the kind of stress that kills you — at least not in modest doses. On the other hand, doing nothing and feeling bored to tears is a form of negative stress.

In this chapter, we talk about how you can control negative stress not only through various yogic-relaxation techniques, but also by cultivating appropriate attitudes and habits.

The Nature of Stress

Stress is a fact of life. Some estimates indicate that 80 percent of all illnesses result from stress. Endocrinologist Hans Selye, who pioneered research on stress, distinguished three phases of the stress syndrome: alarm, resistance, and exhaustion. *Alarm* can be a harmless activity like stepping from a warm house into the cold air or receiving an upsetting phone call. Both situations require the body to make an adjustment, which is a kind of *resistance*. When the demand on the body goes on for too long, the stage of *exhaustion* sets in, which can lead to a complete breakdown of the body and the mind — be it heart disease, hypertension, failure of the immune system, or mental illness.

Bad stress creates an imbalance in the body and the mind, causing you to tense your muscles and breathe in a rapid and shallow manner. Under stress, your adrenal glands work overtime and your blood becomes depleted of oxygen, which starves your cells. Constant stress triggers the fight-or-flight response, putting you in a chronic state of alertness that's extremely demanding on your body's energies.

Because of the relentless demands that modern life makes on us — work, noise, pollution, and so on — most people experience chronic stress. How can you deal with it efficiently? Yoga suggests a three-pronged solution:

- ✔ Correct those *attitudes* that are stress-producing.

- ✔ Change *habits* that invite stress into your life.

- ✔ Release existing *tension* in the body and do so on an ongoing basis.

Stress can occur without any unpleasant stimulus. Even a birthday celebration can cause you stress, usually because of some hidden anxiety (like another year to mark off). Stress is cumulative and can creep up on you so gradually that it's imperceptible — until its acute and adverse symptoms manifest.

Correcting wrong attitudes

Yoga's integrated approach works with both the body and the mind, offering potent antidotes to just the sort of attitudes that make you prone to stress, especially egotism, extreme competitiveness, perfectionism, and the sense of having to accomplish everything right now and by yourself. In all matters, Yoga seeks to replace negative thoughts and attitudes with positive mental dispositions. Yogic practice helps you understand that everything has its proper place and time. Yoga asks you to be kind to yourself.

If you, like so many stress sufferers, have a hard time asking for help, Yoga can give you a real appreciation that we are all interdependent. If you are by nature distrustful of others, Yoga puts you in touch with that part of your psyche that naturally trusts life itself. It shows you that you don't need to feel as if you were under attack, because your real life — your spiritual identity — can never be harmed or destroyed.

Wherever ego, I go

The ultimate source of stress is the ego, or what the Yoga masters call the "I-maker" *(ahamkara)*, from *aham* ("I") and *kara* ("maker"). From the perspective of Yoga, the ego is a mistaken notion in which we identify with our particular body rather than the universe as a whole. Consequently, we experience fear of death and attachment to the body and the mind. This attachment, which is the survival instinct, in turn gives rise to all those many emotions and intentions that make up the game of life. Keeping this artificial center — the ego — going is inherently stressful. The Yoga masters all agree that by relaxing the grip of the ego, you can experience greater peace and happiness.

Changing poor habits

Everything in the universe follows an ebb-and-flow pattern that you can count on. Seasons change, and newborn babies eventually become elderly adults. Yogic wisdom recommends that you adopt the same natural patterns into your personal life. You may spend much of your time being serious, but you need to play, too. In fact, you need to make time to *just be* with no expectations and no guilt. Taking time to *just be* is good for your physical and mental health. Work and rest, tension and relaxation belong together as balanced pairs.

Often, people desperately maintain a hectic schedule because they can't envision an alternative that includes time out. They fear what may happen if they were to slow down. But money and standard of living aren't everything, and the *quality* of your life is far more important. Besides, if stress undercuts your health, you have to go into low gear anyway, and your climb back to health may prove very costly. Yoga gives you a baseline of tranquillity to deal with your fears effectively.

Your inner wisdom tells you that your body and mind are subject to change and that nothing in your environment permanently stays the same. Therefore, there's no point in anxiously clinging to anything. Yoga recommends that you constantly remember your spiritual nature, which is beyond the realm of change and ever blissful. However, Yoga also asks you to care for others and the world you live in, but all the while appreciating that you can't step into the same river twice.

Detach yourself

Yoga shows you how to cultivate the *relaxation response* throughout the day by letting go of your hold on things. This phrase was coined by Herbert Benson, MD, who was among the first to point out the hidden epidemic of hypertension (high blood pressure) as a result of stress. In his #1 national bestseller *The Relaxation Response,* he calls the relaxation response "a universal human capacity" and "a remarkable innate, neglected asset."

Yoga teaches you how to tap into that underused capacity of your own body-mind. The yogic equivalent of the relaxation response is *vairagya,* which means literally "dispassion" or "nonattachment." It is good to feel passionate about what you do rather than have a lukewarm attitude. At the same time, however, you merely invite suffering when you become too attached to people, situations, and the outcome of your actions. Yoga recommends an attitude of inner detachment in all matters. This detachment doesn't spring from boredom, failure, fear, or any neurotic attitude but from inner wisdom.

For example, if you are a mother, you will love and take tender care of your children. But if you also are a *yogini,* you won't succumb to the stress-producing illusion that you *own* your children. Instead, you always remain aware of the fact that your sons and daughters have their own lives to live, which may turn out to be quite different from yours, and that all you can do is guide them as best you can.

Of course, you can do many practical things, which are described in books on stress management, to reduce stressful situations. These suggestions include not waiting until the last minute to start or finish projects, improving your communication with others, avoiding confrontations, and accepting that we live in an imperfect world.

Your daily Hatha Yoga routine, especially the relaxation exercises, can help you extend the feeling of peacefulness or calmness beyond the session to the rest of the day. Pick some activities or situations that you repeat several times a day as reminders to consciously relax, such as when you go to the bathroom, wait at a traffic light, sit down, open or close a door, look at your watch, or hang up the telephone. Whenever you encounter these activities, exhale deeply and consciously relax, remembering the peaceful feeling evoked in your daily session.

Releasing bodily tension

Yoga pursues tension release through all its many different techniques, including breathing exercises and postures (see Part III), but especially relaxation techniques. The former are a form of *active* or *dynamic relaxation*, the latter are a form of *passive* or *receptive relaxation*.

Relaxation Techniques That Work

The Sanskrit word for relaxation is *shaithilya,* which is pronounced *shy-theel-yah* and means "loosening." It refers to the loosening of bodily and mental tension — all the knots that you tie when you don't go with the flow of life. These knots are like kinks in a hose, which prevent the water from flowing freely. Keeping muscles in a constant alert state expends a great amount of your energy, which then is unavailable when your muscles are called upon to really function. Conscious relaxation trains your muscles to release their grip when you don't use them. This relaxation keeps the muscles responsive to the signals from your brain telling them to contract so that you can perform all the countless tasks of a busy day.

Tips for a successful relaxation practice

Relaxation is not quite the same as doing nothing. Often, when we believe we're doing nothing, we are really busy contracting unused muscles — quite unconsciously. Relaxation is a conscious endeavor that lies somewhere between effort and noneffort. To truly relax, you have to understand and practice the skill.

Relaxation doesn't require any gadgets, but you may try the following:

- ✔ Practice in a quiet environment where you are unlikely to be disturbed by others or the telephone.

- ✔ Try placing a small pillow under your head and a large one under your knees for support and comfort in the supine, or lying, positions.

- ✔ Ensure that your body stays warm. If necessary, heat the room first or cover yourself with a blanket. Particularly avoid lying on a cold floor, which isn't good for your kidneys.

- ✔ Don't practice relaxation techniques on a full stomach.

Deep relaxation: The corpse posture

The simplest and yet the most difficult of all Yoga postures is the corpse posture (*shavasana*, from *shava* and *asana*, pronounced *shah-vah ah-sah-nah*), also widely known as the dead pose (*mritasana*, from *mrita* and *asana*). This posture is the simplest because you don't have to use any part of your body at all, and it's the most difficult precisely because you are asked to do nothing whatsoever with your limbs. The corpse posture is an exercise in mind over matter. The only props you need are your body and mind.

Here is how you do the corpse pose:

1. **Lie flat on your back, with your arms stretched out and relaxed by your sides, palms up (or whatever feels most comfortable).**

   Place a small pillow under your head if you need one and another large pillow under your knees for added comfort.

2. **Close your eyes.**

   See Figure 4-1 for a look at the corpse posture.

3. **Form a clear intention to relax.**

   Some people find it helpful to picture themselves lying in white sand on a sunny beach.

4. **Take a couple of deep breaths, lengthening exhalation.**

5. **Contract the muscles in your feet for a couple of seconds and then consciously relax them.**

   Do the same with the muscles in your calves, upper legs, buttocks, abdomen, chest, back, hands, forearms, upper arms, shoulders, neck, and face.

6. **Periodically scan all your muscles from your feet to your face to check that they are relaxed.**

   You can often detect subtle tension around the eyes and the scalp muscles. Also relax your mouth and tongue.

7. **Focus on the growing bodily sensation of no tension and let your breath be free.**

8. **At the end of the session, before opening your eyes, form the intention to keep the relaxed feeling for as long as possible.**

9. **Open your eyes, stretch lazily, and get up slowly.**

Practice 10 to 30 minutes; the longer the duration the better.

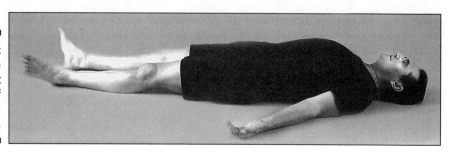

Figure 4-1:
The corpse is the most popular of all Yoga poses.

Ending relaxation peacefully

Allowing relaxation to end on its own is best — your body knows when it has benefited sufficiently and naturally brings you out of relaxation. However, if you only have a limited time for the exercise, set your mental clock to 15, 20, or however many minutes after closing your eyes as part of your intention. If you need to have a sound to remind you to return to ordinary waking consciousness, make sure that your wristwatch or clock isn't so loud that it startles you and provokes a heavy surge of adrenaline.

Staying awake during relaxation

If it looks like you're going to fall asleep while doing the corpse posture, try bringing your feet closer together. Also, periodically pay attention to your breathing, making sure it's even and unforced. Catnaps are generally excellent; if, however, you're experiencing insomnia, we suggest you save your sleep until you go to bed at night. In any case, the benefits of conscious relaxation are more profound than any catnap. The beautiful thing about relaxation is that you are conscious throughout the experience and can control it to some extent. Through relaxation, you become more in touch with your own body, which benefits you throughout the day: You can detect stress and tension in your body more readily and then take remedial action. Also, you avoid the risk of feeling drowsy afterward because you inadvertently entered into a deeper sleep. Remember that sleep is not necessarily relaxing. That's why we sometimes wake up feeling like we've done heavy work in our sleep.

Afternoon delight

When your energies flag in the afternoon, try the following exercise, which is a great stress buster. You can practice it at home or in a quiet place at the office. Just make sure that you won't be interrupted. For this exercise, you need a chair, one or two blankets, and a towel or an eye bag (see the appendix). Allow five to ten minutes.

1. **Lie on your back and put your feet up on the chair, which should face you (see Figure 4-2).**

   Make sure that your legs and back are comfortable. Your legs should be 15 to 18 inches apart. You can also put your legs and feet up on the edge of a bed. If none of the feet-up positions feels good, just lie on your back with your legs bent and feet placed on the floor. If the back of your head is not flat on the floor, and your neck and throat feel tense, or if your chin is pushed up toward the ceiling, raise your head slightly on a folded blanket or firm flat cushion to feel comfortable.

2. **Cover your body from the neck down with one of the blankets.**

   Don't let your body cool down too quickly, which can not only feel uncomfortable and interfere with your relaxation, but also cramp your muscles and harm your kidneys.

3. **Place the eye bag or towel folded lengthwise over your eyes.**

4. **Rest for a few moments and get used to the position.**

5. **Visualize a large balloon in your stomach. As you inhale through your nose, expand the imaginary balloon in all directions. As you exhale through your nose, release the air from the balloon.**

   Repeat several times until the exercise becomes easy for you.

6. **Now inhale freely and begin to make your exhalation longer and longer.**

   Inhale freely, exhale forever.

7. **Repeat at least 30 times.**

8. **When you finish the exercise, allow your breath to return to normal and rest for a minute or so, enjoying the relaxed feeling.**

   Don't rush getting up.

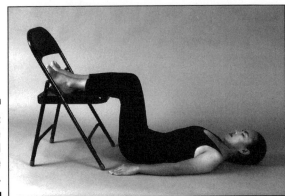

Figure 4-2:
Inhale freely, and then exhale forever.

Magic triangles

The following relaxation technique again utilizes your power of imagination. If you can picture things easily in your mind, you will find the exercise enjoyable and refreshing. For this exercise, you need a chair and a blanket (if necessary). Allow five minutes.

1. **Sit up tall in a chair, with your feet on the floor and comfortably apart and your hands resting palms up on top of your knees (see Figure 4-3).**

   If your feet are not comfortably touching the floor, fold up the blanket and place it under your feet for support.

2. **Breathe through your nose, but allow your breath to move freely.**

3. **Close your eyes and focus your attention on the middle of your forehead, just above the level of your eyebrows.**

   Make sure that you don't crinkle your forehead or squint your eyes.

4. **Visualize as vividly as possible a triangle connecting the forehead point and the palms of both hands.**

   Register (but don't think about) any sensations or colors that appear on your mental screen while you are holding the triangle in your mind. Do this for 8 to 10 breaths and then dissolve the triangle.

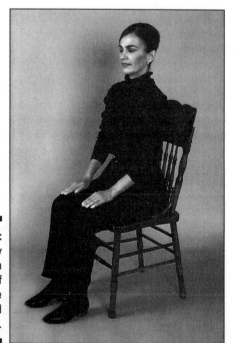

Figure 4-3: Mentally focus on the part of the triangle that is hard to connect.

5. **Visualize a triangle formed by your navel and the big toes of your feet.**

    Retain this image for 10 to 12 breaths. If any part of the mental triangle is difficult to connect, persist in focusing on that part until the triangle fully forms.

6. **This final step is more challenging: Keeping your eyes closed, visualize again the first triangle formed between your forehead and your two palms.**

    When you have a clear image, visualize at the same time the second triangle formed between your navel and your big toes. Picture both triangles together for 12 to 15 breaths and then dissolve them.

Relaxation before sleep

If you want to enjoy deep sleep or are experiencing insomnia (but don't want to count sheep), the following exercise can help you. Many people don't make it to the end of this relaxation technique without falling asleep. For this exercise, you need the following props: a bed or other comfortable place to sleep, two pillows, and one or two blankets. Allow five to ten minutes.

1. **Prepare yourself for sleep and get into bed, lying on your back under the blankets.**

    Your legs can be straight or bent at the knees with your feet flat on the mattress.

2. **Place one pillow under your head and have the other one close by.**

3. **With your eyes closed, begin to breathe through the nose, making your exhalation twice as long as your inhalation.**

    Keep your breathing smooth and effortless. Also, don't try to direct your breath to any part of your body. Let the 1:2 breathing ratio be effortless, something you can keep up.

4. **Remain on your back for eight breaths, then roll over onto your right side and place the second pillow between your knees.**

    Now use the same 1:2 ratio for 16 breaths.

5. **Finally, roll over on to your left side, with the second pillow still between your knees, and use the 1:2 ratio for 32 breaths.**

Yogic Sleep (Yoga Nidra)

Yogic Sleep is a very powerful relaxation technique that you can do after you gain some control over the relaxation response. When practiced successfully, this technique is as restorative as sleep — except you remain fully aware throughout.

Its traditional name — *yoga nidra* (pronounced *yoh-gah nee-drah*)— makes reference to Brahma, the Hindu creator god, who "sleeps" between successive world creations. His sleep is never unconscious.

One feature of this practice is to focus in relatively quick succession on individual parts of the body (as described later). Mentally name each part and then feel it as distinctly as possible.

In the beginning, you may find it difficult to actually feel certain body parts. Don't let this dismay you, but continue to rotate your awareness fairly rapidly. Later, as you become more skilled at this technique, you can slow down the rotation and feel each part ever more distinctly. With practice, you can include in this circuit even the inner organs.

Practicing Yoga Nidra before sleep is best because it's an excellent technique for inducing lucid dreaming and out-of-the-body experiences during sleep. *Lucid dreaming* refers to the kind of dream in which you're aware that you're dreaming. Great Yoga masters remain aware even during deep sleep. Only the body and brain are fast asleep, whereas awareness is continuous.

Yoga Nidra over mind

Using the Yoga Nidra technique serves as a potent tool for reprogramming your brain because you can reach a deep level of the mind. This deep-level reaching is done by formulating an intention. The Sanskrit word for intention is *samkalpa* (pronounced *sahm-kahl-pah*), meaning *intention, desire, wish,* or *will*. An intention may be your aspiration to become enlightened for the benefit of all beings; your wish to overcome anger, jealousy, unkindness, or any other negative emotion; or simply your desire to become or remain healthy. The *samkalpa* should not contradict the high moral values of Yoga, which we cover in Chapter 18. Be sincere about your intention and repeat it at least a dozen times both at the beginning and the end of the exercise.

Here is how you perform Yoga Nidra:

1. **Lie flat on your back, with your arms stretched out by your sides, palms up (or whatever feels most comfortable). Refer to Figure 4-1.**

   Place a pillow behind your neck for support and another pillow under your knees for added comfort.

2. **Close your eyes.**

3. **Form a clear intention.**

4. **Take a couple of deep breaths, emphasizing exhalation.**

5. **Starting with your right side, rotate your awareness through all parts of the body — limb by limb — in fairly quick succession: each finger, palm of the hand, back of the hand, the hand as a whole, forearm, elbow, upper arm, shoulder joint, shoulder, neck, each section of the face (forehead, eyes, nose, chin, and so on), ear, scalp, throat, chest, side of the rib cage, shoulder blade, waist, stomach, lower abdomen, genitals, buttocks, whole spine, thigh, top and back of knee, shin, calf, ankle, top of foot, heel, sole, each toe.**

6. **Be aware of your body as a whole.**

7. **Repeat the rotation one or more times until adequate depth of relaxation is achieved, always ending with whole-body awareness.**

8. **Be aware of the whole body and the space surrounding it.**

   Feel the stillness and peace.

9. **Reaffirm your initial intention.**

10. **Mentally prepare to return to ordinary consciousness.**

11. **Gently move your fingers for a few moments, take a deep breath, and then open your eyes.**

No time limit applies to your Yoga Nidra performance, unless you impose one. Expect to come out of Yogic Sleep naturally, whether you return after only 15 minutes or a whole hour. Or you may just fall asleep. So if you have things to do afterward, make sure you set your wristwatch or clock for a *gentle* wakeup call.

Several good audiotapes for practicing Yogic Sleep are available, but don't be surprised to discover that the instructions vary from tape to tape. For our choice, see the appendix.

Chapter 5

Breath and Movement Simplified

. . . .

In This Chapter

▶ Understanding breathing basics

▶ Detailing the mechanics of breathing

▶ Linking breath and postural movement

▶ Adding sound to postural practice

▶ Introducing traditional methods of breath control

. . . .

*T*he masters of Yoga discovered the usefulness of the breath thousands of years ago and in Hatha Yoga have perfected a system for the conscious control of breathing. In this chapter, we share their secrets with you. In the ancient Sanskrit language, the word for *breath* is the same as the word for *life* — *prana* (pronounced *prah-nah*) — which gives you a good clue about how important Yoga thinks breathing is for your well-being.

In this chapter, we show you how to use conscious breathing in conjunction with the Yoga postures, and we also introduce several breathing exercises that you do while being seated on a chair or, if you are up to it, while assuming one of the Yoga sitting postures. Always combine moving in to and out of the postures with proper breathing, because the mix greatly enhances the effect on your physical health and mental tranquillity. Yoga without *prana* would be like putting an empty pot on the stove and hoping for a delicious meal.

Breathe Your Way to Good Health

Think of your breath as your most intimate friend. Your breath is with you from the moment you're born and stays with you until you die. In a given day, you take between 20,000 and 30,000 breaths. Most likely, though — barring any respiratory problems — you are barely aware of your breathing. This is like taking your best friend so for granted that the relationship gets stale and is put at risk. To be sure, allowing breathing to occur automatically isn't necessarily to your advantage, because automatic doesn't always mean optimal. In fact, most people's breathing habits are quite poor and to their great disadvantage. They accumulate a lot of stale air in their lungs, which become as unproductive as a stale friendship. Poor breathing is known to cause and increase stress. Conversely, stress shortens your breath and increases your level of anxiety.

You can help alleviate stress through the simple practice of yogic breathing. Among other things, breathing loads your blood with oxygen, which, by nourishing and repairing your body's cells, maintains your health at the most desirable level. Shallow breathing, which is widespread, doesn't oxygenate the ten pints of blood circulating in your arteries and veins very efficiently. Consequently, toxins pile up in the cells. Before you know it, you feel mentally sluggish and emotionally down, and eventually organs begin to malfunction. Is it any wonder that the breath is the best tool you have to profoundly affect your body and mind?

Bad breath is improved by brushing your teeth regularly and occasionally sucking on a mint. Bad breathing, however, is a bad habit that requires a bit more to change: You must retrain your body through breath awareness.

In Yoga, consciously regulated breathing has the following three major applications:

- ✔ Use it in conjunction with the various postures to achieve the deepest possible effect and to prepare the mind for meditation.

- ✔ Use it as breath control (called *pranayama,* pronounced *prah-nah-yah-mah*), to invigorate your vitality.

- ✔ Use it as a healing method, in which you consciously direct the breath to a particular part or organ of the body to remove energetic blockages and facilitate healing; this is Yoga's gentle version of acupuncture.

Taking high-quality breaths

Before you jump right in and make drastic changes to your method of breathing, take a few minutes to assess your current breathing style. You may find it helpful to keep a log of your breathing habits over the course of a couple of days, noting how your breathing changes as situations around you occur. Check your breathing by asking yourself the following questions:

- ✔ Is my breathing shallow (my abdomen and chest barely move when I fill my lungs with air)?

- ✔ Do I often breathe erratically (my breathing rhythm is not harmonious)?

The cosmic side of breathing

The Yoga scriptures state that we take an average of 21,600 breaths per day. This number, which falls within the range accepted by modern research, is profoundly symbolic. Here's why: 21,600 is one-fifth of 108,000. The number 108, or multiples of it, is charged with special significance in India. The importance is related to the astronomical fact that the distance between the sun and the earth is 108 times the sun's diameter. Because the sun is symbolic of higher levels of reality, this is the Hindu version of Jacob's Ladder. The symbolism is represented in the 108 beads of the rosary used by many Yoga practitioners in India. A full round on the rosary is a symbolic journey from the earth to heaven, that is, from ordinary consciousness to higher consciousness. And, hardly accidental, the number of breaths per day are one fifth of 108,000, because 5 is the number associated with the air element.

This correlation is one of many that Yoga masters profess between the human body-mind and the universe at large.

> ✔ Do I easily get out of breath?
>
> ✔ Is my breathing labored at times?
>
> ✔ Do I generally breathe too fast?

If your answer to any of these questions is yes, you make an ideal candidate for yogic breathing. Even if you didn't answer yes, practicing conscious breathing still benefits your mind and body.

By the way, men take an average of 12 to 14 breaths per minute, while women take 14 to 15. Breathing at a markedly faster pace — usually associated with *chest breathing* — qualifies as hyperventilation, which leads to carbon dioxide depletion (your body needs some of this gas to maintain the right acid-alkaline balance of the blood).

Relaxing with a couple of deep breaths

Think about the many times you've heard someone say "Now just take a couple of deep breaths and relax." This recommendation is so popular because it really works! Pain clinics across the country use breathing exercises for pain control. Childbirth clinics teach Yoga-related breathing techniques to both parents to aid the birthing process. Moreover, since the 1970s, "Stress Gurus" have taught yogic breathing to corporate America with great success.

Yogic breathing is like sending a fax to your nervous system with the message to relax.

One easy way to experience the effect of simple breathing is to try the following exercise:

1. **Sit comfortably in your chair.**

2. **Close your eyes and visualize a swan gliding peacefully across a crystal-clear lake.**

3. **Now, like the swan, let your breath flow along in a long, smooth, and peaceful movement. Ideally, inhale and exhale through your nose.**

   If your nose is plugged up, try the combination of nose and mouth, or just the mouth.

4. **Extend your breath to its comfortable maximum for 20 rounds; then gradually let your breath return to normal.**

5. **Afterward, take a few moments to sit with your eyes closed and notice the difference in how you feel overall.**

   Can you imagine how relaxed and calm you would feel after 10 to 15 minutes of conscious yogic breathing?

Practicing safe yogic breathing

As you look forward to the calming and restorative power of yogic breathing, take time to reflect on a few safety tips that can help you enjoy your experience.

✔ If you have problems with your lungs (such as a cold or asthma), or if you have a heart disease, consult your physician first before embarking on breath control even under the supervision of a Yoga therapist (unless he or she happens to be a physician as well).

✔ Don't practice breathing exercises when the air is too cold or too hot.

✔ Avoid practicing in polluted air, including the smoke from incense; whenever possible, practice breath control outdoors or with an open window: Negative ions are positive for your health, at least in moderation. These ions are electrically charged atoms with a negative charge. Positive ions are produced by your TV and computer and have been connected with fatigue, headaches, and respiratory problems.

✔ Don't strain your breathing — remain relaxed while doing the breathing exercises.

✔ Don't overdo the number of repetitions. Stay within our guidelines for each exercise.

✔ Don't wear any constricting pants or belts.

Reaping the benefits of yogic breathing

In addition to relaxing the body and calming the mind, yogic breathing has an entire spectrum of other benefits that work like insurance, protecting your investment in a longer and healthier life. Here are six important gains of controlled breathing:

- ✔ It steps up your metabolism (the best manager of weight increase).
- ✔ It uses muscles that automatically help improve your posture so that you can prevent the stiff, slumped carriage characteristic of many older people.
- ✔ It keeps the lung tissue elastic, which allows you to take in more oxygen food for the 50 trillion cells in your body.
- ✔ It tones your abdominal area, which is a common site for health problems, because many illnesses begin in the intestines.
- ✔ It helps strengthen your immune system.
- ✔ It reduces your levels of tension and anxiety.

 The late T. Krishnamacharya of Madras, India — one of the great Yoga masters of the twentieth century — is a classic illustration of the benefits of yogic breathing. On his 100th birthday celebration, he initiated the ceremony by chanting a 30-second-long continuous *om* sound. He also sat up perfectly straight on the floor for many hours every day during the festivities, which lasted several days. Not bad for a centenarian!

 To give another example, Chris Briscoe is a baby-boomer beauty, the mother of two grown boys and a long-time popular resident and community leader in Malibu, California. In her 20s, she developed asthma and for 25 years was on heavy medication and allergy shots. If Chris woke up in the morning wheezing, she could count on being in the hospital by that evening. Aerobic exercise and allergies also induced her asthma. In 1990, Chris attended her first User Friendly Yoga class at the Malibu Community Center, where she learned yogic breathing and the principles of breath and movement. After only three months of attending classes twice a week, practicing yogic breathing at home and taking Chinese herbs, Chris was able to stop taking her asthma medication and allergy shots. She has remained in class and off medication for the past seven years.

Breathing through the nose

No matter what anybody else tells you, yogic breathing is typically done through the nose, both during inhalation and exhalation. For the traditional yogis and yoginis, the mouth is meant for eating and the nose for breathing. We know at least three good reasons for breathing through the nose:

- ✔ It slows down the breath because you are breathing through two small openings instead of the one big opening in your mouth: Slow is good in Yoga.

- ✔ The air is hygienically filtered and warmed by the nasal passages. Even the purest air contains at least dust particles and at worst all the toxic pollutants of a metropolis.

- ✔ According to traditional Yoga, nasal breathing stimulates the subtle energy center — the so-called *ajna-cakra* (pronounced *ah-gyah-chuk-rah*) which is located near sinuses in the spot between the eyebrows. This very important location is the meeting place of the left (cooling) and the right (heating) current of vital energy (*prana*) that act directly on the nervous and endocrine systems. (For the two currents, see the "Alternate nostril breathing" section, later in this chapter.)

Folk wisdom knows that every rule has an exception, which is definitely the case with the yogic rule of breathing through the nose. A few classical yogic techniques for breath control require you to breathe through the mouth. When presenting a mouth-breathing technique, we alert you to that fact.

What if I can't breathe through my nose?

Some of you may suffer from various physiological conditions that prevent you from breathing through the nose. Of course, Yoga is flexible. If you have difficulty breathing when lying down, try sitting up. The time of day can also make a difference in your ability to breathe. For example, you may be more congested or allergic in the morning than in the afternoon. You, of course, can detect the differences. If you're still not sure how to settle on a comfortable breathing method, first try inhaling through the nose and exhaling through the mouth and, failing this, just breathe through your mouth and don't worry for now. Worry is always counterproductive.

How about breathing through my nose all the time?

Many Americans participate in more than one kind of physical activity or exercise discipline. Each has its own guidelines and rules for breathing, which we suggest you follow. For example, the majority of aerobic activities — running, walking, weight lifting, and so on — recommend that you inhale through the nose and exhale through the mouth. The reason: You need to move a lot of air quickly in and out of your lungs. And breathing only through the nose while swimming can be very dangerous. In fact, we don't recommend underwater *pranayama* unless you enjoy a snootful of water making its way to your lungs.

In the beginning, save yogic breathing for your Yoga exercises. Down the line, when you become more skillful at it, you may want to adopt nasal breathing during all normal activities. You can then benefit from its calming and hygienic effects throughout the day.

Taking your breath away (and giving it back)

According to Yoga, controlled breathing has four aspects:

- Inhalation *(puraka, pronounced poo-rah-kah)*

- Retention or holding after inhalation *(antar-kumbhaka, pronounced ahn-tahr-koom-bhah-kah)*

- Exhalation *(recaka, pronounced reh-chah-kah)*

- Retention or holding after exhalation *(bahya-kumbhaka, pronounced bah-yah-koom-bhah-kah)*

In this book, we emphasize exhalation. Some classical Yoga authorities also refer to a type of retention that occurs spontaneously and effortlessly in some higher states of consciousness. This retention is known as *kevala-kumbhaka* (pronounced *keh-vah-lah-koom-bhah-kah*), or absolute retention.

The Mechanics of Yogic Breathing

Most people are either shallow-chest breathers or shallow-belly breathers. Yogic breathing incorporates a complete breath that expands both the abdomen and the chest on inhalation either from the abdomen up or the chest down. Both are valid techniques. (See Figures 5-2 and 5-3.)

Yogic breathing involves breathing much deeper than usual, which in turn brings more oxygen into your system. Don't be surprised if you feel a little light-headed or even dizzy in the beginning. If this happens during your Yoga practice, just rest for a few minutes or lie down until you feel like proceeding. Remind yourself that there's no rush.

Some Yoga practitioners think that it is the breath that flows either down into the chest or upward. Not so. The breath obviously always comes from above (either the nose or the mouth) and then expands into the lungs, depending on the contraction of the muscles in the upper torso. Any suggestion of an up or down movement of the breath is due entirely to the sequence of your muscular control and the flow of your attention.

In both chest and abdominal breathing, the abdomen draws in on exhalation. From a mechanical standpoint, Yoga breathing moves the spine and works the muscles and organs of respiration, which primarily include the diaphragm, intercostal (between the ribs) and abdominal muscles, and the lungs and heart. When the diaphragm contracts, it is pulled down, which creates more space for the lungs during inhalation. The chest noticeably widens. When the diaphragm relaxes, it moves back into its upward curve, forcing the air out of the lungs.

The *diaphragm* is a vaulted muscle sheath that separates the lungs and heart from the stomach, liver, kidneys, and other abdominal organs. It is attached all around the lower border of the rib cage and, by a pair of powerful muscles, to the first through fourth lumbar vertebrae. The diaphragm and the chest muscles activate the lungs, which don't have muscles themselves.

The diaphragm and your emotions

Psychologically, people tend to use the diaphragm as a "lid" by which they bottle up their "undigested" or unwanted emotions of anger and fear. Chronic contraction of the diaphragm makes it inflexible and blocks the free flow of energy between the abdomen and the chest (the nether region of the bowels and the feelings associated with the heart). Yogic breathing helps restore flexibility and function to the diaphragm and removes obstructions to the flow of psychosomatic energy (the life force). You can then experience liberation of your emotions, which can lead you to integrate them with the rest of your life.

Deep breathing not only affects the organs in your chest and abdomen, but also reaches down into your "gut" emotions. Don't be surprised if sighs and perhaps even a few tears accompany the tension release your breath work achieves. These are welcome signs that you are peeling off the muscular armor you have placed around your abdomen and heart. Instead of feeling concerned or embarrassed, rejoice in your newly gained inner freedom! Yoga practitioners know that real men do cry.

Appreciating the complete yogic breath

If shallow or erratic breathing put your well-being at risk, the complete yogic breath is your ticket to excellent physical and mental health. If you do no other Yoga exercise, the complete Yoga breath— integrally combined with relaxation — will still be of inestimable benefit to you. It's your secret weapon, except Yoga doesn't believe in the use of force.

Belly breathing

Before you jump into practicing the complete yogic breath, try out this exercise:

1. **Lie flat on your back and place one hand on your chest, the other on your abdomen. (See Figure 5-1.)**

   Place a small pillow or folded blanket under your head if you have tension in your neck or if your chin tilts upward. Place a large pillow under your knees if your back is uncomfortable.

2. **Take 15 to 20 slow, deep breaths.**

   During inhalation, expand your abdomen, during exhalation contract your abdomen but keep your chest as motionless as possible. Your hands will act as motion detectors.

3. **Pause for a couple of seconds between inhalation and exhalation keeping the throat soft.**

Figure 5-1:
Belly
breathing
exercises
the
diaphragm
and
prepares
you for the
complete
yogic
breath.

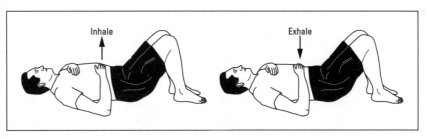

Inhale

Exhale

Belly-to-chest breathing

In belly-to-chest breathing, shown in Figure 5-2, you really exercise your chest and diaphragm muscles, as well as your lungs, and treat your body with oodles of oxygen and life force (*prana*). Your cells will be humming with energy and your brain will be very grateful to you for the extra boost. You can use this form of breathing before you begin your relaxation practice, before and where indicated during your practice of the Yoga postures, and in fact whenever you feel so inclined throughout the day. You don't necessarily have to lie down, as stipulated for the following exercise. You can be seated or even walking. After practicing this technique for a while, you may find that it's become second nature to you.

1. **Lie flat on your back with your knees bent and the feet on the floor at hip width and relax.**

   Place a small pillow or folded blanket under your head if you have tension in your neck or if your chin tilts upward. Place a large pillow under your knees if your back is uncomfortable.

2. **Inhale while expanding the abdomen, and then the ribs, and finally the chest.**

   Pause for a couple of seconds.

3. **Exhale while releasing chest and shoulder muscles, gently and continuously contracting or drawing the abdomen in.**

   Pause again for a couple seconds.

4. **Repeat the sequence.**

You can greatly enhance the value of this and other exercises by fully participating with your mind. *Feel* the air fill your lungs. *Feel* your muscles work. *Feel* your body as a whole. *Visualize* precious life energy entering your lungs and every cell of your body, rejuvenating and energizing you. To help you experience this exercise more profoundly, keep your eyes closed. You also can place your hands on your abdomen and feel it expand upon inhalation.

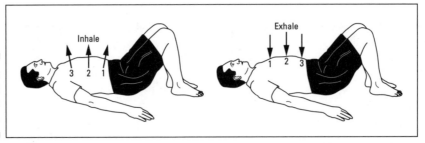

Figure 5-2:
This is the classic Yoga breath.

Chest-to-belly breathing

Classically, yogic breathing was taught from the abdomen up on inhalation, which you can see in numerous publications on Yoga (refer to Figure 5-2). This method works very well for a lot of people. However, in the 1960s, Yoga master T. K. V. Desikachar, with the guidance of his father, the late T. Krishnamacharya, began to adapt the traditional yogic breathing to the needs of their Western students.

Think about it! In the West, we sit in chairs and bend forward too much. Our daily sitting routine begins in the early morning when we go to the bathroom. Then we lean over the sink to brush our teeth and do whatever else we do to our faces. We sit at the breakfast table, and then we sit again while we commute to our workplace. At work we clock a lot more time sitting, perhaps slouching, in front of a computer or typewriter, or bending over a machine. Finally, in the evening, we come home and sit down for dinner and afterward, perhaps, sit in front of the television or our personal computer until our eyes get blurry.

The chest-to-belly breathing emphasizes arching the spine and the upper back to compensate for all this bending forward throughout the day, and it also works very well for moving in and out of Yoga postures. Chest-to-belly breathing is also an excellent energizer in the morning and can be done even before you hop out of bed. We don't recommend this exercise late at night, though, because it's likely to keep you awake.

The following exercise complements the belly-to-chest breathing (illustrated in Figure 5-2). As with the belly-to-chest breathing technique, you can practice the following exercise lying down or while you're walking.

1. **Lie flat on your back, with your knees bent and the feet on the floor at hip width and relax.**

   Place a small pillow or folded blanket under your head if you have tension in your neck or if your chin tilts upward. Place a large pillow under your knees if your back is uncomfortable.

2. **Inhale while expanding the chest from the top down and continuing this movement downward into the belly (see Figure 5-3a).**

   Pause for a couple of seconds.

3. **Exhale while gently contracting and drawing the belly inward, starting just below the navel (see Figure 5-3b).**

   Pause for a couple of seconds.

4. **Repeat the sequence.**

Figure 5-3:
The new
Yoga
breath.

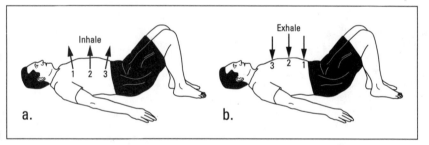

Starting out with focus breathing for beginners

If you're having a little difficulty synchronizing yourself with the rhythm of the complete Yoga breathing techniques, you may want to try a simpler method we call *focus breathing* first. Focus breathing is a great stepping stone to all the other techniques and may be just what you need for a confidence-builder.

Phase one

During your Yoga practice, simply follow the directions we give you about when to inhale and exhale for each posture, breath only through the nose and make the breath a little longer than normal. That's all you have to do! Don't worry about where the breath is starting or ending, just breathe slowly and evenly. (We present the postures in Part III.)

Phase two

After you are used to the phase one practice, just add a short pause of one or two seconds after inhalation and another one after exhalation.

Phase three

When you are comfortable with the practices of phase one and phase two, add drawing the belly in during exhalation — without force or exaggeration.

Taking a pause

During your normal shallow breathing, you will notice a slight natural pause between inhalation and exhalation. This pause becomes very important in yogic breathing. Even though the duration is usually only one or two seconds, this pause is a natural moment of stillness and meditation. If you pay attention to this pause, it can help you become more aware of the unity between body, breath, and mind — all of which are key elements in your Yoga practice. With the help of a teacher, you also can learn to lengthen the pause during various Yoga postures to heighten its positive effects.

Partners in Yoga: Breath and Postural Movement

In Hatha Yoga, breathing is just as important as the postures, which we describe in Part III. How you breathe when you're moving in to, holding, or moving out of any given posture can greatly increase the efficiency and the benefits of your practice.

Think of the breath as "mileage plus." The more you use breathing consciously, the more mileage you gain for your health and longevity. Here are some basic guidelines:

✔ Let the breath surround the movement. The breath leads the movement by a couple of seconds; that is, you initiate breathing (both inhalation and exhalation), and then you make the movement.

- When you inhale, the body opens or expands.

- When you exhale, the body folds or contracts.

✔ Both inhale and exhale end with a natural pause.

✔ In the beginning, let the breath dictate the length of the postural movement. For example, if you are raising your arms as you inhale and you run out of breath before you reach your goal, just pause your breathing for a moment and then bring your arms back down as you exhale. With practice, your breath will gradually get longer.

✔ Let the breath itself be your teacher. When your breath sounds labored, it's time to back off or come out of a posture.

✔ Try to sense the breath flowing into the area you're working with any given posture.

Breathing in four directions

You can move your body in four natural directions:

✔ **Flexion:** Bending forward.

✔ **Extension:** Bending backward.

✔ **Lateral flexion:** Bending sideways.

✔ **Rotation:** Twisting your body.

Normally, when people move they tend to hold or strain their breath. In Yoga, you simply follow the natural flow of the breath. As a rule, adopt this pattern:

✔ Inhale when moving into back bends (as shown in Figure 5-4a).

✔ Exhale when moving into forward bends (see Figure 5-4b).

✔ Exhale when moving into side bends (see Figure 5-4c).

✔ Exhale when moving into twists (as shown in Figure 5-4d).

Understanding the roles of movement and holding in Yoga postures

Most Yoga books talk about *stationary* or *held* Yoga postures (*asanas*). We suggest that before learning to hold a posture, you first become acquainted with moving in and out of most of the postures we recommend in this book. Always, of course, follow the rules of breath and movement given in the immediately preceding section on inhalation and exhalation. Then, when you can move in and out of a given posture easily and confidently, try holding the posture for a short period *without* retaining or straining your breath. You can tell you're straining when your face is turning into a grimace or you feel it going red like a tomato. Learning to move in to and out of the postures before adding the element of holding is important for three reasons:

✔ It helps to prepare your muscles and joints by bringing circulation to the area. It's like "juicing your joints" which adds a safety factor.

✔ It helps you experience the intimate connection between body, breath, and mind.

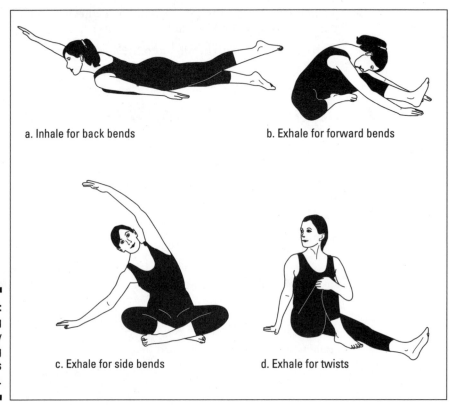

a. Inhale for back bends

b. Exhale for forward bends

c. Exhale for side bends

d. Exhale for twists

Figure 5-4:
Breathing
properly
during
postures is
important.

✔ In the case of stretching postures, moving in and out of a given posture before holding the posture supports the concept of *Proprioceptive Neuromuscular Facilitation* (PNF). If you tighten a muscle before stretching it either by gentle resistance (isotonic) or by pushing against a fixed force (isometric), the subsequent stretch is deeper than just using a static pose. Scientific research now supports this phenomenon; numerous physical therapy texts refer to it as PNF. If you want to experience this phenomenon for yourself, try the following exercise with a partner (see Figure 5-5).

The Yoga Miracle

1. **Lie on your back, with your left leg bent and your left foot on the floor; your right leg is up in the air and slightly bent.**

   Ask your partner to stand near your feet and test the flexibility of your hamstrings by holding the back of your right heel and pushing it gently towards you until you reach the first resistance point. The partner on the floor is relaxed and does not resist. (See Figure 5-5a.) Be sure not to force anything.

2. **Now bring your right leg back to the starting point again and then begin to push against the standing partner's hand (see Figure 5-5b).**

   The standing partner now takes a wider stance, bends his or her knees a little for support and gently resists your right foot either completely (*isometrically*) or allows your foot to move a little with resistance (*isotonically*).

   Both tests produce the same effect As you push against your partner's hand, your right hamstring muscles tighten. You want these muscles to tighten for about ten seconds.

3. **After approximately ten seconds the partner on the ground relaxes the right leg and then allows the standing partner to stretch the right leg and the hamstrings further for a comparison to Step 1 (see Figure 5-5c).**

   Behold the Yoga Miracle!

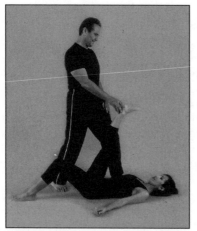

a. Test the flexibility of your hamstring.

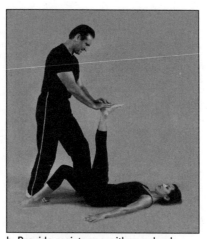

b. Provide resistance with your heel.

Figure 5-5:
Test your
new
flexibility
and behold
the Yoga
Miracle!

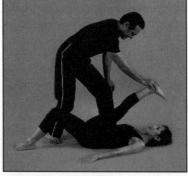

c. Experience the results.

Don't try to push your partner over, just push until you feel your leg muscles tighten. Next, after about ten seconds, release your leg and allow your partner to stretch you again by gently pushing against your heel, causing your leg to move toward you in a stretch that's not forced, as shown in Figure 5-5c. See how far you can extend this time. You may be pleasantly surprised!

How much should I move and how long should I hold?

We note the number of repetitions and how long to hold them in all our recommended programs. With practice, you develop an idea of what's right for you. A lot depends on how you feel at any given moment. In general, we suggest *at least three but no more than eight repetitions* for a *dynamic* or a *moving posture*. You can put together a program that has only moving postures, but normally we recommend a combination of both static and dynamic postures.

We often ask you to hold a posture for 6 to 8 breaths, which translates to roughly 30 seconds. Keep breathing when you hold a posture — don't hold your breath.

What about bouncing when I hold a stretching posture?

Now and then, we still see eager Yoga practitioners seeking to achieve better flexibility by bouncing during the holding phase of a stretching posture. This practice is part of Old School training, which is really not such a good habit after all. Bouncing not only tends to disconnect you from the breath, but it also can be risky, especially if your muscles are stiff or not adequately warmed up. Be kind to yourself!

How do I start combining breath with movement?

The arrows in the following exercise and wherever they appear in this book tell you the direction of postural movement and the part of the breath that goes with the movement. *Inhale* means inhalation; *Exhale* means exhalation; *breaths* means the number of breaths defining the length of a postural hold.

1. **Lie on your back comfortably, with your legs straight or bent.**

   Place your arms at your sides near your hips with the palms turned down (see Figure 5-6a).

2. **Inhale through your nose and after one or two seconds begin to slowly raise your arms up over your head — in sync with inhalation — until they touch the ground behind you (see Figure 5-6b).**

   Leave your arms slightly bent.

3. **When you reach the end of inhalation, pause for one or two seconds even if your arms don't make it to the floor. Then exhale slowly through your nose and bring your arms back to your sides along the same path (as in Step 1).**

4. **Repeat this movement with a nice slow rhythm.**

   Remember, open or expand as you inhale, fold or contract as you exhale.

After you become comfortable with this exercise, combine it with each of our recommended breathing techniques: Use either focus breathing (refer to "Starting out with focus breathing for beginners" earlier in this chapter), belly breathing (refer to Figure 5-1), belly-to-chest breathing (refer to Figure 5-2), or chest-to-belly breathing (refer to Figure 5-3). You can decide which technique you prefer as you begin combining breathing with movement.

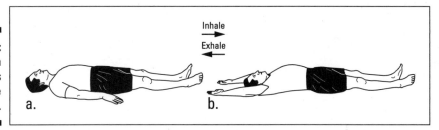

Figure 5-6:
The breath surrounds the movement.

Inhale

Exhale

a.

b.

Sounding Off: Yogic Breathing

Sound, which is a form of vibration, is one of the means that Yoga employs to harmonize the vibration of your body and mind. In fact, the repetition of special sounds is one of the older and more potent techniques of Yoga. Here, we show you how to try this technique in conjunction with conscious breathing. A good way to start is to use the soft-sounding syllables *ah, ma,* and *sa.* (We're not asking you to chant, although chanting can be a great and useful experience as well.) Try the following exercise while sitting in a chair or on the floor:

1. **Take a deep breath, and then as you exhale make a long *ah* sound in a way that you find pleasing and comfortable.**

   Continue the same sound for as long as your exhalation lasts. Then take a resting breath in between and repeat the exercise a total of five times.

2. **Relax for a few moments and next do five repetitions with the sound *ma.***

   Relax again and conclude by using the sound *sa* five times. After you complete the full cycle, just sit quietly for a few minutes and notice how relaxed you feel.

Good vibes

Yoga masters have long known that the universe is an ocean of vibrations. Some have maintained that even the ultimate reality is a state of continuous vibration — but a vibration that exceeds the three dimensions of space. Some quantum physicists call this a *holomovement.* The Sanskrit word for vibration is *spanda* (pronounced *spun-dah*). According to Yoga, the human body and mind are constantly vibrating. However, this vibration is more or less disharmonious and out of sync with the supervibration of the *ultimate reality,* (which we cover in Chapters 1 and 20). This disharmony creates unhappiness, alienation, and a sense of being separate from the world we inhabit. The purpose of Yoga is to remove this disharmony and syncronize the body and mind with the ultimate reality, thereby restoring joy and the sense of being connected with everyone and everything.

True yogic breathing also includes the *throat sound,* which forms part of the traditional practice of *ujjayi,* or "victorious" breath control (pronounced *ooh-jah-yee*). This more advanced technique is often mistakenly identified as sound breathing. The *ujjayi* sound is produced by slightly constricting the throat during inhalation and exhalation, which produces a soft hissing sound similar to a baby's breathing or a very gentle snore. This technique is easiest to learn during exhalation; then you can gradually apply it to the inhalation phase. If you're making the sound properly, you notice a slight contraction of your abdomen. The sound should be audible to you, but not to someone standing four feet away from you. Certainly don't strain to the point where you make a grimace! If the throat sound doesn't happen for you right away, just leave it until later — no need to rush.

The *ujjayi* sound is produced with the mouth closed and by breathing through the nose.

Sound, or sonar, breathing stimulates the energetic center at the throat and is quite relaxing. Some evidence states that sound breathing slows down the heart rate, lowers blood pressure, and induces a deeper and more restful sleep.

Practicing Breath Control the Traditional Way

Hatha Yoga includes various methods of breath control, all of which belong to the more advanced practices and traditionally follow extensive purification of body and mind. Some Western teachers have incorporated these methods into their beginner's classes, but our experience shows us that they are best taught at the intermediary to advanced levels. There are, however, three methods that we believe are suitable for beginners, if you practice them with the necessary modifications and precautions.

Traditional Hatha Yoga emphasizes holding the breath — not a good idea for beginners. In this section, we focus on techniques that are safe for any healthy person to practice.

Alternate nostril breathing

Researchers have demonstrated in the lab what Yoga masters have known for hundreds, if not thousands, of years: We don't breathe evenly through both nostrils. In a two-to-three-hour cycle, the nostrils become alternately dominant. It appears that left-nostril breathing is particularly connected with functions of the left cerebral hemisphere (notably verbal skills), while right-nostril breathing seems to connect more with the right hemisphere (notably spatial performance).

Expanding the life force through Yoga

According to Yoga, the breath is only the material aspect of an energy that is far more subtle and universal. They call it *prana* (pronounced *prah-nah*), which means both "breath" and "life." The term corresponds to the Chinese concept *chi,* which is known to a growing number of Westerners from acupuncture and Far Eastern martial arts.

This life force underlies everything that exists and, ultimately, is the power *(shakti,* pronounced *shuk-tee)* aspect of the spirit itself. When *prana* leaves the body, we die. Thus, the practitioners of Hatha Yoga seek to carefully preserve the life force and enhance or expand it as much as possible. The most significant practice for doing so is breath control, which is named *pranayama* (pronounced *prah-nah-yah-mah*).

This Sanskrit term is often incorrectly explained as being composed of *prana* and *yama* ("control"). The correct derivation is from *prana* and *ayama* (pronounced *ah-yah-mah*) — the expansion or extension of the life force. The term is conveniently translated as breath control, but much more is implied by it.

Science has solved many mysteries, but is still as puzzled about life itself. Some scientists now believe that a subtle, vital energy that can't be reduced to biochemistry does indeed operate in the body. They have named it *bioenergy* or *bioplasma.* Through Yoga, especially yogic breathing, you can learn to control that energy, whatever you wish to call it, in your own body. Some Yoga masters can even influence the life force in someone else's body, helping them to heal or speeding up their spiritual awakening.

The technique called *alternate nostril breathing* goes by various others names, including *nadi-shodhana* ("channel cleansing," pronounced *nah-dee-shod-hah-nah*). Here's how you do it at the beginning level:

1. **Sit comfortably, with your back straight, on a chair or in one of the yogic sitting postures (see Chapter 7).**

2. **Check which nostril has the most air flowing through it and begin alternative breathing with the open nostril.**

   If both are equally open, all the better. In that case, begin with the left nostril.

   You can check which nostril is dominant simply by breathing through one nostril and then the other and comparing the two flows.

3. **Place your right hand so that your thumb is on the right nostril and the little and ring fingers are on the left nostril, with the index and middle fingers tugged against the ball of the thumb.**

   Note: According to some authorities, you should place the index and middle fingers on the spot between the eyebrows (known as the "third eye"). We recommend the other method if it feels comfortable to you.

4. **Close the blocked nostril and, mentally counting to 5, inhale gently but fully through the open nostril — don't strain (see Figure 5-7).**

5. **Open the blocked nostril and close the other nostril and exhale, again mentally counting to 5.**

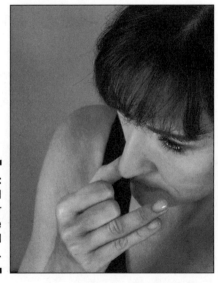

Figure 5-7:
Hand
position for
alternate
nostril
breathing.

6. **Inhale through the same nostril to the count of 5, and exhale through the opposite nostril, and so on.**

Repeat 10 to 15 times.

As your lung capacity improves, you can make your inhalations and exhalations longer, but *never* force the breath. Gradually increase the overall duration of the exercise from, say, 3 minutes to 15 minutes.

The cooling breath

This technique, which in Sanskrit is called *shitali* (pronounced *sheet-ah-lee*), gets its name from the cooling effect that it has on the body and the mind. Traditionally, the cooling breath is believed to remove fever, still hunger, quench thirst, and alleviate diseases of the spleen. Here is how you practice it:

1. **Sit in a comfortable Yoga posture or on a chair and relax your body.**

2. **Curl your tongue lengthwise and let its tip protrude from your mouth.**

3. **Then slowly suck in the air through the tube formed by your tongue and exhale gently through the nose (see Figure 5-8).**

Repeat this 10 to 15 times.

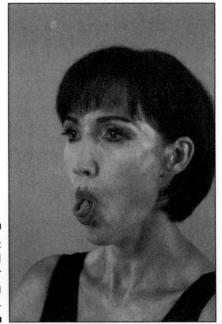

Figure 5-8:
Curled
tongue for
cooling
breath.

If you can't curl your tongue — some people can't for genetic reasons — then you can practice the Crow's Beak instead. This technique is technically known as *kaki-mudra* ("crow's gesture," pronounced *kah-kee-moo-drah*). Here you pucker your mouth, leaving just a small space for the air to pass through. Inhale through the mouth and exhale through the nose as with *shitali*.

Shitkari — inhaling through the mouth

Shitkari (pronounced *sheet-kah-ree*) is another technique that calls for inhalation through the mouth. The term means "that which makes a sucking sound." Its effects are similar to the cooling breath. Sitting upright and relaxed, move through the following routine:

1. **Open your mouth but keep your teeth closed, as if you were going to brush your front teeth.**

2. **Place the tip of the tongue against the palate behind the upper teeth.**

   Keep your eyes closed and make sure that you don't squint your face.

3. **Inhale through your teeth and breathe out through your nose.**

   Repeat the inhalation and exhalation 10 to 15 times.

If your gums are sensitive or a visit to the dentist is long overdue, avoid doing this practice when the air is cool. For anyone, this and the other cooling methods are best done in warm weather.

Kapala-bhati — frontal brain cleansing

Kapala-bhati (pronounced *kah-pah-la-bhah-tee*) means literally "skull luster," is also known as *frontal brain cleansing*. The curious Sanskrit name is explained by the fact that the technique causes a sense of luminosity in the head, as well as light-headedness, especially when you are overdoing it. Sometimes this breathing method is wrongly equated with *bhastrika* ("bellows"), which is a more advanced technique of rapid breathing. *Kapala-bhati* belongs to the preparatory practices of traditional Hatha Yoga. The technique requires rapid inhalation and exhalation through the nose with short staccato breaths, with emphasis on exhalation. *Kapala-bhati* is a very energizing technique that you can use to combat physical or mental fatigue or to warm your body (but be careful to avoid practicing this technique in cold air!). If you value your sleep, don't practice *kapala-bhati* at night. Before attempting the following exercise, learn to relax your abdomen during inhalation and to pull it in during exhalation. Gradually shorten the exhalations.

1. Sit, if you can, in a comfortable cross-legged posture, holding your spine straight, and with your hands resting in your lap.

2. Take a few deep breaths and, after your last inhalation, do 15 to 20 fast exhalations each followed by a short inhalation, using the nose to inhale and exhale.

   Repeat twice. With each exhalation, which lasts only for half a second, pull in your abdomen.

If you're contracting your facial or shoulder muscles during *kapala-bhati,* you're not practicing correctly. Remember to stay relaxed and let the abdominal muscles do most of the work.

I've got the whole world in my breath

According to Yoga, we all are interconnected and part of the same single reality. You can make this abstract fact more concrete and personal when you consider the breath. Each breath you take contains about ten sextillion atoms, which is the number 1 followed by 22 zeros. Every time you take a breath, you inhale an average of 1 atom from each of the ten sextillion breaths in the atmosphere. Upon exhalation, you release 1 atom to each of these breaths. Consequently the breath you just took contains a quadrillion (the number 1 followed by 15 zeros) atoms breathed during the past few weeks by the other 5 billion people of the human family.

We literally share each other's breaths and life energy.

Part III
Postures for Health Maintenance and Restoration

The 5th Wave   By Rich Tennant

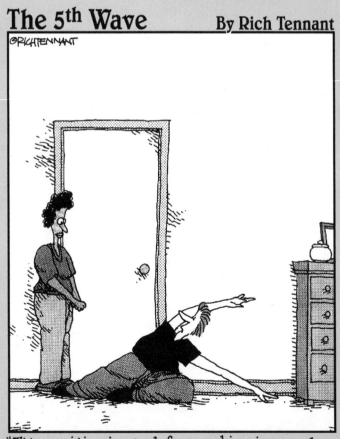

"This position is good for reaching inner calm, mental clarity, and things that roll behind the refrigerator."

In this part . . .

This part, as they say, is where the action is. We trust you actually read the chapters at least of Part II, so that you are now properly prepared for the ten chapters of this meaty part.

Here we introduce dozens of Hatha Yoga postures for a rounded and varied exercise program. For your convenience, we have organized the Yoga postures into basic categories, such as sitting, standing, bending, twisting, balancing, inverted, and dynamic postures. We even have put together several routines that you can use to vary your program and make it enjoyable as well as specific to your needs.

Chapter 6

What to Do When — The Importance of Sequencing

*T*he art and science of sequencing in Yoga is called *vinyasa-krama* (pronounced *veen-yah-sah-krah-mah*). In the Sanskrit language, the word *vinyasa* means "placement" and *krama* means "step" or "process." Before you experiment with various Yoga postures, you need to know how to combine postures correctly. The flow of postures is very important, and paying attention to proper sequencing can help you derive maximum benefit from your Hatha Yoga session.

Some Yoga teachers are quite skilled and knowledgeable about sequencing while others, unfortunately, are not. So the more you know about sequencing, the better. Understanding sequencing is like figuring out how to open the door of a bank vault. You may have a list of all of the correct numbers, but if you don't know the correct combination, you will never open the door to the treasures hidden in the vault. In this chapter, we give you the secret combination, the essential rules for postural sequencing.

Framing Your Practice with Awareness

The sequence of postures depends on the overall format of your Yoga session, which in turn depends on your specific goals. What do you have in mind for your Yoga practice? What do you expect to accomplish? Are you interested in a simple stress reduction program, or do you want to put together a routine for general conditioning? After you establish your goal, you need a plan that can bring you safely and intelligently to your goal. A good plan includes these considerations:

- ✔ Your starting point
- ✔ Your next activity
- ✔ Your available time

Where'd you come from?

Nothing stands still; every moment is unique. The same principle applies to the condition of your body-mind, which is in constant flux. To practice Yoga intelligently, you need to observe yourself. What is your physical, mental, and emotional state as you prepare for a Yoga session? For instance, if you're sore from intense physical activity, you may want to spend more time warming up. Or, if you just finished an emotionally challenging phone call, you may want to lie down and relax before you begin. Many personal factors determine the best approach to your Yoga practice. Be aware of the quality of your present moment and tailor your session according to your needs.

Where are you off to?

Just as your starting point is important, so is the context in which you create a session. In other words, what do you plan to do after your session? Are you off work, or do you have an important appointment to keep?

Early in my teaching career, before I (Larry Payne) had learned sequencing, I received a call from a high-level executive at a major corporation. He had heard about me through a relative and asked me to come to his office in the afternoon to give him a private Yoga lesson. His major complaint was that he was stressed out. So, for about 30 minutes I taught him various postures and then I asked him to lie on the floor and put his feet up on a chair. I covered his eyes, recommended long exhalations, and then gave him a long, guided relaxation. He became so relaxed and looked so comfortable that I didn't want to disturb him when it was time for me to leave. He had already paid me, so I left thinking he would appreciate continuing the relaxation on his own. Unfortunately, he had neglected to tell me that he was giving a presentation at a board meeting shortly after the class. His secretary had to wake him in a hurry, and he was so spaced out for his presentation that he was even accused of being on drugs. The moral of the story: Never pay your Yoga instructor ahead of time. Just kidding. The true moral is that you should always take your next activity into account when designing your Yoga session.

Give me a little practice time, will ya?

One of the great obstacles for most beginners is creating the time for their Yoga sessions, whether the preferred practice is in a group class or a personal exercise. In Chapter 5, we emphasize the importance of never rushing your practice or surrounding it with anxiety. We recommend that you're realistic about what you can do without thinking about the clock ticking. Create for yourself a time-free zone — however short — in which all you think about is your Yoga practice. Savor each moment. Become involved in what you do, knowing that you can then find greater enjoyment in it.

If you go to a group class, expect to be there for at least 60 to 90 minutes. If you have a personal practice, which we highly recommend, allow at least 15 to 30 minutes but, if you can, treat yourself to a full hour of Yoga as well.

Whatever the duration of your session, leave room for relaxation or rest. In fact, for an extremely busy person, just 3 to 5 minutes of relaxation breathing can be a valuable practice session. Good discipline in one area of your life can empower you to exercise discipline in other areas. When you see all the positive results from your Yoga sessions, you will soon find ways of creating more time for practice.

After you establish your goals (see Chapter 2), you're ready to apply the rules of sequencing to achieve the best possible flow of exercises. This section introduces the principles of the art and science of sequencing; let the concepts take firm root in your mind. Sequencing has many approaches, and we encourage you to consult a qualified teacher (see Chapter 2). However, you cannot go wrong when you bear in mind the following four basic categories:

- ✔ Warm-up or preparation
- ✔ Main postures
- ✔ Compensation
- ✔ Rest

Follow each step-by-step instruction carefully to avoid injuring yourself and also to enjoy maximum benefits. Always move into and out of the posture slowly, and pause after the inhalation and exhalation (see the details on correct breathing in Chapter 5).

We include some sample warm-up, compensation, and rest postures in this chapter. The main postures are covered in the other chapters in this part of the book.

Get Ready for Exercise with Warm-Ups

Any physical exercise requires adequate warm-up, and Yoga is no exception. If you have a trainer at the gym, he or she probably suggests that you step on the treadmill before doing weight training. If you visit any of the top health retreats in the United States and sign up for a hike, the leader is likely to first ask you to perform a set of stretching and warm-up exercises. The purpose of warm-up exercises is to increase circulation to the parts of your body that you're about to use and also to make you more aware of those areas of your physical self. What's different about the Yoga warm-up is that it is done slowly and deliberately, with conscious breathing and awareness. Here are some of the benefits of yogic warm-up:

- ✔ Brings awareness and presence of mind
- ✔ Allows you to test your body before executing the postures
- ✔ Increases the temperature and blood supply to your muscles, joints, and connective tissue
- ✔ Prepares your body for more challenging demands and reduces the possibility of muscle tear or strain. Enhances the supply of oxygen and nutrients, thus providing more stamina for the practice
- ✔ Prevents muscle soreness

Yoga warm-up postures are also called *preparation postures,* which are usually done *dynamically* and are performed before other exercises begin. In general, the safest Yoga warm-ups before you begin are simple forward bends and easy sequences that fold and unfold the body. Figure 6-1 shows some of our recommended warm-up exercises. You may select from the various reclining, sitting, and standing positions in this chapter. Warm-up doesn't have to be monotonous or dull!

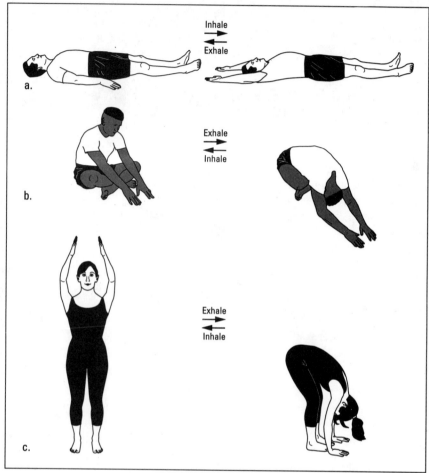

Figure 6-1:
Simple
forward
bends and
easy
opening
and folding
sequences
are good
preparations,
whether
you're lying
down (a),
sitting (b),
or standing
(c).

If you have disc problems in your lower back, forward bends may not be a good way to warm-up. Check with your doctor.

In addition to warming up at the beginning of a session, preparation postures are used throughout a given routine to precede and enhance the effect of the main postures (see Figure 6-2 for some samples). For example, the leg lift is used to stretch the hamstrings just before a seated forward bend. The bridge posture works well just prior to a shoulder stand.

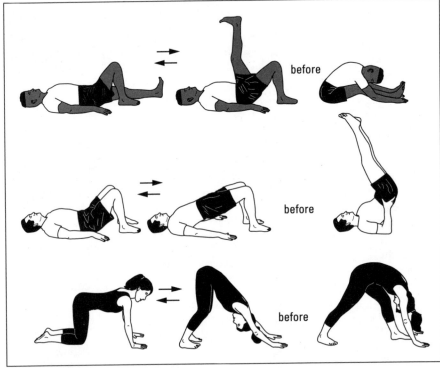

Figure 6-2:
Warm-up postures help you prepare for specific main postures.

Beware of using full neck rotations as a warm-up. They are done by letting your head flop forward, then rolling it to the one side, then backward, next to the other side, and finally returning to the starting position. Although turning your head from side to side or forward and backward is usually no problem, we consider full rotations to be risky. If you're having neck problems, we recommend that you avoid rotations altogether. Over the last 100 years, Westerners' necks (like Westerners' backs) have become quite weak and vulnerable from a cushy lifestyle, poor posture, and all too many whiplashes from car accidents. In addition, neck rotations can compress or obstruct important arteries that bring blood to the brain. If your neck makes a grating sound when you turn your head to either side, your cervical spine isn't in mint condition. A full neck rotation would only aggravate rather than remedy the situation.

Avoid warming up with more complex postures such as shoulder stands (see Figure 6-3a), advanced back bends (shown in Figure 6-3b), or deep twists (see Figure 6-3c). Also, we suggest avoiding a heavy cardiovascular workout before a strenuous Yoga practice because you can experience muscle cramps.

Figure 6-3:
Avoid
warming up
with
complex
postures,
like these.

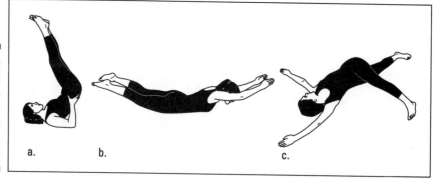

a. b. c.

Reclining postures

Most Yoga practitioners enjoy reclining (supine) exercises because they are intrinsically relaxing. When you pair them with warm-ups, you're enjoying the benefits of having your cake and eating it, too. The combination effectively allows you to warm-up specific muscles or muscle groups while keeping the other muscles at rest.

Lying arm raise

The following eight warm-up exercises requires you to start with the corpse posture (or dead pose), which we describe in Chapter 4. These exercises help revive you even when you start your Yoga session dead-tired (pun intended).

1. **Lie flat on your back in the corpse posture, arms relaxed at your sides, palms turned down (see Figure 6-4a).**

2. **As you inhale, slowly raise your arms over your head and touch the floor (see Figure 6-4b).**

3. **As you exhale, bring your arms back to your sides as in Step 1.**

4. **Repeat the sequence 6 to 8 times.**

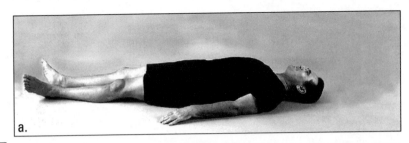

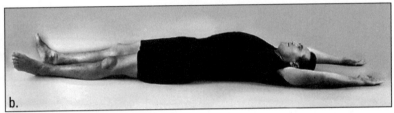

Figure 6-4:
Arm raises
stretch the
back and
warm up
the neck.

The double breath

If you like to double your pleasure, the double breath definitely gives you multiple relief from tension in your body and prepares your muscles for the main postures.

1. **Repeat Steps 1 and 2 of the lying arm raise in the previous exercise.**

2. **After you raise your arms overhead on the inhalation, leave them on the floor above your head and fully exhale.**

   Your arms should remain where they are for another inhalation while you deeply stretch your entire body, from the tips of your toes to your fingertips.

3. **On the next exhalation, return your arms to your sides and relax your legs; repeat 3 to 4 times.**

Knee-to-chest

Use this exercise for either warm-up or compensation. The knee-to-chest pose is also a classic in low back programs.

1. **Lie on your back, knees bent, feet flat on the floor.**

2. **As you exhale, bring the your right knee into your chest. Hold your shin just below your knee (see Figure 6-5a).**

   If you have knee problems, hold the back of your thigh rather than your shin (see Figure 6-5b).

3. **If you can do so comfortably, straighten your left leg on the floor.**

   If you have back problems, though, keep your left knee bent.

4. **Stay on each side for 6 to 8 breaths.**

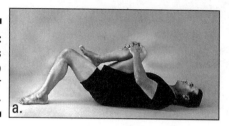
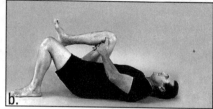

Figure 6-5: Use this posture to tune your back.

Double leg extension

This exercise, which uses both legs simultaneously, has a dual function. It prepares the lower back and gently stretches the hamstrings. The double leg extension can also be used for warm-up or compensation

1. **Lie on your back and bring your bent knees toward your chest.**

2. **Hold the backs of your thighs at arms' length (see Figure 6-6a).**

3. **As you inhale, straighten both legs perpendicular to the floor; as you exhale, bend both legs again (see Figure 6-6b).**

4. **Repeat Steps 2 and 3 six to eight times.**

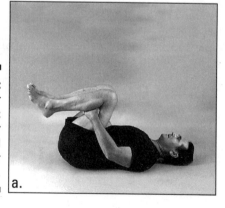
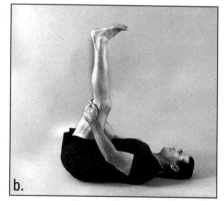

Figure 6-6: Double your pleasure; stretch your back and your hamstrings.

Hamstring stretch

Without the hamstrings (both muscles and associated tendons), you would have to let your fingers do all the walking. The hamstrings are an important part of your anatomy, and it pays to prepare them properly for exercise. When the hamstring muscles aren't warmed up, you can injure them quite easily, especially when you are prone to overexertion (never a good idea).

1. Lying on your back with your legs straight, place your arms along your sides, palms down.

2. Bend just your left knee and put the foot on the floor (see Figure 6-7a).

3. As you exhale, bring your right leg up as straight as possible (see Figure 6-7b).

4. As you inhale, return your leg to the floor.

   Keep your head and your hips on the floor.

5. **Repeat Steps 3 and 4 three times.**

   Then with your hands interlocked on the back of your raised thigh, just above your knee, hold your leg in place (see Figure 6-7c) for 6 to 8 breaths and repeat the sequence on the other side.

Lift your head on a pillow or folded blanket if the back of your neck or your throat tenses when you raise or lower your leg.

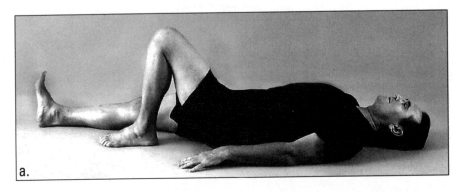

a.

Figure 6-7: Unlock your hamstrings, and you open the door to many Yoga postures.

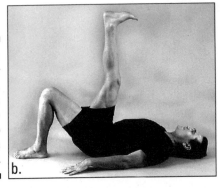

b.

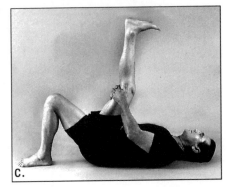

c.

Dynamic bridge — dvipada pitha

You can use this exercise for warm-up and compensation. The Sanskrit term *dvipada* means "two-footed" and *pitha* means "seat," which is a synonym for *asana.* (The pronunciation is *dvee-pah-dah* and *peet-hah,* respectively.)

1. Lie on your back, knees bent, feet flat on the floor at hip width.

2. Place your arms at your sides, palms turned down (see Figure 6-8a).

3. As you inhale, raise your hips to a comfortable height (see Figure 6-8b).

4. As you exhale, return your hips to the floor.

5. Repeat Steps 3 and 4 six to eight times.

Figure 6-8:
A frequently used posture for preparation, compensation, or as a main posture.

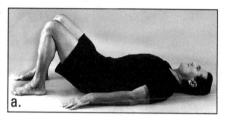 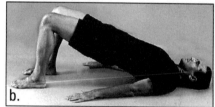

Bridge variation with arm raise

This posture is another good candidate for warm-up and compensation.

1. Lie on your back, knees bent, feet flat on the floor at hip width.

2. Place your arms at your sides, palms turned down (see Figure 6-9a).

3. As you inhale, raise your hips to a comfortable height and, at the same time, raise your arms overhead to touch the floor (see Figure 6-9b).

4. As you exhale, return your hips to the floor and your arms to your sides.

5. Repeat Steps 3 and 4 six to eight times.

Figure 6-9:
A nice variation for the bridge posture.

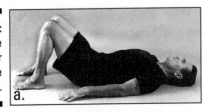
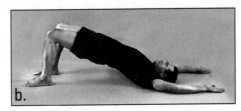

Dynamic head-to-knee

Dynamic had to knee is a little more vigorous kind of warm-up. Do not perform this sequence if you're having neck problems.

1. **Lie flat on your back in the corpse posture, arms relaxed at your sides, palms turned down (refer to Figure 6-4a).**

2. **As you inhale, raise your arms slowly overhead and touch the floor (see Figure 6-10a).**

3. **As you exhale, draw your right knee toward your chest, lift your head off the floor, and then grasp your right knee with your hands.**

   Keep your hips on the floor. Bring your head as close to your knee as possible, but don't force it (see Figure 6-10b).

4. **As you inhale, release your knee and return your head, arms, and straightened right leg to the floor, as in Step 2.**

5. **Repeat Steps 2–4 six to eight times on each side, alternating right and left.**

To make the sequence a little easier, keep your head on the floor, as in Step 3.

Standing postures

The standing postures are probably the most diverse of all the groups. They can be used for warm-up/preparation, compensation, or as a main postures. As a warm-up, use standing postures when the next part of your routine is also performed from a standing position.

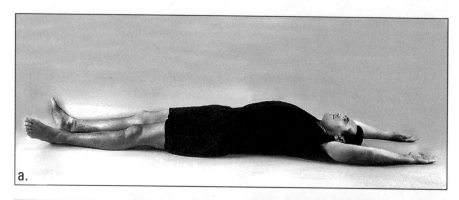

a.

Figure 6-10:
Use this
sequence
before a
slightly
more
physical
routine.

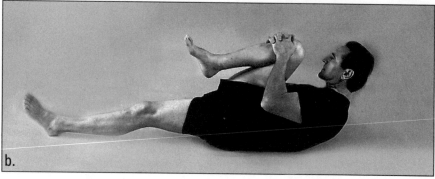

b.

Standing arm raise

You can perform this versatile warm-up almost anywhere that you want to enjoy a complete break from sitting. Try it at the office and start a new trend.

1. **Stand tall, but relaxed, with your feet at hip width (see Figure 6-11a).**

2. **Hang your arms at your sides, palms turned back.**

   Look straight ahead.

3. **As you inhale, raise your arms forward and then up overhead (see Figure 6-11b).**

4. **As you exhale, bring your arms down and back to your sides.**

5. **Repeat Steps 3 and 4 six to eight times.**

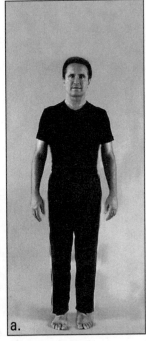
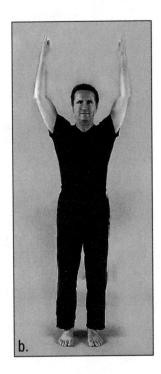

Figure 6-11:
Release the
most
frequent
site of
tension: the
neck and
shoulders.

a.

b.

The head turner

Think of your entire upper body, all the way out to your hands, as part of
your wingspan. Sequences like the head turner, which combine breath and
movement in the parts of the upper body with breath and movement,
stretch, strengthen, and heal your entire wingspan.

1. **Stand tall, but relaxed, with your feet at hip width.**

2. **Hang your arms at your sides, palms turned back.**

   Look straight ahead.

3. **As you inhale, raise your right arm forward and up overhead as you
   turn your head to the left (see Figure 6-12).**

4. **As you exhale, bring your arm down and turn your head forward.**

5. **As you inhale, raise your left arm forward and up overhead while
   turning your head to the right.**

6. **Repeat Steps 3–5 six to eight times on each side, alternating right
   and left.**

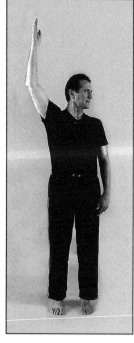

Figure 6-12:
This posture is great for minor stiff necks.

Shoulder rolls

You can use shoulder rolls in many types of exercise routines. The major difference here is that we move slowly, with awareness, coordinating with the breath.

1. **Stand tall, but relaxed, with your feet at hip width.**

2. **Hang your arms at your sides, palms turned back.**

   Look straight ahead.

3. **As you inhale, roll your shoulders up and back (see Figure 6-13); as you exhale, drop the shoulders down.**

4. **Repeat Step 3 six to eight times.**

   Reverse the direction 6 to 8 times.

Dynamic standing forward bend

You can use this exercise for warm-up, and compensation.

1. **Stand tall, but relaxed, with your feet at hip width.**

2. **Hang your arms at your sides, palms turned back.**

3. **As you inhale, raise your arms forward and up overhead (refer to Figure 6-11b).**

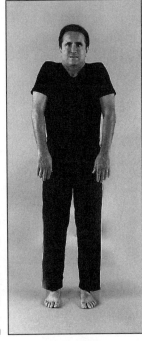

Figure 6-13:
Move
slowly,
coordinating
breath and
movement.

4. **As you exhale, bend forward and when you feel a pull in the back of your legs, bend your legs and arms slightly — this is called "Forgiving Limbs" (see Figure 6-14).**

5. **As you inhale, roll up slowly, stacking the bones of your spine one at a time from bottom to top, and then raise your arms overhead.**

   Finally, release the arms back to your sides.

6. **Repeat Steps 3–5 six to eight times.**

Rolling up in Step 5 is the safest way to come up. If you do not have back problems, after a few weeks you may want to try two more advanced techniques: As you come up, sweep your arms out and up from the sides like wings then overhead; Or, as you inhale, extend your slightly bent arms forward and up until they are parallel with your ears. Then raise your upper back, your mid back, and then your lower back, until you are all the way up and your arms are overhead.

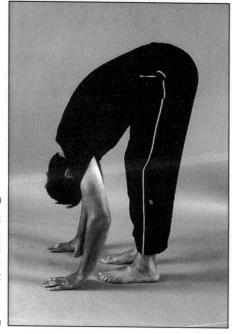

Figure 6-14:
How you
come back
up is just as
important
as how you
go down.

Sitting postures

Yoga postures have a very broad spectrum of possibilities. As a practitioner, you can do an entire routine from a sitting position, including forward bends, back bends, side bends, and twists. In this section, we show you how to prepare for the main postures from a sitting position.

Sitting fold

The sitting fold is a very simple way to warm-up or prepare your back for forward bends or to compensate after sitting twists.

1. **Sit on the floor with your legs crossed in the easy posture,** *sukhasana* **(see Chapter 7).**

2. **Place your hands on the floor in front of you, palms down (see Figure 6-15a).**

3. **As you exhale, slide your hands out along the floor and bend forward at the hips.**

   If possible, bring your head down to the floor or just come as close as you comfortably can (see Figure 6-15b).

4. **As you inhale, roll your torso and head up and return to the starting position in Step 2.**

5. **Repeat Steps 3 and 4 four to six times; then switch your legs and repeat four to six times.**

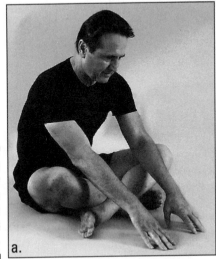 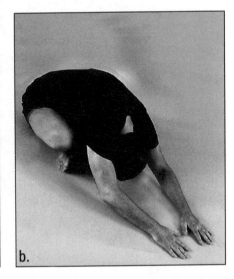

Figure 6-15:
Slide your hands forward on the floor as you exhale.

a.

b.

Sitting wing-and-prayer

The wing-and-prayer is an excellent way to decompress the upper spine and open the chest.

1. **Sit on the floor with your legs crossed in the easy posture (see Chapter 7).**

2. **Join your palms in the prayer position, thumbs at the breastbone (see Figure 6-16a).**

3. **As you inhale, raise your joined hands overhead.**

   Follow your thumbs with your eyes (see Figure 6-16b).

4. **As you exhale, bring your hands back to your breastbone (refer to Figure 6-16a).**

5. **As you inhale, separate your hands and stretch your arms like wings to your sides at shoulder height.**

   Look straight ahead (see Figure 6-16c).

6. **As you exhale, join your palms again at the breastbone (refer to Figure 6-16a).**

7. **Repeat Steps 3–6 six to eight times.**

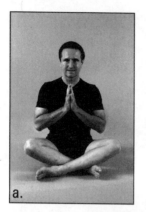
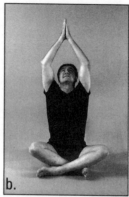
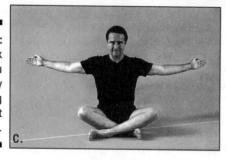

Figure 6-16: For a quick break, you can also try this sitting in a chair at the office.

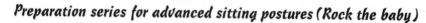

Preparation series for advanced sitting postures (Rock the baby)

If you cannot do the following sequence without pain, do not try the more advanced sitting postures in Chapter 7. Moreover, we don't recommend the rock the baby sequence if you have knee problems.

1. **Sit on the floor with your legs stretched out in front of you.**

   Press your hands on the floor behind you for support (see Figure 6-17a).

2. **Shake your legs out.**

3. **Bend your right knee and place your right foot just above your left knee, right ankle to the outside of the knee.**

4. **Stabilize your right foot with your left hand and your right knee with your right hand; swing your right knee up and down 6 to 8 times by gently pressing, and then releasing, the inner right thigh (see Figure 6-17b).**

5. **Carefully lift your right foot up and cradle it in the crook of your left elbow.**

6. **Cradle your right knee in the crook of your right elbow and, if you can, interlock your fingers.**

7. **Lift your spine and rock your right leg gently side to side 6 to 8 times (see Figure 6-17c).**

   Repeat with the left leg (reversing the cradle).

8. **Shake your legs out.**

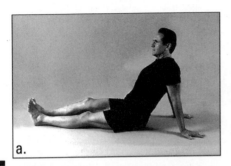
a.

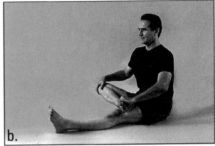
b.

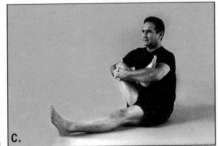
c.

Figure 6-17:
Make sure you're comfortable with Steps 1–4 before you move on to 5–7.

Get Set to Select Your Main Postures

The main postures are the standard *asanas* you find featured in the classical Yoga texts and modern manuals. These *asanas* are the stars of your routine, requiring you to work a little harder. In the other chapters of Part III, we describe many of the main postures that we recommend for beginners. Whichever *asanas* you select, remember to match them with your specific goals.

Whenever possible, a warm-up posture precedes and a compensation posture follows each category of main postures.

Go Back to the Start with Compensation Exercises

The reason for doing compensating postures is to ensure that you emphasize the positive effects of Yoga postures and neutralize tension and strain. For example, if you do a strenuous back bend like the cobra and experience tightness in your lower back, you want to be sure to follow up with a simple compensating folding posture, such as the child's posture. You not only need to explore the main Yoga postures, but also to understand how to compensate or bring your body back to where you started. The following anecdote makes this point in a graphic way:

When I (Larry Payne) was a little boy, my father often took me fishing. It was a time for us to be together and just talk about life. One weekend we went fishing for trout in a very rocky, mountainous area. In our quest for ideal fishing spots, we had to climb a very high, steep grade in order to continue down the river. When my father saw that things could get a little tricky, he told me to wait while he checked out the area ahead. I watched him climb higher and higher until he was out of sight. I waited for more than an hour, and finally I heard his voice from far away: "Get help!" He had climbed so high that he couldn't get down. My father was stuck on the side of the mountain for many hours before the sheriff's rescue squad was able to help him return to safer ground. If you move ahead with the main postures without knowing about the compensation postures, you may find yourself in a similar sticky situation.

Most established Yoga centers teach good compensating postures. We provide the information about compensation here to protect you from teachers who are not well-trained.

Here are some basic guidelines for using compensation exercises:

✔ Use one or two simple compensating postures to neutralize tension you feel in any area of the body after a Yoga posture or sequence.

✔ Compensating postures are normally done dynamically with a few exceptions, but always with conscious breathing (see Chapter 5).

✔ Perform compensating postures that are simpler or less difficult than the main posture, right after the main posture (see Figure 6-18).

✔ Do not follow a strenuous posture by another strenuous posture in the opposite direction. Some Yoga instructors teach the fish posture as compensating for the shoulder stand. However, this combination can cause problems especially for beginners, and therefore we recommend the less strenuous cobra posture instead.

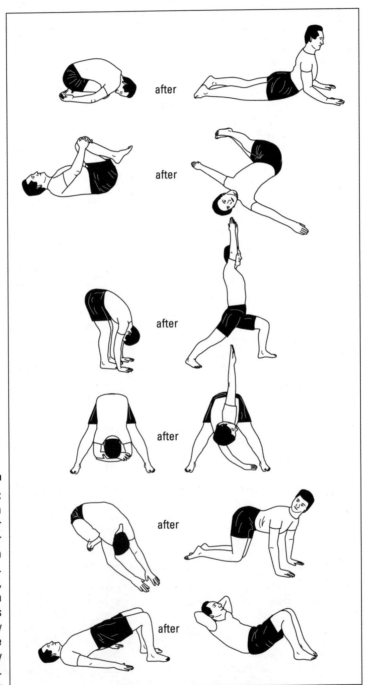

Figure 6-18:
Compensation
postures for
many of our
main Yoga
postures.
Remember,
compensation
postures
are usually
done
dynamically
(moving).

REMEMBER

✔ Practice compensating postures even when you feel no immediate need for them. This tandem plan applies especially to deep back bends, twists, and inverted postures.

✔ Back bends, twists, and side bends are usually followed with gentle forward bends.

✔ Many forward bends are self-compensating, but sometimes we follow with gentle back bends.

✔ Rest after strenuous postures, such as inverted postures or deep back bends, before beginning the compensating postures.

Compensation postures

Use compensation postures to unwind or bring your body back into neutral, especially after strenuous postures. Compensation is part of bringing you back into balance, which is a key concept in Yoga.

The dynamic cat

You can use the dynamic cat for both compensation and warm-up.

EXERCISE

1. **Starting on your hands and knees, look straight ahead.**

2. **Place your knees at hip width, hands below the shoulders.**

   Straighten but don't lock your elbows (see Figure 6-19a).

3. **As you exhale, sit back on your heels and look at the floor (see Figure 6-19b).**

4. **As you inhale, slowly return to the starting position.**

   Again, look straight ahead.

5. **Repeat Steps 3 and 4 six to eight times.**

Figure 6-19: You don't have to sit all the way back, just a comfortable distance.

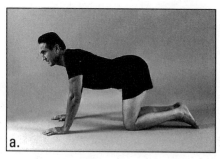
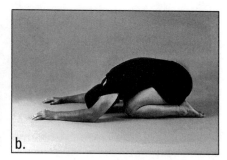

Thunderbolt posture — vajrasana

This exercise is useful for compensation or warm-up. *Vajra* (pronounced *vahj-rah*) means both "diamond/adamantine" and "thunderbolt."

1. **Kneel on the floor, knees and feet at hip width.**

2. **Sit back on your heels, and hang your arms close to your sides (see Figure 6-20a).**

3. **As you inhale, lift your hips back up, and sweep your arms up over your head.**

   Lean back and look up (see Figure 6-20b).

4. **As you exhale, sit on your heels again, fold your chest to your thighs, and bring your arms behind your back (see Figure 6-20c).**

5. **Repeat Steps 3 and 4 six to eight times.**

Don't perform the thunderbolt if you have knee problems.

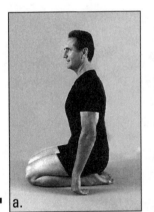
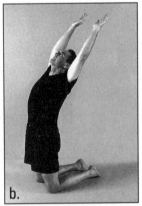
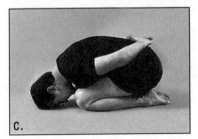

Figure 6-20: Get into a nice flow. Inhale when you open and exhale when you fold.

Dynamic knees-to-chest

You can find many variations of knees to chest. This variation is especially good after back bends.

1. **Lie on your back and bend your knees toward your chest.**

2. **Hold your legs just below your knees, one hand on each knee (see Figure 6-21a).**

   If you have any knee problems, be sure to hold the backs of your thighs.

3. **As you exhale, draw the knees toward your chest (see Figure 6-21b).**

4. **As you inhale, move your knees away from your chest.**

5. **Repeat Steps 3 and 4 six to eight times.**

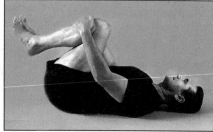
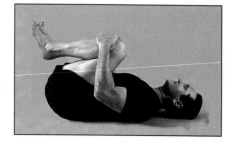

Figure 6-21: Hold each leg separately.

Rest and Relaxation

Rest periods during your routine are an indispensable part of any good Yoga program. Rest is not just zoning out at the end of a session. In Yoga, a quiet interval is an active tool for enhancing the quality of your practice at the following times, in these ways:

- Before the beginning of a class to shift gears and establish a union between your body, breath, and mind
- Between postures to renew and prepare for the next posture
- As part of compensation after strenuous postures
- To restore proper breathing
- For self-observation
- To prepare for relaxation techniques

Knowing when to rest and when to resume

The two best indicators of the need to rest are your *breath* and *energy level*. Continue to monitor yourself throughout the session. If your breath is not deep and even, rest. If you feel a little tired after a posture, rest. Figure 6-22 shows you some recommended rest postures.

No die-cast formula can prescribe how long you need to rest. Simply rest whenever you need until you're ready for the next exercise. Don't cheat yourself out of well-deserved rest periods between the postures and at the end of a session. Many practitioners relish them greatly!

Of course, if you start out really tired, with a sleep deficit, then you probably sleep or mainly rest during your session. If you allow 30 to 60 minutes for your routine, start with rest and some breathing exercises, which can help resuscitate your energies quickly.

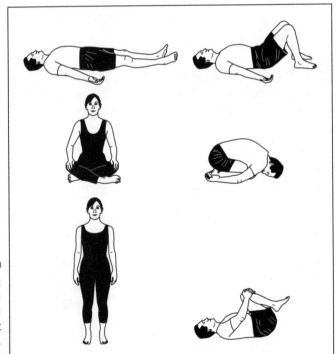

Figure 6-22:
Some recommended rest positions.

Rest postures

You can stay in any rest pose for 6 to 12 breaths or as long as it takes to feel rested, which may depend on how much time you have and where you are in the sequence of the routine. Keep in mind that Yoga should never feel like you are in a hurry.

Corpse posture — *shavasana*

The word *shava* (pronounced *shah-vah*) means "corpse;" this posture is also called the dead pose or *mritasana,* from *mrita* (pronounced *mree-tah*) meaning "dead" and *asana* meaning "posture."

1. **Sit on the floor with your knees bent, feet flat on the floor.**

   Press your palms on the floor behind you for support.

2. **Slide your hips forward slightly and lean back onto your forearms.**

3. **Bring your upper back and head to the floor.**

4. **Straighten your legs, and then separate your feet to hip width and turn your feet out.**

5. **Cross your arms over your chest and hug yourself, widening your upper back.**

6. **Release your arms to the floor, rolling out from the shoulders and down to the hands.**

   Turn your palms up (see Figure 6-23).

7. **Slowly turn your head from side to side a few times, coming to rest on the middle of the back of your head.**

8. **Close your eyes and relax.**

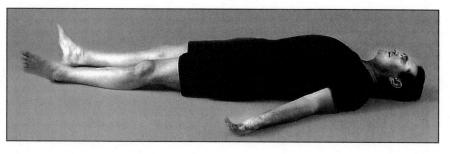

Figure 6-23: The most popular of all Yoga postures.

Shavasana variation with bent legs

Follow the steps for *shavasana* but keep your knees bent, feet on the floor at hip width (see Figure 6-24).

Figure 6-24:
Use this variation for any back problems.

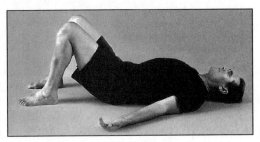

If your back is uncomfortable, place a pillow or blanket roll under your knees. If your neck or throat is tense, place a folded blanket or small pillow under your head.

Easy posture — sukhasana

The word *sukha* means "easy" or "pleasant." Compared to some of the other sitting postures, this one is indeed easy as pie.

1. **Sitting on the floor with your legs straight out in front of you, place your hands, palms down, fingers pointing forward, on the floor beside your hips.**

2. **Shake your legs out.**

3. **Cross your ankles, with the left ankle on top and the right ankle on the bottom.**

4. **Press your palms down and cross your legs a little further until your right foot is underneath your left knee and your left foot is underneath your right knee.**

5. **Rest your hands on the top of your knees, palms down, right hand on your right knee, left hand on your left knee.**

   If your knees are higher than your hips, sit on a folded blanket or cushion.

6. **Bring your back, neck, and head up nice and tall and look straight ahead (see Figure 6-25).**

   You can keep your eyes open or closed.

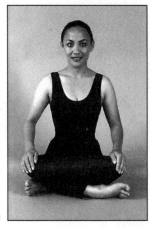

Figure 6-25:
Most
beginners
use this
sitting
posture.

Mountain posture — tadasana

The Sanskrit word *tada* (pronounced *tah-dah*) actually means "palm tree"; hence, this exercise is also called the palm tree posture.

1. **Stand tall, but relaxed, with your feet at hip width.**

   Arms are at your sides, palms turned toward the sides of the legs.

2. **Visualize a vertical line connecting the hole in your ear, your shoulder joint, and the sides of your hip, knee, and ankle.**

3. **Look straight ahead, with your eyes open or closed (refer to Figure 6-11a, earlier in this chapter).**

Child's posture — balasana

The Sanskrit word *bala* (pronounced *bah-lah*) means "child."

1. **Start on your hands and knees.**

2. **Place your knees about hip width, hands just below your shoulders.**

   Keep your elbows straight but not locked.

3. **As you exhale, sit back on your heels; rest your torso on your thighs and your forehead on the floor.**

4. **Lay your arms on the floor beside your torso, palms up (see Figure 6-26).**

5. **Close your eyes and breathe easily.**

Child's posture with arms in front

Follow the steps for the child's posture, but extend your arms forward at Step 4, spreading your palms on the floor (see Figure 6-27).

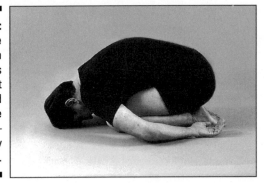

Figure 6-26:
This is the position most of us first experienced in the womb — very nurturing.

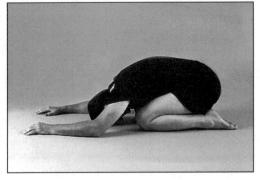

Figure 6-27:
With your arms in front, you will feel more stretch in your upper back.

Knees-to-chest posture — *apanasana*

The Sanskrit word *apana* (pronounced *ah-pah-nah*) refers to the downward-going life force or exhalation.

1. **Lie on your back and bend your knees in toward your chest.**

2. **Hold your shins just below the knees (see Figure 6-28).**

   If you have any knee problems, hold the backs of your thighs instead.

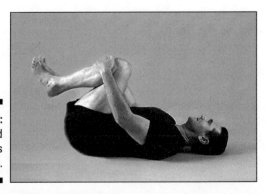

Figure 6-28:
Just hold your legs and relax.

Chapter 7

Sitting Made Easy

● ●

● ●

*T*he culture around us greatly influences the way we humans sit. People in the Eastern hemisphere favor squatting on their haunches or sitting cross-legged on the floor, while most Westerners are only comfortable sitting on chairs — as you're probably doing right now as you read this book. Actually, our everyday sitting preferences have a decided effect on our capacity to feel steady and comfortable in the Yoga postures, whether standing or sitting.

If you are new to Yoga and its sitting postures, you'll soon discover that a lifetime of chair-sitting exacts a stiff price. Your work with the postures in this book can help you gradually improve your floor sitting. But until you are ready to make the transition to the floor, use a chair when you sit for formal practice. After all, two of the larger Yoga organizations in the world, The Self-Realization Fellowship (SRF) and Transcendental Meditation (TM), encourage their Western practitioners to use a chair for meditation and breathing exercises.

In this chapter, we describe the following sitting postures that you can use for relaxation, meditation, breath control, various cleansing practices, or as a starting point for other postures:

✔ Chair sitting posture

✔ Easy posture

✔ Thunderbolt posture

✔ Auspicious posture

✔ Perfect posture

Many other sitting postures exist in Yoga; you can gradually add to your basic repertoire as your joints become more flexible and your back muscles gain strength.

Understanding the Philosophy of Postures

Postures, or *asanas* (pronounced *ah-sah-nah*) in Sanskrit, are probably the part of Yoga that you're most familiar with. They're those poses that look impossible, but that are done with ease by many Yoga students. Beyond stretching and increasing strength and flexibility, Yoga postures help you get in tune with yourself, your body, and your environment. Through *asanas,* you can begin to see yourself as one with your environment.

For traditional Yoga masters, *asanas* are just one part of the yogic system. Postures are the basis of the third limb of the classical eightfold path of Yoga formulated by Yoga master Patanjali (see Chapter 18).

Yogic postures are more than mere bodily poses. They are also expressions of your state of mind. An *asana* is poise, composure, carriage — all words suggesting an element of balance and refinement. The postures demonstrate the profound connection between body and mind.

Traditional Yoga adepts view the body as a temple dedicated to the spirit. They believe that the body must be kept pure and beautiful to honor the spiritual reality it houses. Each posture is another way of remembering that higher principle — commonly called the *spirit, divine, or transcendental Self* — that the body enshrines. If you prefer to practice Yoga without such ideas, you can still see in posture a means of connecting with nature at large because your body is not totally isolated from its environment. Where *exactly* does your body end, and where *exactly* does the surrounding space begin? How much does your body's electromagnetic field extend beyond your skin? How far away did the oxygen particles that are now part of your body originate?

According to traditional Yoga manuals, the main purpose of *asana* is to prepare the body to sit quietly, easily, and steadily for breathing exercises and meditation. The way we sit is, in fact, an important foundation technique for these practices; when you perform them properly, the sitting postures act as natural "tranquilizers" for the body, and when the physical vehicle is still, the mind soon follows.

Chuck and Maty, a leading Yoga couple in Los Angeles, are owners of one of the larger Hatha Yoga centers in the world. One location serves over 1,100 students a week. Because they're both teachers of advanced Yoga asanas, they need to keep their hips and legs flexible. So they avoid chair sitting — and encourage floor sitting — by having almost no furniture in their apartment.

Asana by any other name

The term *asana* simply means "seat." It can denote both the surface on which the Yoga practitioner sits and the bodily posture. Some postures are called *mudras* (pronounced *moo-drahs*) or "seals," because they are especially effective in keeping the life energy *(prana)* sealed within the body. This leads to greater vitality and better mental focusing. Life energy is everywhere, both inside and outside our bodies, but it must be properly harnessed within the body in order to promote health and happiness.

If your knees are more than a few inches higher than your hips when you sit cross-legged on the floor, it's an indication that your hip joints are tight. If you try to sit for a long while like this for meditation or breathing exercises, you may very well end up with an aching back. Don't feel bad, you're not alone. Accept your current limitations in this area and use a prop, like a firm cushion or thickly folded blanket, to raise your buttocks off the floor high enough to drop your knees at least level with your hips.

If you attend a lecture or other special gathering at a Hatha Yoga center, remember that few, if any, chairs are usually available, so be prepared to sit on the floor. If you are not accustomed to sitting cross-legged on the floor with an unsupported back, bring along a prop, such as a firm cushion or a blanket, to raise your buttocks (see Chapter 17). Arrive early so that you can find a wall or post to sit against to support your back. If none of these ideas sits well with you (no pun intended), just bring your own folding chair and sit near the rear of the room.

Trying Out Sitting Postures

Some contemporary Hatha Yoga manuals feature more than 50 sitting postures, which demonstrate not only the inventiveness of Yoga practitioners, but also the body's amazing versatility. Yet, all you may ever need or want are perhaps half a dozen yogic sitting postures. If you, like most Westerners, are accustomed to sitting on furniture rather than the floor, you may find sitting cross-legged for more than a few minutes uncomfortable. In that case, practice yogic sitting on a chair for a while.

Chair-sitting posture

Because cultural habits inspire most Westerners to sit in a chair when they meditate, floor sitting is usually something we have to work up to with practice. Over time, your *asana* practice can help you build comfort with sitting on the floor for exercises (see Figure 7-1).

1. **Use a sturdy armless chair and sit near the front edge of the seat, without leaning against the chair back.**

   Make sure that your feet are flat on the floor. If they don't quite reach, support them with a phone book.

2. **Rest your hands on your knees, palms down, and then close your eyes.**

3. **Rock your spine a few times, alternately slumping forward and arching back, to explore its full range of motion.**

   Settle into a comfortable upright position, midway between the two extremes.

4. **Lift your chest, without exaggerating the gentle inward curve in your lower back, and balance your head over the torso.**

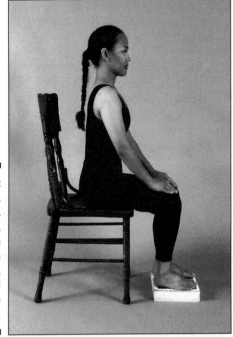

Figure 7-1: Ideally, your ear, shoulder, and hip are in alignment, as viewed from the side.

The easy posture — sukhasana

According to Yoga master Patanjali, posture should be "steady" *(sthira)* and "easy, pleasant, comfortable" *(sukha)*. The basic Yoga sitting position is called, appropriately, the easy posture *(sukhasana),* which Westerners sometimes call the *tailor's seat.* We strongly recommend that beginners start their floor sitting practice with the easy posture (see Figure 7-2).

The easy posture is a steady and comfortable sitting position for meditation and breathing exercises. The posture also helps you become more aware of, and actually increase, the flexibility in your hips and spine and, therefore, is a good preparation for more advanced postures.

In this posture, and the ones that follow, raising the buttocks off the floor on a firm cushion or thickly folded blanket is helpful, as it allows you to sit comfortably and stably.

1. **Sit on the floor with your legs straight out in front of you.**

   Place your hands on the floor beside your hips, palms down and fingers pointing forward; shake your legs up and down a few times to get the kinks out.

2. **Cross your legs at the ankles with the left leg on top, the right leg below.**

3. **Now press your palms on the floor and slide each foot toward the opposite knee, until the right foot is underneath the left knee and the left foot is underneath the right knee.**

4. **Lengthen the spine by stretching your back in an upward motion and balance your head over the torso.**

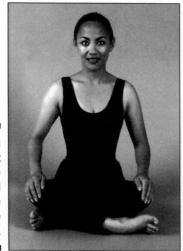

Figure 7-2:
Be sure that
you are
steady and
comfortable
in the
posture.

Note: In the classic posture, you drop your chin to your chest and extend your arms and lock your elbows; we suggest, however, that you rest the hands on the knees, palms down and elbows bent, and keep the head upright, which is more relaxing for beginners.

Be sure to alternate the cross of the legs from day to day when practicing any of the sitting postures because you don't want to become lopsided.

The thunderbolt posture — Vajrasana

The thunderbolt posture is one of the safer sitting postures for students with back problems. *Vajrasana* increases flexibility of the ankles, knees and thighs, improves circulation to the abdomen, and is good for digestion.

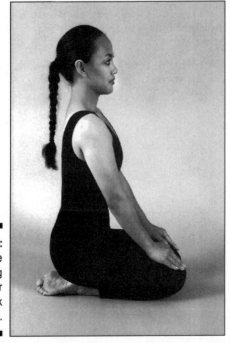

1. **Kneel on the floor and sit back on your heels.**

   Position each heel under the buttock on the same side and rest your hands on the tops of your knees, elbows bent, palms down.

2. **Lengthen your spine by stretching your back in an upward motion, balance your head over your torso, and look straight ahead (see Figure 7-3).**

Figure 7-3:
A safe sitting posture for lower back problems.

Note: In the classic posture, which we don't recommend for beginners, you rest your chin on your upper chest and extend your arms until your elbows are locked and your hands are on your knees.

If you have trouble sitting back on your heels, either because of tightness in your thigh muscles or pain in your knees, put a cushion or folded blanket between your thighs and calves. Increase the thickness of your lift until you can sit down comfortably. If you feel discomfort in the fronts of your ankles, put a rolled-up towel or blanket underneath them.

The Sanskrit word *vajra* (pronounced *vahj-rah*) means "thunderbolt" or "adamantine."

The auspicious posture — svastikasana

Before its perversion in Nazi Germany, the *svastika* served as a solar symbol for good fortune. This is also its meaning in Yoga.

The *svastikasana* improves the flexibility of the hips, knees and ankles, and strengthens the back.

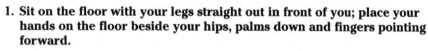

Use the "Preparation series for advanced sitting postures" (see Chapter 6) to improve your performance for this posture.

1. **Sit on the floor with your legs straight out in front of you; place your hands on the floor beside your hips, palms down and fingers pointing forward.**

   Shake your legs up and down a few times to get the kinks out.

2. **Bend your left knee and place the left foot sole against the inside of your right thigh with the left heel close to the groin. (If this step is difficult, don't use this pose.)**

3. **Bend your right knee toward you and take hold of the right foot with both hands.**

4. **Grip the front of the ankle with your right hand and the ball of the big toe with your left.**

   Now slide the little-toe side of the foot between the left thigh and calf until only the big toe is visible. If you can, wiggle the big-toe side of the left foot up between the right thigh and calf.

5. **Rest your hands on your knees, arms relaxed, palms down.**

6. **Lengthen your spine by stretching your back in an upward motion, balance your head over your torso and look straight ahead (see Figure 7-4).**

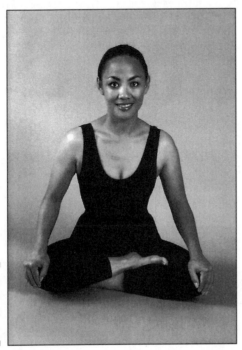

Figure 7-4:
The good
luck
posture.

Note: In the classic posture, the chin rests on the chest with the arms straight down and palms open in *jnana mudra* at the knees. The bottom or left foot is pulled up and wedged between the right calf and thigh.

Jnana mudra (pronounced *gyah-nah moo-drah*) meaning "wisdom seal," is one of a number of hand positions used in Yoga. To do this mudra, bring the tip of your index finger to the tip of your thumb to form a circle; extend the three remaining fingers, keeping them close together (as shown in Figure 7-5). This hand gesture makes a nice circuit, sealing off the life energy *(prana)* in your body (see Chapter 5).

The perfect posture — siddhasana

The Sanskrit word *siddha* (pronounced *sidd-hah*), means both "perfect" and "adept." Many Yoga masters in bygone ages preferred this posture and used it often in place of the lotus posture. We don't cover either the half lotus or the full lotus position in this book because they're suitable only for more experienced students.

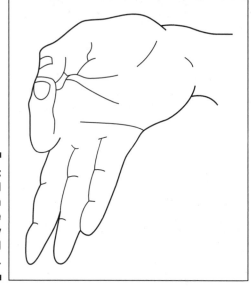

Figure 7-5:
This hand
position
seals off life
energy
called
prana.

The *siddhasana* improves the flexibility of the hips, knees and ankles, and strengthens the back. The posture is considered the perfect meditation posture for those practicing celibacy. Siddhasana is also beneficial for men with various prostate problems.

Use the "Preparation series for advanced sitting postures" (see Chapter 6) to improve your performance for this posture.

1. **Sitting on the floor with your legs straight out in front of you, place your hands, palms down, at your sides, fingers forward, with your hands close to your hips.**

   Shake your legs out in front of you a few times.

2. **Bend your left knee and bring the left heel into the groin, near the** *perineum* **(the area between the anus and the genitals).**

   Stabilize your left ankle with your left hand.

3. **Bend your right knee and slide your right heel towards the front of your left ankle.**

4. **Lift your right foot and position your right ankle just above your left ankle and bring your right heel into the genital area.**

5. **Tuck the little-toe side of your right foot between your left thigh and calf.**

6. **Place your hands palms down on the same-side knee with arms relaxed.**

7. **Straighten and extend your back and neck, bringing your head up nice and tall; look straight ahead (see Figure 7-6).**

   You can use a cushion to raise your hips, so that they are level with your knees.

   Note: In the classic posture, which we don't recommend for beginners, your chin rests on your chest, your arms are straight down, elbows locked, with your palms open in *jnana mudra* (refer to the description in "The auspicious posture — *svastikasana*" section earlier in this chapter) at your knees. The big-toe side of your left foot is pulled up and wedged between your right calf and thigh.

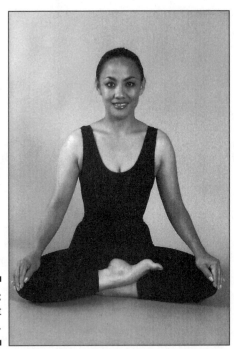

Figure 7-6:
The perfect
posture.

Chapter 8

Standing Tall

· ·

In This Chapter
▶ Standing as an art
▶ Singing praises of standing postures
▶ Practicing standing postures

· ·

*S*tanding upright is a uniquely human trait, and Yoga is a uniquely human practice. In this chapter, we discuss standing from the Yoga perspective, with an emphasis on the difference between just standing and the more quintessential version of *standing*. The simple act of standing upright depends on your spine, muscles, tendons, and ligaments. Ordinarily, these do their assigned tasks quite automatically. But in order to stand efficiently and elegantly you also need to bring awareness to the act. This is where Yoga comes into play.

We give you ten of the more common and favored Yoga standing postures to practice. They will help you discover the art of standing consciously, efficiently, and beautifully.

Identifying That Two-Legged Creature

We are human, in large part, because hundreds of thousands of years ago our ancestors figured out how to "stand on their own two feet." Appropriately, the yogic standing postures are considered to be the foundation of *asana* practice. One of the capacities that makes us most human — standing — also prepares us for that most human of endeavors: Yoga.

The way that you stand tells a lot about you. These days, a person who stands tall usually sucks in the belly and sticks out the chest and chin in military fashion. But you can stand tall and straight and be relaxed at the same time.

You're grounded!

Calling yogic standing posture an *asana* ("seat") may seem contradictory, but the posture actually helps you become firmly grounded. In Yoga, grounding is as important as reaching up. You can reach the heights of Yoga only when you are as sturdy as a mountain or a sequoia.

Remember, body and mind form a unit; they're the outside and the inside of the same person: you. In a way, your body is a map of your mind.

Through regular Yoga practice, you can use the feedback from your body to discipline your mind, and the feedback from your mind (particularly your emotions) to train your body.

Standing Tall

The standing postures are a kind of microcosm of the practice of *asana* as a whole (except for inversions, or upside-down postures, described in Chapter 11); you may hear that you can derive everything you need to know to master your physical practice from the standing postures. The standing postures help you strengthen your legs and ankles, open your hips and groin, and improve your sense of balance. In turn, you develop ability to "stand your ground" and to "stand at ease," which is an important aspect of the yogic lifestyle.

The standing postures are very versatile. They can be used in the following ways:

- ✔ As a general warm-up for your practice.
- ✔ In preparation for a specific group of postures (we like to think of the standing forward bends, for example, as a kind of "on-ramp" to the seated forward bends).
- ✔ For compensation (or to counterbalance another posture, such as a back bend or side bend). For more information, see Chapter 6.
- ✔ For rest.
- ✔ As the main body of your practice.

ANECDOTE

Now, that's a stretch!

A beautiful young woman named Heather came to a Larry Payne's User Friendly Yoga class in Brentwood, California, for her "first ever" Yoga class. It was clear right away that she was not very flexible; in fact, she was perhaps the most inflexible young person I had ever seen. When I led the class in seated forward bends, for example, she literally could not touch her knees. In that moment, when she realized how tight she really was, she began to cry. I spoke to her after class and learned that she had been involved in competitive sports since age 5, and that now, at 17, she played on a state champion volleyball team. As athletic as she was, she had done very little stretching over the years . . . and it showed.

I recommended that she lean her buttocks against a wall, with her feet about 3 feet away from the wall, and just hang down, keeping her knees "soft," as in Forgiving Limbs (see Chapter 6). In this modified standing posture, she had an easy angle to bend forward and release her back and hamstrings. She practiced this standing posture every day and within three weeks, she experienced a dramatic change. For the first time, she could sit with her legs extended and reach her toes. With the entire class spontaneously applauding, Heather cried again, but this time out of joy.

TIP

You can creatively adapt many postures from other groups to a standing position, which you can then use as a learning (or teaching) tool, or for therapeutic purposes. Take, for example, the well-known cobra posture, a back bend that many beginning students find hard on the lower back (see Chapter 12). By performing this same posture in a standing position near a wall, you can use the changed relationship to gravity, the freedom of not having your hips blocked by the floor and the pressure of the hands on the wall, to free the lower back. Then you can apply this newly won understanding about the back in your practice of the more demanding traditional form of the cobra posture or any other posture that you choose to modify at the wall.

Exercising Your Options

In this section, we introduce you to ten standing postures and describe the step-by-step process for each exercise. We also discuss the benefits and the classical version of the posture. We do not recommend the classical version for beginners because, in most cases, the postures are more difficult and sometimes risky. Before attempting any of these postures, check out the information in Chapters 5, 6, and 16.

Note: When you try the postures on your own, follow the instructions for each exercise carefully, including the breathing. Always move into and out of the posture slowly and pause after the inhalation and exhalation (see Chapter 5). Complete each posture by relaxing and returning to the starting place.

When you bend forward from all of the standing postures, start with the legs straight and then soften your knees when you feel the muscles pulling in the back of your legs.

When you come up out of a standing forward bend, choose one of three ways:

- ✔ The easiest and safest way is to roll the body up like a rag doll, stacking the vertebrae one on top of other.

- ✔ The next level of difficulty is to bring your arms up from the sides like wings as you inhale and raise your back.

- ✔ The third and most desirable way, if possible, is to start with the inhalation and extend your arms forward and up along side of the ears. Then continue raising the upper, mid and lower back until you are straight up and your arms are over head.

Mountain posture (tadasana) — building block for other stances

The mountain posture is the foundation for all the standing postures. *Tadasana* aligns the body, improves posture and balance, and facilitates breathing. Although this exercise is commonly called the mountain posture, the name for this position is actually "palm posture," from the Sanskrit word *tada* (pronounced *tah-dah*). Some authorities also refer to this exercise as the tree posture.

1. **Stand tall but relaxed with your feet at hip width.**

   Hang your arms at your sides, palms turned toward your legs.

2. **Visualize a vertical line connecting the hole in your ear, your shoulder joint and the sides of your hip, knee, and ankle.**

   Look straight ahead, with your eyes open or closed (see Figure 8-1).

3. **Remain in this posture for 6 to 8 breaths.**

Note: In the classical version of this posture, the feet are together, and the chin *rests* on the chest.

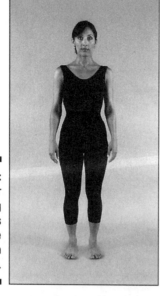

Figure 8-1:
Start your
standing
postures
with the
mountain
posture.

Standing forward bend — uttanasana

The standing forward bend stretches the entire back of the body and decompresses (makes space between the vertebrae) the neck (see Figure 8-2). In the upright posture, the cervical spine and the neck muscles have to work hard to balance the head. Because we generally don't pay enough attention to this part of our anatomy, we tend to accumulate a lot of tension in the neck, which can lead to headaches. This posture frees the cervical spine and allows the neck muscles to relax. It also improves overall circulation and has a calming effect on the body and mind.

Be very careful of all forward bends if you are having a disc problem. If you are unsure, check with your doctor or health professional.

1. **Start in mountain posture (refer to Figure 8-1) and, as you inhale, raise your arms forward, and then up overhead (see Figure 8-2a).**

2. **As you exhale, bend forward from your hips.**

   When you feel a pull in the back of your legs, soften your knees (see coverage of Forgiving Limbs in Chapter 6) and hang your arms.

3. **If your head is not close to your knees, bend your knees more.**

   If you have the flexibility, straighten your knees but keep them soft.

   Relax your head and neck downward (see Figure 8-2b).

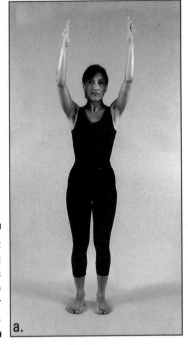

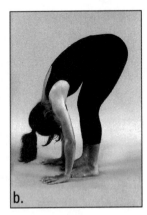

Figure 8-2:
Bending
your knees
can help
stretch your
back.

a.   b.

4. **As you inhale, roll up slowly, stacking the bones of your spine one at a time from bottom to top, and then raise your arms overhead.**

5. **Repeat Steps 1–4 three times, and then stay in the folded position (Step 3) for 6 to 8 breaths.**

Note: In the classical posture, the feet are together and the legs are straight. The forehead presses against the shins, and the palms are on the floor.

Rolling up in Step 4 is the safest way to come up. If you do not have back problems, after a few weeks you may want to try two more advanced techniques: As you come up, sweep your arms out and up from the sides like wings then over your head; Or, as you inhale, extend your slightly bent arms forward and up until they are parallel with your ears. Then raise your upper back, then your lower back until you are all the way up and your arms are overhead.

The Sanskrit word *uttana* (pronounced *oo-tah-nah*) means "extended."

Half standing forward bend — ardha uttanasana

The half standing forward bend strengthens the legs, the back, shoulders and arms, and improves stamina.

1. **Start in the mountain posture (refer to Figure 8-1) and as you inhale, raise your arms forward, and then up overhead (refer to Figure 8-2a).**

2. **As you exhale, bend forward from your hips.**

   Soften your knees and hang your arms.

3. **Bend your knees, and as you inhale, raise your torso and arms up from the front, to parallel to the floor (see Figure 8-3).**

   If you have any back problems, keep your arms back by your sides, and then over a period of time gradually stretch them out in front of you to parallel.

4. **Bring your head to a neutral position, so that your ears are between your arms.**

   Look down and a little forward. To make the posture easier, move your arms back toward your hips — the further back, the easier.

5. **Repeat Steps 1–4 three times, and then stay in Step 4 for 6 to 8 breaths.**

Note: In the classical version of this posture, the feet are together and the legs and arms are straight.

The Sanskrit word *ardha* (pronounced *ahrd-ha*) means "half."

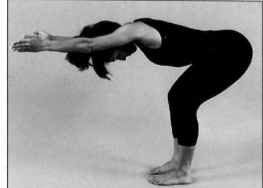

Figure 8-3:
This posture is great for stamina.

Asymmetrical forward bend — parshva uttanasana

The asymmetrical forward bend stretches each side of the back and hamstrings separately. The posture opens the hips, tones the abdomen, decompresses the neck, improves balance, and increases circulation to the upper torso and head (see Figure 8-4).

1. **Stand in the mountain posture, and as you exhale, step forward about 3 to 3½ feet (or the length of one leg) with your right foot.**

   Your left foot will turn out naturally, but if you need more stability turn your left foot out more (so that the toes point to the left.)

2. **Place your hands on the top of your hips and square the front of your pelvis; then release your hands and hang your arms.**

3. **As you inhale, raise your arms forward and then overhead (see Figure 8-4a).**

4. **As you exhale, bend forward from the hips, soften your right knee and both arms, and hang down (see Figure 8-4b).**

   If your head is not close to your right knee, bend your knee more. If you have the flexibility, straighten your right knee but keep it soft.

Figure 8-4:
This exercise stretches each side of the back and hamstrings separately.

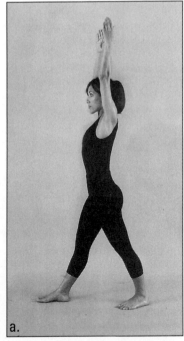

a.

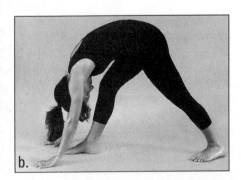

b.

5. **As you inhale, roll up slowly, stacking the bones of your spine one at a time from the bottom up, and then raise your arms overhead.**

   Relax your head and neck downward.

6. **Repeat Steps 3–4 three times, and then stay in Step 4 for 6 to 8 breaths.**

   Repeat the same sequence on the left side.

Note: In the classical version of this posture, both legs are straight and the forehead presses against the forward leg.

Rolling up in Step 4 is the safest way to come up. If you do not have back problems, after a few weeks you may want to try two more advanced techniques: As you come up, sweep your arms out and up from the sides like wings then over your head; Or, as you inhale, extend your slightly bent arms forward and up until they are parallel with your ears. Then raise your upper back, then your lower back until you are all the way up and your arms are overhead.

The Sanskrit word *parshva* (surprisingly, pronounced just like it looks *pahr-shvah*) means "side" or "flank."

Triangle posture — utthita trikonasana

The triangle posture stretches the sides of the spine, the backs of the legs and the hips. This posture also stretches the muscles between the ribs (the intercostals) which opens the chest and improves breathing capacity (see Figure 8-5).

1. **Stand in the mountain posture (refer to Figure 8-1), exhale, and with your right foot, step out to the right about 3 to 3$^1/_2$ feet (or the length of one leg).**

2. **Turn your right foot out 90 degrees and your left foot 45 degrees.**

   An imaginary line drawn from the right heel (toward the left foot) should bisect the arch of the left foot.

3. **Face forward and, as you inhale, raise your arms out to the sides parallel to the line of the shoulders (and the floor), so that they form a "T" with the torso (see Figure 8-5a).**

4. **As you exhale, reach your right hand down to your right shin as close to the ankle as is comfortable for you;. then reach and lift your left arm up.**

   Bend your right knee slightly if the back of your leg feels tight (see Figure 8-5b).

   As much as you can, bring the sides of your torso parallel to the floor.

5. **Soften your left arm and look up at your left hand.**

   If your neck hurts, look down at the floor.

6. **Repeat Steps 3–5 three times, and then stay in Step 5 for 6 to 8 breaths.**

   Repeat the same sequence on the left side.

Note: In the classic version of this posture, the feet are parallel, the arms and legs are straight, and the trunk is parallel to the floor. The right hand is on the floor outside the right foot.

The Sanskrit word *utthita* (pronounced *oot-hee-tah*) means "raised" and *trikona* (pronounced *tree-ko-nah*) means "triangle."

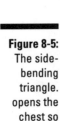

Figure 8-5: The side-bending triangle. opens the chest so you can breathe deeply.

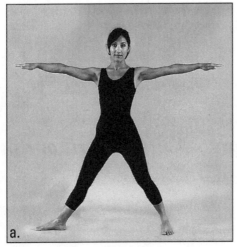

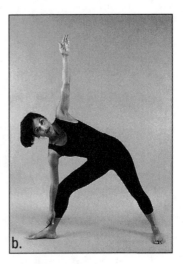

a. b.

Reverse triangle posture — parivritta trikonasana

The action of twists, including the reverse triangle, on the discs between the spinal vertebrae (intervertebral discs) is often compared to squeezing and then releasing a wet sponge: First you squeeze the dirty water out, and then you "sponge" up the clean water. The twisting-untwisting action increases circulation of fresh blood to these discs and keeps them supple as you grow older. The reverse triangle also stretches the backs of your legs, opens your hips, and strengthens your neck, shoulders, and arms (see Figure 8-6).

1. Standing in the mountain posture (refer to Figure 8-1), exhale and, with the right foot, step out to the right about 3 to 3¹/₂ feet (or the length of one leg).

2. As you inhale, raise your arms out to the sides parallel to the line of the shoulders (and the floor), so that they form a "T" with the torso (see Figure 8-6a).

3. As you exhale, bend forward from the hips and then place the right hand on the floor near the inside of the left foot.

4. Raise your left arm toward the ceiling and look up at your left hand.

   Soften your knees and your arms. Bend your left knee or move your right hand away from your left foot (and more directly under the torso), if necessary (see Figure 8-6b).

5. Repeat Steps 2–4 three times, and then stay in Step 4 for 6 to 8 breaths.

   Repeat the same sequence on the left side.

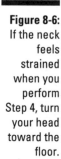

Figure 8-6: If the neck feels strained when you perform Step 4, turn your head toward the floor.

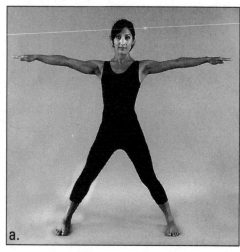
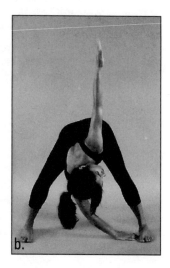

a. b.

Note: In the classic version of this posture, the feet are parallel and the legs and arms are straight. The torso is parallel to the floor and the bottom hand rests lightly outside the opposite side foot.

The Sanskrit word *parivritta* (pronounced *pah-ree-vree-tah*) means "revolved."

Warrior posture — vira bhadrasana

The warrior posture strengthens your legs, back, shoulders and arms, opens your hips, groin and chest, increases strength and stamina, and improves balance (see Figure 8-7). As its name suggests, this posture instills a feeling of fearlessness and inner strength.

1. **Stand in the mountain posture (refer to Figure 8-1) and, as you exhale, step forward approximately 3 to 3¹/₂ feet (or the length of one leg) with your right foot (see Figure 8-7a).**

   Your left foot will turn out naturally, but if you need more stability, turn your left foot out more (so that the toes point to the left).

2. **Place your hands on the top of your hips and square the front of your pelvis; then release your hands and hang your arms.**

3. **As you inhale, raise your arms forward and overhead and bend your right knee to a right angle (so that the knee is directly over the ankle and the thigh is parallel to the floor). See Figure 8-7b.**

   If your lower back is uncomfortable, lean the torso slightly over the forward leg until you feel a release of tension in your back.

4. **As you exhale, return to the starting place as in Figure 8-7a. Soften your arms and face your palms toward each other. Look straight ahead.**

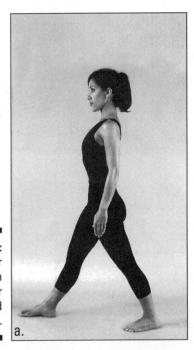
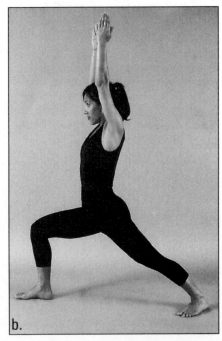

Figure 8-7:
The warrior
is a position
of power
and
strength.

a.

b.

5. **Repeat Steps 3 and 4 three times, and then stay in Step 4 for 6 to 8 breaths.**

   Repeat the same sequence on the left side. When you stay in the posture, if your lower back is uncomfortable, lean the torso slightly over the forward leg until you feel a release of tension in your back.

The Sanskrit word *vira* (pronounced *vee-rah*) is often translated as "hero" and *bhadra* (pronounced *bhud-rah*) means "auspicious."

Standing spread leg forward bend — prasarita pada uttanasana

This posture, also called the wide leg standing forward bend stretches the hamstrings and the adductors (on insides of the thighs) and opens the hips. The hanging forward bend increases circulation to the upper torso and lengthens the spine.

1. **Stand in the mountain posture, exhale, and, with your right foot, step out to the right about 3 to 3½ feet (or the length of one leg).**

2. **As you inhale, raise your arms out to the sides parallel to the line of the shoulders (and the floor) so they form a "T" with the torso (refer to Figure 8-6.)**

3. **As you exhale, bend forward from the hips and soften the knees.**

4. **Hold your bent elbows with the opposite-side hands, and hang your torso and arms (see Figure 8-8).**

5. **Stay in Step 4 for 6 to 8 breaths.**

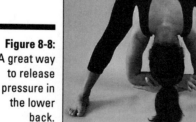

Figure 8-8:
A great way to release pressure in the lower back.

Note: In the classic version of this posture, the legs are straight, the head is on the floor (and the chin presses the chest), and the arms reach back between the legs, palms on the floor.

The Sanskrit word *prasarita* (pronounced *prah-sah-ree-tah*) means "outstretched" and *pada,* (pronounced *pah-dah*) means "foot."

Half chair posture — ardha utkatasana

The half chair posture strengthens the back, legs, shoulders and arms, and builds overall stamina. If you find this posture difficult, or have "problem knees," you may want to skip this position for now and return to it after your leg muscles become a little stronger. Don't overdo this exercise (either by holding the position or by repeating it more than we recommend), or you'll have sore muscles the next day. But there is no harm in experiencing some muscle soreness either, especially if you haven't done any exercise in a long time.

1. **Start in the mountain posture (refer to Figure 8-1), and as you inhale, raise your arms forward and up overhead, palms facing each other (refer to Figure 8-2a).**

2. **As you exhale, bend your knees and squat halfway to the floor.**

3. **Soften your arms but keep them overhead (see Figure 8-9).**

   Look straight ahead.

4. **Repeat Steps 1–3 three times, and then stay in Step 3 for 6 to 8 breaths.**

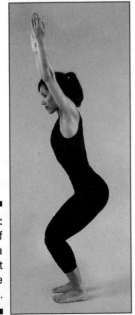

Figure 8-9: The half chair is a great posture for skiers.

Note: In the classic version of this posture, the feet are together and the arms are straight, with the fingers interlocked and the palms turned upward. The chin rests on the chest.

The Sanskrit word *ardha* (pronounced *ahrd-ha)* means "half," while *utkata,* (pronounced *oot-kah-tah*) is translatable as "extraordinary."

Downward facing dog posture — adhomukha shvanasana

The practice of downward facing dog stretches the entire back of your body, and strengthens your wrists, arms, and shoulders. This posture is a good alternative for beginning students who are not yet ready for inversions like handstand and headstand. Because the head is lower than the heart, this *asana* circulates fresh blood to the brain, and acts as a quick "pick-me-up" when you're fatigued (see Figure 8-10).

1. **Start on your hands and knees, straighten your arms, but don't lock your elbows (see Figure 8-10a).**

   Be sure that your hands are directly under your shoulders, palms spread on the floor, and knees directly under your hips.

2. **As you exhale, lift and straighten (but don't lock) your knees.**

   As your hips lift, bring your head to a neutral position so that your ears are between your arms.

3. **If possible, press your heels to the floor and your head toward your feet (see Figure 8-10b).**

   Do not complete Step 3 if doing so strains your neck.

4. **Repeat Steps 1–3 three times, and then stay in Step 3 for 6 to 8 breaths.**

Note: In the classical posture, the feet are together and flat on the floor, the legs and arms are straight, and the top of the head is on the floor with the chin pressed to the chest.

Be careful not to hold this posture too long if you have problems with your neck, shoulders, wrists, or elbows.

The Sanskrit work *adhomukha* (pronounced *ahd-ho-mook-hah*) means "downward facing," and *shvan* (pronounced *shvahn*) means "dog."

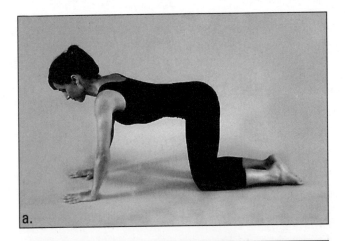

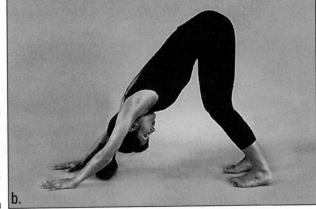

Figure 8-10:
Challenge
yourself,
but don't
strain.

Chapter 9

Steady as a Tree: Mastering Balance

- -

In This Chapter

▶ The psychology of balance

▶ Six balancing exercises

- -

Balance (called *samata* or *samatva* in Sanskrit and pronounced *sah-mah-tah* or *sah-mah-tvah*) is fundamental to Yoga. A balanced approach to life includes being even-tempered and seeing the great unity behind all diversity. Balance translates to being nonjudgmental and treating others with equal fairness, kindness, and compassion.

One way to begin to gain this balance is to practice balancing postures. Remember, according to Yoga, body and mind form a working unit. Imbalances in the body are reflected in the mind, and vice versa. This chapter emphasizes the importance of balance in Yoga and offers six postures that provide you with a *samata* sampling.

Getting to the Roots of the Posture

When you look at a tree, you see only what is above ground — the vertical trunk with its crown of branches and foliage and maybe a few chirping birds. Trees appear to just perch atop the soil, and you wonder how in the world such a top-heavy thing can stay upright.

Well, everyone knows that the secret of the tree's equilibrium is its underground network of roots that anchor the visible part of the plant solidly into the earth. In the balancing postures, you too can discover how to grow your "roots" into the earth and stand up as steady as a tree.

For us, the balancing postures can be the most fun and the most dramatic of all the postures. Although they are relatively simple, the postures can produce profound effects. As you may expect, they work to improve your overall sense of physical balance, coordination, and grounding. With awareness in these three areas, you can move more easily and effectively, whether you're going about your daily business or are engaged in activities calling for great coordination, such as sports or dance. The yogic balancing postures also have therapeutic applications, such as with back problems or retraining whole muscle groups.

When you improve your physical balance naturally, you can expect to enjoy improved mental balance. The balancing postures are exceptional "seeds" for concentration, and when they're mastered, they create confidence and a sense of accomplishment.

Balancing Postures for Graceful Strength

Contemporary life is highly demanding and stressful; if you're not properly grounded, you face a constant risk of being pushed out of balance. *Grounding* means being centered and firm, without being inflexible; and it means knowing who you are and what you want, and feeling that you are empowered to achieve your life goals. A good way to begin your grounding work is by improving your physical sense of balance, which helps you synchronize the movement of your arms and legs, giving you poise. When you can stand and move in a more balanced manner, your mind is automatically affected. You *feel* more balanced.

A sense of balance is connected with the inner ears. Your ears tell you where you are in space. The ears are also connected with *social space;* if you aren't well-balanced, you may feel — or actually *be* — a bit awkward in your social relationships. Balancing and grounding work can remedy this discomfort. Only when you can stand still — in balance — can you also move harmoniously in the world.

Imagine yourself as a tree and ask yourself the following questions:

- ✔ Where are my roots?
- ✔ Are my roots nourishing me?
- ✔ Are my roots strong?
- ✔ Are my roots entangled with other competing roots?

According to Yoga, the best roots are those that are anchored in the domain of the spirit. This is the traditional image of the upside-down tree, which derives its sustenance from above and spreads its fruit down below.

Now ask yourself these questions:

- ✔ Do I feel supported?
- ✔ Do I feel able to grow?
- ✔ What, if anything, is blocking my further growth?
- ✔ How do I want to grow?
- ✔ What must I do to grow even more?

The following postures appear in order of easier to more advanced exercises. We recommend that if you try the postures individually rather than as part of a sequence, you hold each posture for 6 to 8 breaths. Breathe freely through the nose and pause briefly after inhalation and exhalation.

Warrior at the wall (vira bhadrasana III variation)

This posture improves your overall balance and stability. It strengthens the legs, arms, and shoulders and stretches the thighs — both front and back — and the hips. As with the other one-leg balancing poses, this posture enhances focus and concentration.

1. **Stand in the mountain posture (see Chapter 8), facing a blank wall about three feet away.**

2. **As you exhale, bend forward from the hips and extend your arms forward until your fingertips are touching the wall.**

   Adjust yourself so that your legs are perpendicular and your torso and arms are parallel with the floor.

3. **As you inhale, raise your left leg back and up until it's parallel to the floor (see Figure 9-1).**

4. **Stay in Step 3 for 6 to 8 breaths; then repeat with the opposite leg.**

The Sanskrit word *vira* (pronounced *vee-rah*) means "hero." *Bhadra* (pronounced *bhud-rah*) means "auspicious."

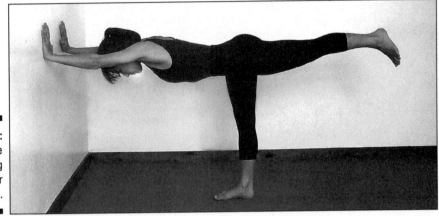

Figure 9-1:
A safe
balancing
posture for
beginners.

Balancing cat

Balancing cat strengthens the muscles along the spine *(paraspinals)*, the arms, and the shoulders, and it opens the hips. The posture enhances focus and concentration and also builds confidence.

1. **Beginning on your hands and knees, position your hands directly under your shoulders, palms spread on the floor, with your knees directly under your hips.**

   Straighten your arms, but don't lock your elbows.

2. **As you exhale, slide your right hand forward and your left leg back, keeping your hand and your toes on the floor.**

3. **As you inhale, raise your right arm and left leg to a comfortable height, or as high as is possible for you (see Figure 9-2).**

4. **Stay in Step 3 for 6 to 8 breaths, and then repeat with opposite pairs (left arm and right leg).**

This posture is a variation of *cakravakasana* (pronounced *chuk-rah-vahk-ah-sah-nah*). The *cakravaka* is a particular kind of goose, which in India's traditional poetry is often used to convey "love bird." Apparently, when these birds have paired up and then are separated, their heartache causes them to call to each other.

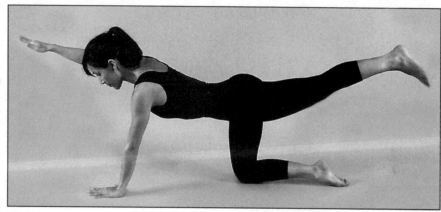

Figure 9-2:
Extend your arm and leg fully on the ground before you lift them up.

The tree — vrikshasana

The tree posture improves overall balance, stability, and poise. It strengthens the legs, arms, and shoulders, and "opens" (relaxes and loosens up) the hips and groin. The posture, like the other one-leg balancing poses, enhances focus and concentration and produces a calming effect on the body and mind.

1. **Stand in the mountain posture (see Chapter 8).**

2. **As you exhale, bend your left knee and place the sole of your left foot, toes pointing down, on the inside of your right leg between your knee and your groin.**

3. **As you inhale, bring your arms over your head and join your palms together.**

4. **Soften the arms and focus on a spot 6 to 8 feet in front of you on the floor (see Figure 9-3).**

5. **Stay in Step 4 for 6 to 8 breaths and then repeat with the opposite leg.**

Note: In the classical version of this posture, the arms are straight and the chin rests on the chest.

The Sanskrit word *vriksha* (pronounced *vrik-shah*) means "tree."

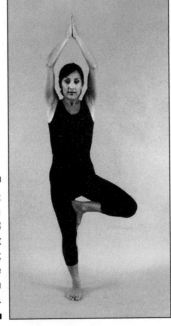

Figure 9-3:
Focus on a
spot 6 to 8
feet in front
of you;
concentrate
and breath
slowly.

The karate kid

The karate kid improves overall balance and stability. It strengthens the legs, arms and shoulders, and opens the hips. As with the other one-leg balancing postures, the karate kid enhances focus and concentration.

1. **Stand in the mountain posture, which we describe in Chapter 8.**

2. **As you inhale, raise your arms out to the sides parallel to the line of your shoulders (and the floor) so that they form a "T" with the torso.**

3. **Steady yourself and focus on a spot on the floor 10 to 12 feet in front of you.**

4. **As you exhale, bend your left knee, raising it toward your chest.**

   Keep your right leg straight (see Figure 9-4).

5. **Stay in Step 4 for 6 to 8 breaths; then repeat with the right knee.**

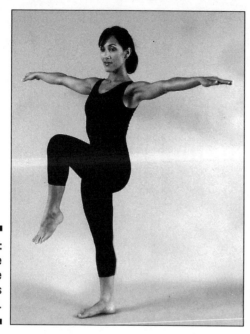

Figure 9-4:
The Karate Kid of movie fame was also a yogi.

Standing heel-to-buttock

The standing heel-to-buttock posture improves your overall balance and stability. This posture strengthens the legs, arms, and shoulders, and stretches the thighs. As with the other one-leg balancing poses, this posture enhances focus and concentration.

1. **Stand in the mountain posture (see Chapter 8).**

2. **As you inhale, raise your right arm forward and overhead.**

3. **Steady yourself and focus on a spot on the floor 10 to 12 feet in front of you.**

4. **As you exhale, bend your left knee and bring your left heel toward the left buttock, keeping the right leg straight.**

   Grasp the left ankle with the left hand (see Figure 9-5).

5. **Stay in Step 4 for 6 to 8 breaths; then repeat with the right foot.**

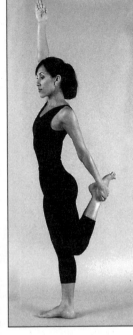

Figure 9-5:
This pose can improve your balance for the more advanced postures.

Scorpion

The scorpion posture improves overall balance and stability. This posture, which is a variation of *cakravakasana,* strengthens the shoulders, improves the flexibility of the hips, legs, and shoulders, and enhances focus and concentration.

1. **While on your hands and knees, place your hands directly under your shoulders, palms spread on the floor, and knees directly under your hips.**

   Straighten your arms, but don't lock your elbows.

2. **Place your right forearm on the floor, right hand just behind the left wrist.**

   Reach behind you with your left hand, twisting the torso slightly to the left, and grab your right ankle.

3. **As you inhale, lift your right knee off the floor, raise your chest until it is parallel to the floor, and look up.**

   Find a comfortable height for your chest and raised leg, Steady yourself by pressing your right forearm and thumb on the floor (see Figure 9-6).

4. **Stay in Step 3 for 6 to 8 breaths, and then repeat on the opposite side (left forearm and left foot).**

Figure 9-6: Steady yourself by pressing your right forearm and thumb into the floor.

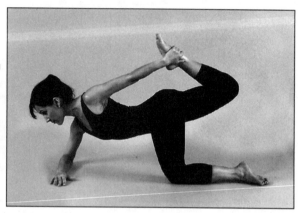

Chapter 10

Absolutely Abs

- -

In This Chapter

▶ Centering on the significance of the belly

▶ Enjoying the rewards of six simple abdominal exercises

▶ Sounding off during exhalation

- -

*M*any Eastern systems of spiritual exercise and healing consider the lower abdomen to be the vital center of your whole being — body, mind, and spirit. The Japanese call this potent area *hara,* which appropriately enough means "belly." As Westerners, we think much differently about our bellies.

Many people have a love-hate relationship with their bellies. Although people may be obsessed with having the "perfect" midriff, they tend to neglect or even abuse this area of their bodies. On the inside, they stuff the belly with junk food, and way too much of it. On the outside, they let it grow slack. But, as the Yoga masters warn, when this area is "polluted" by impurities, it becomes a seat of sickness.

Apart from diseases, weak bellies (and belly muscles) make a significant contribution to the well-documented epidemic of lower back problems. Studies indicate that 80 percent of the American population has had, is having, or will have back problems, and that back-related problems are the second-leading cause of missed workdays, trailing only respiratory problems or the common cold.

In this chapter, we describe exercises that work with three sets of abdominal muscles:

✔ The *rectus abdominis,* which is strung vertically along the front of the belly from the bottom of the sternum to the pubis.

✔ The internal and external *obliques,* which, as their name suggests, take an "oblique" course along the side of the belly from the lower ribs to the top rim of the pelvis.

✔ The *transversalis abdominis,* which lies behind the internal obliques.

You may hear these three abdominals called the "stomach muscles," which is really a misnomer. The actual stomach muscles line the baglike stomach and are active only during digestion. Of course, the yogic exercises also positively affect the abdominal organs — stomach, spleen, liver, and intestines. If you take care of your abdominal muscles and the organs they protect — through exercise and proper diet — you have accomplished 90 percent of the work to stay healthy.

Taking Care of the Abdomen: Your Busy "Corporation"

The abdomen is an amazing enterprise, with its complex food-processing plant (the stomach), several subsidiary operations (liver, spleen, kidneys, and so on), and a 25-foot-long sewer system (the intestines). As long as the sum and its parts are not overburdened and no negative genetic predisposition exists, everything will stay in fine working order for most of your life. However, because most people follow a poor diet and have poor eating habits, breakdowns occur quite frequently: constipation, diarrhea, irritable bowel syndrome, stomach ulcers, and colon cancer. Regular Yoga practice ensures that your abdominal organs perform their various duties well throughout your life. You won't need antacids, digestive enzyme supplements, or laxatives.

The secret of the navel

After a doctor severs a child's umbilical cord, thus creating his navel, no one pays much attention to this birth socket. Yet the navel is a very important feature of your anatomy. According to Yoga, a special psychoenergetic center is located at the navel.

This center is known as the *manipura-cakra* (pronounced *mah-nee-poo-rah-chuk-rah*) which means literally "center of the jeweled city." The center corresponds to (but isn't identical with) the *solar plexus*, which is a large network of nerves that has been called the body's "second brain." It controls the abdominal organs and regulates the flow of energy through the entire body. The navel center is associated with emotions and the will. You can have "too much navel" (be pushy) or "not enough navel" (be a pushover).

Exercising Those Abs

Our yogic postures for the abdominal muscles incorporate a "team approach" that values slow, conscious movement, proper breathing mechanics, and the use of sound. The emphasis here is on the quality of the movement rather than sheer quantity — we believe that a few movements done with diligent attention are much safer and more effective than dozens, even hundreds of mindless repetitions. We also believe that conscious breathing, especially the gentle tightening of the front belly on each exhale, can encourage and then sustain the strength and tone of the abdominals. The use of sound, which we discuss later in this chapter, further enhances this kind of breathing.

Exploring push-downs

Push-downs strengthen the abdomen, especially the lower abdomen. In addition to a floor exercise, you can do push-downs in a seated position by pushing your lower back against the back of your chair. You can perform this exercise sitting in a car, on a plane, or at the office.

1. **Lie on your back, knees bent, feet on the floor at hip width.**

   Rest your arms near your sides, palms down.

2. **As you exhale, push your lower back down to the floor for 3 to 5 seconds (see Figure 10-1).**

3. **As you inhale, release the back.**

4. **Repeat Steps 2 and 3 six to eight times.**

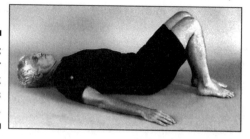

Figure 10-1: Push your lower back down as you exhale.

ANECDOTE

Producing the yogic sound

A well-known movie producer from Malibu was referred to me (Larry Payne) by his physician. The producer suffered from a chronic neck and stress condition. He also had a girlfriend who constantly teased him about his "little jelly belly." His personal trainer had given him regular sit-ups, which just aggravated his neck problem. To make matters worse, he was in the middle of a big film project and had very little time to practice. I gave him a 12-minute, twice-a-day Yoga routine that included the yogi sit-back and the use of sound. The exercises worked like a miracle. His neck problem went away. His belly firmed up nicely, and he liked using sound so much that many of the members of his movie crew joined him in the afternoon for "a little sound."

Trying yogi sit-ups

Yogi sit-ups strengthen the abdomen, especially the upper abdomen, the adductors (insides of your legs), the neck, and the shoulders.

1. **Lie on your back, knees bent, feet on the floor at hip width.**

2. **Turn your toes in "pigeon-toed" and bring the inner knees together.**

3. **Spread your palms on the back of your head, fingers interlocked and keep your elbows wide.**

4. **As you exhale, press the knees firmly, tilt the front of the pelvis toward your navel and, with the hips on the ground, slowly sit up halfway.**

   Keep your elbows out to the sides in line with the tops of your shoulders. Look toward the ceiling. *Don't pull your head up with your arms;* rather, support your head with your hands and come up by contracting the abdominal muscles (see Figure 10-2).

5. **As you inhale, slowly roll back down.**

6. **Repeat Steps 4 and 5 six to eight times.**

Figure 10-2: Let your eyes follow the ceiling as you sit up.

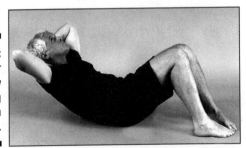

Strengthening with yogi sit-backs

Yogi sit-backs strengthen both the lower and upper abdomen (see Figure 10-3). This posture is a variation of *navasana*. The Sanskrit word *nava*, pronounced *nah-vah*, means "boat."

1. **Sit on the floor with your knees bent, feet on the floor at hip width.**

2. **Place your hands on the floor, palms down, near your hips.**

3. **Bring your chin down and round your back in a "C" curve (see Figure 10-3a).**

4. **As you inhale, roll slowly onto the back of your pelvis, dragging your hands along on the floor.**

   Keep the rest of your back off the floor to maintain the contraction of the abdominals, but *don't strain* to hold this position; if you feel strain, lift out of the sit-back slightly (see Figure 10-3b).

5. **As you exhale, roll up again, sliding your hands forward.**

6. **Repeat Steps 4 and 5 six to eight times.**

Figure 10-3: Bring your chin down and keep your back rounded in a "C" curve.

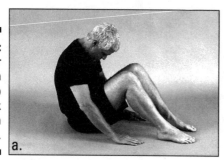
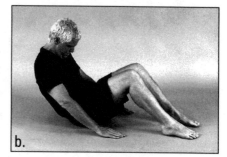

Sit-backs are easier on the neck than most sit-ups. However, if you have lower back problems, be cautious with sit-backs. If you notice any pain in your back, just stop. Work with the other exercises in this chapter instead.

Working with extended leg slide-ups

A variation of *navasana*, the extended leg slide-ups strengthen both the upper and lower abdomen, as well as the neck (see Figure 10-4).

If this pose bothers your neck, support your head by putting both hands behind it. If the problem persists, stop.

1. **Lie on your back with your knees bent and feet flat on the floor at hip width.**

2. **Bend the left elbow and place your left hand on the back of your head, just behind the left ear.**

   Raise the left leg as close to vertical (90 degrees) as possible, but keep your knee slightly bent.

3. **Draw the top of the foot toward your shin to flex the ankle and place your right palm on your right thigh near the pelvis (see Figure 10-4a).**

4. **As you exhale, sit up slowly halfway and slide your right hand toward your knee.**

   Keep your left elbow back in line with your shoulder and look at the ceiling. Don't throw your head forward (see Figure 10-4b).

5. **Repeat Steps 1 – 4 six to eight times, and then repeat the sequence on the other side.**

Figure 10-4:
Work the abs and the hamstrings.

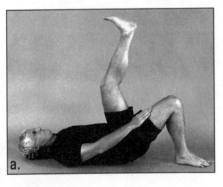
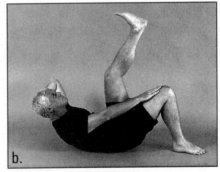

Arching with the suck 'em up posture

The suck 'em up posture strengthens and tones the abdominal muscles and the internal organs. The posture is especially beneficial for relieving constipation.

1. **Start on your hands and knees, with your hands just below the shoulders and your knees at hip width.**

2. **Inhale deeply through the nose.**

3. **Exhale through your mouth and hump your back like a camel as you bring your chin down.**

   When you have fully exhaled, hold your breath and then suck your belly up towards your spine (see Figure 10-5).

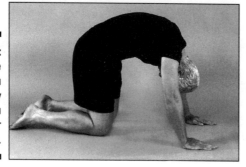

Figure 10-5:
Make sure that you exhale fully before you suck your belly up.

Wait two to three seconds with the belly up and breath restrained, providing you don't end up gasping for air.

4. **As you inhale, return to the starting position.**

5. **Repeat Steps 2 – 4 four to six times, pausing for a breath or two between each repetition.**

Do this exercise only on an empty stomach, and avoid it if you are having stomach pain or cramps of any kind. Avoid this exercise during menstruation.

Exhaling "soundly"

The use of sound exercise strengthens and tones the abdomen and its internal organs, in addition to strengthening the muscles of the diaphragm.

1. **Sit in a chair or on the floor with your spine comfortably upright.**

2. **Place the palm of your right hand on your navel so that you can feel your belly contracting as you exhale.**

3. **Take a deep inhalation through the nose and, as you exhale, make the sound *ah, ma,* or *sa*.**

   Continue sounding this consonant for as long as you can do so comfortably.

4. **Repeat Steps 2 and 3 six to eight times.**

   Pause for a resting breath or two between each sound.

If you are on a detox program of any kind and the use of sound gives you a headache, work with the other exercises in this chapter instead.

Chapter 11

Looking at the World Upside Down

housands of years ago, the Yoga masters made an amazing discovery: By tricking the force of gravity with the help of inversion exercises, you can reverse the effects of aging, improve your health, and add years to your life.

To picture how inversions work, take a look at a jug of unfiltered apple juice sitting on the grocery store shelf. Gravity has pulled solids in the juice to the bottom of the jug, diluting the liquid near the top. If you turn the bottle upside down, gravity pulls the bottom sediment toward the top of the inverted jug, remixing the juice with the pulp of the apples.

In a similar way, when you turn yourself upside down, the sediments that have collected in your lower limbs — mostly blood and lymph — during a long day of uprightness sink toward your head and revitalize your entire body and mind.

If you're wondering what lymph is, it's a clear yellowish fluid similar to blood plasma. It contains mainly lymphocytes (a type of white blood cell) and fats and has its own system of pathways. Draining the lymphatic vessels periodically through inversion exercises helps keep them fit.

You can make gravity work to your advantage in more than one way: to keep you in a practical posture for everyday activities and to neutralize gravity's detrimental effects on your body.

The Sanskrit name for the general category of postural inversions is *viparita karani* (pronounced *vee-pah-ree-tah kah-rah-nee*) or "reverse process." This is also the particular name of the three shoulder stand variations we describe in this chapter. Strictly speaking, these inversions are not a regular posture or *asana* at all, but a *mudra* (pronounced *mood-rah*). A *mudra* is far more powerful than a regular *asana,* because it keeps the life energy sealed in your body.

Of all the different types of Yoga postures, inversions are perhaps the most effective for influencing overall change in your body and mind through the endocrine system. In addition to rejuvenating and strengthening your body, the yogic inversions also help you face your fears and actually reverse the tide of stagnation and mental negativity.

The widespread notion that the headstand is the only yogic inversion that can make you a "real yogi" is mistaken. In fact, we recommend that you avoid the headstand unless an experienced teacher supervises your work. The neck is designed to support the 8 pounds of the head, not the 100 or more pounds of the body. Therefore, you should approach the headstand cautiously and only after proper preparation.

The more advanced inverted postures are a frequent source of injuries for overly enthusiastic beginners working without a teacher. However, you can practice many safe inversions without risk and so receive the tremendous benefits of the yogic "reverse process." In this chapter, we treat you to several effective and safe inversion exercises.

Turning Attention to the Inversion Postures

Accomplished hatha yogi Theos Bernard, who vanished in the Himalayas in 1947, was able to stand on his head for three hours at a time. He learned to relax his mind sufficiently to overcome boredom and restlessness. We don't expect you to do the same. In fact, we recommend against you even trying. If you practice the following exercises instead, we promise you'll enjoy the benefits of inversion, without any risk.

You can boost the beneficial effect of the exercises described in this chapter by using yogic breathing (see Chapter 5). Make sure, however, that you can breathe easily. If necessary, use a prop to facilitate the posture and your breathing (see Chapter 17).

Avoid all inverted postures if you have an acute headache or if you experience sudden pain while performing the exercise.

Legs up on a chair

The legs up on a chair posture improves circulation to your legs, hips, and lower back and has a calming effect on your nervous system. It also helps alleviate symptoms of PMS in women and prostatitis in men.

1. **Sit on the floor in a simple cross leg position facing a sturdy chair and then lean back onto your forearms.**

2. **Slide your buttocks along the floor toward the chair until they are just under the front edge of the chair seat.**

3. **While exhaling, lift your feet off the floor and place your heels and calves on the chair seat.**

   Make sure that the front edge of the seat is close to the backs of your knees.

4. **Lie back on the floor with your arms near your sides, palms down or up (see Figure 11-1).**

5. **Stay in Step 4 for 2 to 10 minutes. Use any of the recommended Yoga breathing techniques (see Chapter 5).**

This posture is a variation of the classical posture of *urdhva prasarita padasana* (pronounced *oord-hvah prah-sah-ree-tah pahd-ah-sah-nah*) which means "upward extended foot posture."

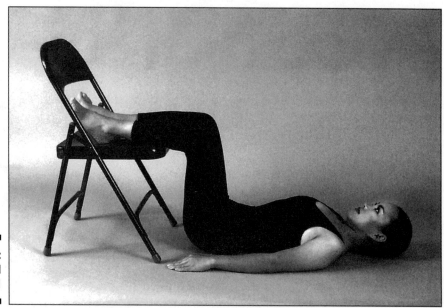

Figure 11-1:
You can all
do this!

Legs up against the wall

Legs up on the wall, which is a variation of *urdhva prasarita padasana,* improves circulation to the legs, hips, and lower back and has a calming effect on the nervous system (see Figure 11-2). It also helps alleviate symptoms of PMS in women and prostatitis in men.

1. **Sit sideways with your right side as close to the wall as possible, with both legs extended forward (see Figure 11-2a).**

2. **As you exhale, swing both legs up on the wall and lie flat on your back.**

   Extend your legs up as far as possible. Extend your arms out comfortably at your sides, palms down, and relax (see Figure 11-2b).

3. **Stay in Step 2 for 2 to 10 minutes; use any of the recommended Yoga breathing techniques (see Chapter 5).**

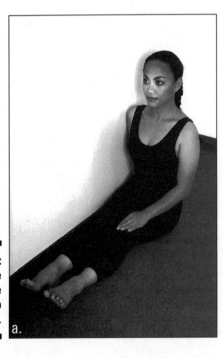
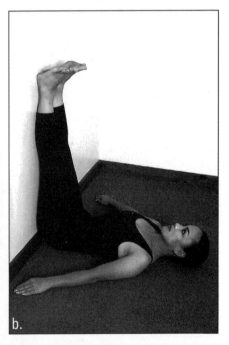

Figure 11-2: This posture will give you a leg up on gravity.

a.

b.

The dying bug

A variation of *urdhva prasarita padasana,* the dying bug posture — excuse the image — improves circulation in the legs, arms, hips, and lower back, and has a calming effect on the nervous system. It also improves the range of motion of the ankles, toes, wrists, and fingers.

1. **Lying on your back with your knees bent and feet flat on the floor, place your arms at your sides, palms down.**

2. **As you exhale, extend your legs and arms up vertically.**

   Keep the limbs relaxed (see "Forgiving Limbs" in Chapter 6) as you hold them up (see Figure 11-3).

3. **With your feet, toes, hands, and fingers draw circles in the air both clockwise and counterclockwise. If you want, you can make your hands and feet go in different directions at the same time.**

   Breathe freely. Keep your arms and legs up as long as you feel comfortable, and then return to the starting position.

4. **Repeat Steps 2 and 3 three to five times, but do not hold the limbs up for more than a total of 5 minutes; you don't want to tire yourself out or strain your back.**

Avoid this posture if you have lower back problems.

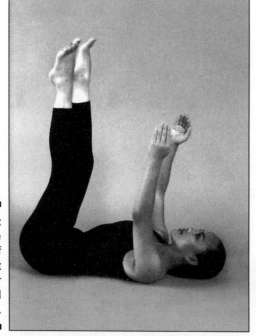

Figure 11-3:
Enjoy the
freedom of
movement
in your
ankles and
wrists.

Standing spread leg forward bend at the wall

The standing spread leg forward bend at the wall improves circulation in the head and stretches the spine and hamstrings.

This posture is a variation of *prasarita pada uttanasana* described in Chapter 8.

1. **Stand with your back 2 to 3 feet from a sturdy wall, separate your feet to a comfortably wide stance, and then lean your buttocks back against the wall.**

2. **As you exhale, bend forward from the hips and hang the arms and head down.**

   If your hands touch the floor, grasp your elbows with opposite-side hands and let your forearms hang. Keep your knees soft and relax your neck and head (see Figure 11-4).

3. **Stay in Step 2 for 2 to 3 minutes; use any of the Yoga breathing techniques (see Chapter 5).**

If you feel light-headed when doing this or any other inversion exercise, reduce the duration and increase the time gradually.

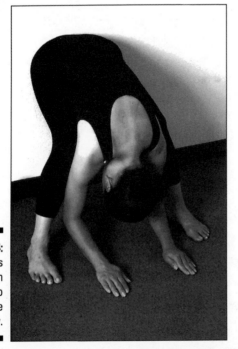

Figure 11-4: There's more than one way to reverse gravity.

A trio of shoulder stands — from easiest to toughest

Each of these three shoulder stands provides common benefits: improved circulation to the legs, hips, back, neck, heart, and head. The postures all stimulate the endocrine glands and improve lymphatic drainage, enhance elimination, and produce a calming and rejuvenating effect on the nervous system. The wall provides a useful prop for the easier two variations; when you're ready, you can then advance with confidence to *viparita karani,* the half shoulder stand.

Due to the neck's vulnerability, we recommend that you *precede* these postures with a dynamic (or moving) bridge posture (see Chapter 6) to prepare the neck and *follow* it with a short rest and then a dynamic cobra posture (see Chapter 12) to compensate.

Do not attempt any of these postures if you're pregnant, have high blood pressure or a hiatal hernia, are moderately overweight, have glaucoma or neck problems, or are in the first few days of your period. Also, do not use a mirrored wall, because you can injure yourself if you fall.

Half shoulder stand at the wall

This posture is a variation of *viparita karani* and is perhaps the easiest way to learn the half shoulder stand in a step-by-step method (see Figure 11-5). The wall provides support as you build experience with the shoulder stand exercises.

1. **Lie on your back, knees bent, feet flat on the floor, with the toes just touching the base of a sturdy wall, Extend your arms along the sides of your torso, palms down.**

2. **Place your soles up on the wall with your knees at a right angle (with your thighs parallel, and your shins perpendicular to the wall).**

   You may need to slide your buttocks closer to or farther away from the wall to get the angle just right (see Figure 11-5a).

3. **As you inhale, press down with your hands, push your feet to the wall, and lift your hips as high as you comfortably can (see Figure 11-5b).**

4. **Bend your elbows and bring your hands to your lower back.**

   Press your elbows and the backs of your upper arms on the floor for support. Relax the neck (see Figure 11-5c).

5. **As you exhale, take one foot off the wall and extend the leg until you are looking straight up at the tip of your big toe (see Figure 11-5d).**

   You can use just one leg and switch or raise both legs. If you alternate legs, divide the time evenly between each leg.

When you want to come back down, slowly place one foot on the wall first, then the other, and finally lower your pelvis slowly to the floor.

6. **Stay in Step 4 or 5 for as long as you feel comfortable, or up to 5 minutes; use Yoga breathing (see Chapter 5).**

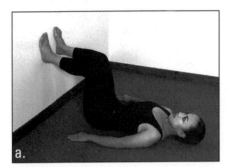
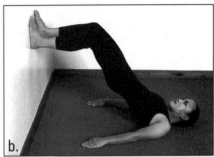
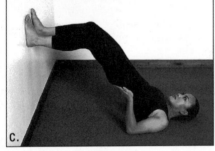
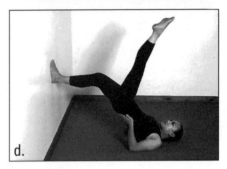

Figure 11-5:
Using the wall gives you support and variety.

Reverse half shoulder stand at the wall

The reverse half shoulder stand at the wall (see Figure 11-6) is also a variation of *viparita karani*. Some people find this exercise easier than the half shoulder stand at the wall. Try them both and see which one is more comfortable for you.

1. **Lie on your back with your head toward the wall at a full arms distance from the wall. Bend your knees and place your feet flat on the floor at hip width (see Figure 11-6a). Then bring your arms back and rest your arms along the sides of your body, palms down.**

Finding the correct distance from the wall can depend on the length of your arms. Try these three different measurements: touching the wall with the fingers extended; touching with the knuckles of the fists; and touching with the backs of your hands.

2. **As you exhale, push your palms down , draw the bent knees in and up and raise your hips to a comfortable angle of 45 to 75 degrees.**

   Be sure that your legs are straight but not locked and your feet are directly above your head.

3. **Bend your elbows and bring your hands to the back of your pelvis and then slide your hands up to your lower back.**

   Press your elbows and the backs of your upper arms on the floor for support.

4. **Let your toes slowly and gently touch the wall for support; relax your neck (see Figure 11-6b).**

5. **When you want to come down, first ease your hips to the floor with the support of your hands, and then bend your knees and lower your feet to the floor.**

6. **Stay in Step 4 for as long as you feel comfortable, or up to 5 minutes.**

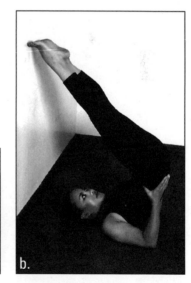

Figure 11-6: Another way to use the wall as a prop.

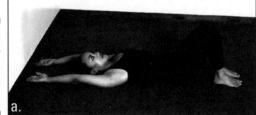

a.

b.

Half shoulder stand — viparita karani

You can work up to this posture by developing comfort with the half shoulder and reverse half shoulder stands at the wall.

The Sanskrit word *viparita* (pronounced *vee-pah-ree-tah*) means "inverted, reversed" and *karani* (pronounced *kah-rah-nee*) means "action, process." Some authorities call this practice *sarvangasana,* meaning "all limbs posture." The word is composed of *sarva* (pronounced *sahr-vah*) and *anga* (pronounced *ahn-gah*) followed by *asana.*

1. Lie on your back with your knees bent and the feet flat on the floor at hip width, rest your arms along the sides of your body, palms down.

2. As you exhale, push the palms down, draw the bent knees in and up, and then straighten your legs as you raise your hips (see Figure 11-7a). Then raise the hips to a comfortable angle of 45 to 75 degrees.

3. Bend your elbows and bring your hands to the back of your pelvis and then slide the hands up to the lower back. Be sure that your legs are straight but not locked and your feet are directly above your head.

   Press your elbows and the backs of your upper arms on the floor for support. Relax your neck (see Figure 11-7b).

4. Stay in Step 3 for as long as you feel comfortable, or up to 5 minutes.

5. When you want to come down, first ease the hips to the floor with the support of your hands, and then bend the knees and lower the feet to the floor.

Figure 11-7:
You can enjoy the benefits of inversion without compressing your neck.

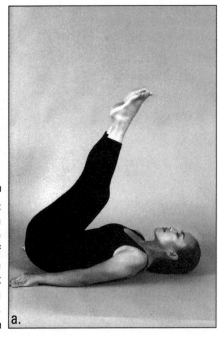

a.

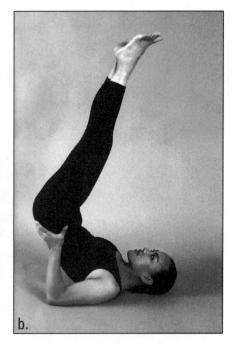

b.

Chapter 12

Easy 'Round the Bends

*T*his chapter presents a variety of yogic bends: Think of them as simple extensions of the breath. Inhalation takes you naturally into a back bend, exhalation into a forward bend (for more explanation, see Chapter 5). You can perform bending postures in Yoga practice from many different positions — standing, kneeling, sitting, lying, or even turned upside-down (see Chapter 11). Because we cover the upright bending postures in Chapter 8 and the most popular bends for warm-up in Chapter 6, this chapter highlights the classic bending postures that you do on the floor.

Gaining a Strong Backbone (And Some Insight)

Without the spinal column, you couldn't walk upright — but then again, you'd never experience back pain, either! Standing erect seems a reasonable tradeoff for risking aches associated with the spine, especially since back pain is preventable. The backbone enables you to bend forward, backward, and sideways, and it also allows you to twist. You perform all these motions every day, but you may do them unconsciously and without adequate muscular support. Yoga uses the natural movements of the spine to train the various muscles supporting it, which contributes to a healthy back.

Although the spinal column, with its elegant curvature, is well-designed for the upright position, people are not always very clever about using it correctly. Above all, many people don't realize that their 33 vertebrae, or backbones (24 of which comprise the flexible part of the spine), are held in place by a series of powerful muscles and ligaments that require regular exercise to maintain top working order.

Many muscles, which are arranged in several layers in the front, back, neck, and perineum, maintain the spine in position. When they become weak from inadequate use or damage through improper use or injury, any of these muscles can pull the spine out of alignment. This misalignment can cause discomfort, pain, and inadequate nerve communication to the organs and other parts of the body, which may lead to further complications.

The spinal column is so important because it protects the spinal cord — a bundle of nerves that runs through the bony tower, your backbone. The nerves feed the trunk and limbs with information from the brain, and the brain returns the favor. If the nerve connection is severed at any point, you lose conscious control of the affected part of your body.

The spine also has psychological significance. A person of integrity and strength of character is said to "have backbone" and a coward is said to be "spineless." Because people believe that outside presentation reflects inside influences, they tend to judge a person's mental state from his bodily demeanor. If you are chronically hunched over, you signal to others that you are also inwardly collapsed. On the other hand, if you stand straight and tall, you give others the impression of self-assuredness, energy, and courage.

From a yogic point of view, the spine is important for another reason: It is the physical aspect of a subtle energetic pathway that runs from the base of the spine to the crown of the head. This pathway is known as the *central channel* or *sushumna-nadi* ("gracious conduit," pronounced *soo-shoom-nah nah-dee*). In traditional Hatha Yoga and Tantra Yoga, the awakened "serpent power," or *kundalini-shakti,* rises through this channel. When this power of pure consciousness reaches the crown of the head, you experience a sublime state of ecstasy. We say more about the central channel in Chapter 20.

The spine as the axis of your world

According to Yoga symbolism, the spine corresponds to the axis of the universe, which is pictured as a gigantic mountain called *Mount* *Meru*. At the top of this mountain (that is, in your head) resides heaven where all the deities are seated.

Bending Over Backwards

Whether you realize it or not, you do a lot of forward bending while going about your everyday business. Putting on a pair of pants, tying shoelaces, picking things up from the floor, sitting at a desk while typing on a computer, working in the garden, even many of the sports you play involve varying degrees of forward bending.

In life, too much of anything can lead to problems. A forward bend tends to close the front of the torso (and so shorten the front of the spine) and round the back. This closing and rounding is exaggerated by the unhealthy habit of bending forward from the waist, rather than from the hip joints.

To personally experience the difference between the bending from the waist and bending from the hips, sit upright in a chair with your feet flat on the floor and place your hands on the outside of your hip bones with the fingers turned inward. As you inhale, move your spine upward, lift your chest and look straight ahead. As you exhale, keep the chest lifted, bend forward: You will experience bending forward from the hips. In contrast, sit in the chair and move your hands up a few inches, until they are just under your rib cage. As you exhale, bring your chin to your chest and your head down toward your thighs, bowing your spine backwards. This is bending forward from the waist. Over the years, this bending habit inevitably leads to what is often called a *stoop,* characterized by a sunken chest and forward leaning head — and all the attendant aches, pains, and shallow breathing.

The antidote for the cumulative effects of forward bending is the regular practice of Yoga back bends, which stretch the front of the torso (and spine). Appropriately, back bends are performed with an inhalation, the active, opening phase of the breathing cycle. Take a deep inhale right now and notice how your torso (and spine) naturally extends, inviting you to bend backwards. Back bends are known as expansive, "extroverted" postures that can trigger powerful emotions. The major back bends are usually done toward the middle of a routine, so that you have plenty of time at the start for preparation and compensation afterwards (see Chapter 6). In this chapter, we present some of the classic floor back bends.

Move slowly and cautiously in all of the cobra and locust postures. Avoid any of the postures that cause pain in your lower back, upper back, or neck.

When you lie face down on the floor and raise your chest and head and use any combination of the arms, you are doing some form of the cobra posture; when you raise your legs, or a combination of your legs, chest, and arms, you are performing some form of the locust posture.

Cobra 1

The cobra posture increases the flexibility and strength of the muscles of the arms, chest, shoulders, and back. Cobra 1 especially emphasizes the upper back (see Figure 12-1). The cobra opens the chest, increases lung capacity, and stimulates the kidneys and the adrenals.

1. **Lie on your abdomen with your legs spread at hip width and the tops of your feet on the floor.**

2. **Rest your forehead on the floor and relax your shoulders; bend your elbows and place your forearms on the floor, palms turned down and positioned near the sides of your head (see Figure 12-1a).**

3. **As you inhale, engage your back muscles, press your forearms against the floor, and raise your chest and head.**

   Look straight ahead, as shown in Figure 12-1b. Keep your forearms and the front of your pelvis on the floor as you continue to relax your shoulders.

4. **As you exhale, lower your torso and head slowly back to the floor.**

5. **Repeat Steps 3 and 4 three times; then stay in Step 3 (the last raised position) for 6 to 8 breaths.**

If you have lower back problems, separate your legs wider than your hips and let your heels turn out.

This posture is also called The Sphinx. It is a variation of the modified version of *bhujangasana,* which we describe in the next section.

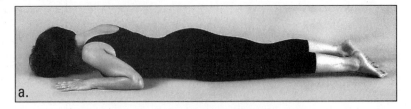

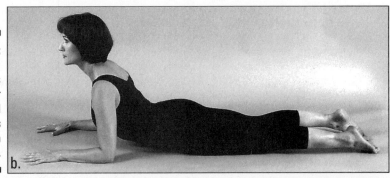

Figure 12-1:
Cobra 1 emphasizes the upper back and is less difficult than Cobra 2.

Cobra 2 — bhujangasana

This posture rewards you with most of the same benefits as the Cobra 1, which we describe in the preceding section. In addition, Cobra 2 emphasizes flexibility in the lower back (see Figure 12-2).

1. **Lie on your abdomen with your legs spread at hip width and the tops of your feet on the floor.**

2. **Bend your elbows and place your palms on the floor with the thumbs near the armpits.**

   Rest your forehead on the floor and relax your shoulders, as shown in Figure 12-2a.

3. **As you inhale, engage your back muscles, press your palms against the floor, and raise your chest and head.**

   Look straight ahead (see Figure 12-2b). Keep the top front of your pelvis on the floor and your shoulders relaxed. Unless you are very flexible, keep your elbows slightly bent.

4. **As you exhale, lower your torso and head slowly back to the floor.**

5. **Repeat Steps 3 and 4 three times; then stay in Step 3 (the last raised position) for 6 to 8 breaths.**

Note: In the classic posture, the inner legs are joined and the knees are straight. The head is in alignment with the spine and the eyes look forward. The palms are on the floor close to the sides of the torso near the navel, the elbows are slightly bent and the shoulders relaxed.

If you move your hands further forward, the cobra is less difficult; if you move your hands further back, to the sides of your navel, you increase the difficulty.

The Sanskrit word *bhujangasana* is composed of *bhujanga* (pronounced *bhooj-ahng-gah)* meaning "serpent" and *asana* or "posture."

Clench those cheeks . . . or maybe not

In the Yoga world, you can find weekend workshops on back bends that focus entirely on the question "Should the buttocks be firm or soft in the cobra?" (What a way to spend a weekend!) The traditional instruction is to firm the buttocks. However, in the last 15 years, the work of New Zealand-born physiotherapist Robin McKenzie has revolutionized back care — and our ideas about back bends. In his own version of the cobra, called *The McKenzie Technique,* McKenzie suggests that the buttocks be soft, to facilitate the healing of numerous lower back ailments. Try the cobra both ways, with the buttocks firm or soft, and see what feels best to you!

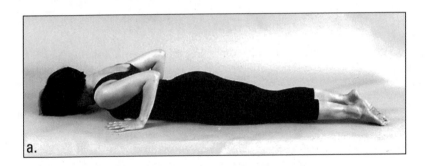

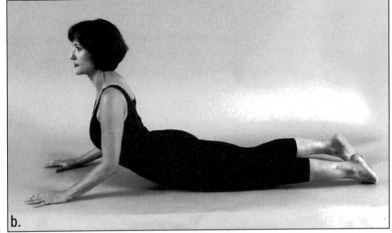

Figure 12-2:
Cobra 2
emphasizes
flexibility in
the lower
back.

Cobra 3

Cobra 3, which is another version of the classic *bhujangasana,* is unique in that it does not call for placing the hands on the floor. The emphasis is on strengthening both the lower and upper back (see Figure 12-3).

1. **Lie on your abdomen, with your legs spread at hip width and the tops of your feet on the floor; rest your forehead on the floor.**

2. **Extend your arms back, along the sides of your torso, palms on the floor (see Figure 12-3a).**

3. **As you inhale, raise your chest and head, and sweep your arms like wings out to the sides and then all the way forward.**

   Keep your legs on the floor, as shown in Figure 12-3b.

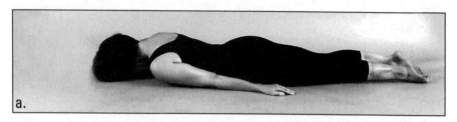

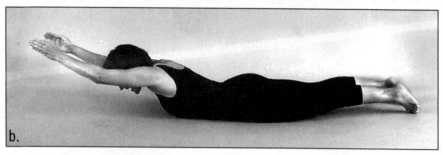

Figure 12-3: Cobra 3 strengthens the lower and upper back and the neck.

4. **As you exhale, sweep your arms back, and lower your torso and your head slowly to the floor.**

5. **Repeat Steps 3 and 4 three times; then stay in Step 3 (the last raised position) for 6 to 8 breaths.**

Locust 1 — shalabhasana

The locust posture strengthens the entire torso including the lower back and the neck (see Figure 12-4). In addition, it strengthens the buttocks, the legs, and improves digestion and elimination.

1. **Lie on your abdomen, with your legs spread at hip width and the tops of your feet on the floor.**

   Rest your forehead on the floor (refer to Figure 12-3a).

2. **Extend your arms along the sides of your torso, palms on the floor.**

3. **As you inhale, raise your chest, head, and one leg up and away from the floor as high as is comfortable for you (see Figure 12-4a).**

4. **As you exhale, lower your chest, head, and leg together slowly to the floor.**

   Repeat with the other leg.

5. **Repeat Steps 3 and 4 three times; then stay in Step 3 (the last raised position) for 6 to 8 breaths.**

You can increase the level of difficulty by raising both legs at the same time in Step 3.

Note: In the classic posture, the inner legs are joined, the knees are straight.

To make this posture and all the other variations of the locust and cobra easier, place a small pillow or a folded blanket underneath you, between your abdomen and your chest. You can move the blanket a little forward or backward to fit your needs (see Figure 12-4b).

The Sanskrit word *shalabha* (pronounced *shuh-lub-ha*) means "locust."

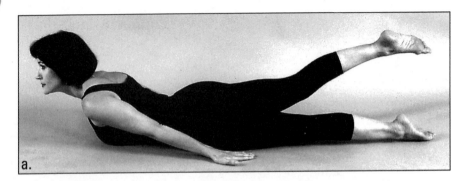

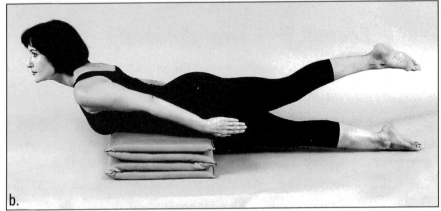

Figure 12-4:
Try this posture with and without blankets to gauge personal comfort.

Locust 2

The locust posture strengthens your back, neck, buttocks, and legs This posture, which is another variation of *shalabhasana,* also teaches the two sides of the body how to work independently of each other. Many back problems are due to imbalances in the musculature on each side of the spine. Health professional circles often call this situation an asymmetrical problem. Locust 2 helps bring your back into symmetry again and also improves your coordination (see Figure 12-5).

1. **Lie on your abdomen, with your legs spread at hip width and the tops of your feet on the floor.**

   Rest your forehead on the floor.

2. **Extend your right arm forward with the palm resting on the floor; bring your left arm back along the left side of your torso, with the back of your hand on the floor (see Figure 12-5a).**

3. **As you inhale, slowly raise your chest, head, right arm, and left leg up and away from the floor as high as is comfortable for you.**

   Try to keep the upper right arm and ear in alignment, and raise your left foot and right hand to the same height above the floor (see Figure 12-5b).

4. **As you exhale, lower the right arm, chest, head, and left leg slowly to the floor at the same time.**

5. **Repeat Steps 3 and 4 three times; then stay in Step 3 for 6 to 8 breaths.**

6. **Repeat the same sequence with opposite pairs (left arm and right leg).**

Locust 2 features some interesting biomechanics. When you raise the chest and the right arm, you strengthen the right side of your upper back. When you raise the left leg, you strengthen the right side of your lower back. So even though this posture uses opposite arms and legs, it strengthens one side of the upper and lower back at a time.

Avoid locust variations that lift just the legs. Lifting the legs alone increases chest pressure, heart rate, and tension in the neck.

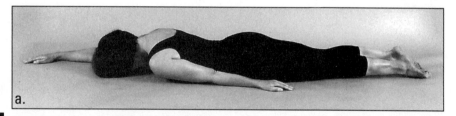

a.

Figure 12-5:
This posture balances the muscles on each side of your back.

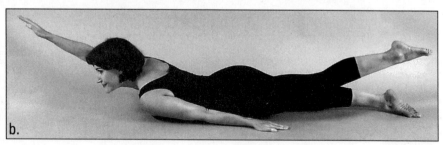

b.

Locust 3 — Superman posture

This posture, a further variation of *shalabhasana,* gets its name from the image of Superman flying through the air at warp speed, with his arms extended out in front leading the way. This is our most strenuous back bend. Full extension of arms and legs puts quite a load on the entire back (see Figure 12-6). Use this pose only after you are comfortable with locust 1 and 2.

This posture is physically challenging. Don't attempt it if you are having back or neck problems.

1. **Lie on your abdomen, with your legs spread at hip width and the tops of your feet on the floor, extend the arms back along the sides of your torso, palms on the floor; rest your forehead on the floor (see Figure 12-6a).**

2. **As you inhale, raise your chest, legs and head, and sweep your arms like wings out to the sides, and then all the way forward (see Figure 12-6b).**

3. **As you exhale, sweep your arms back and lower the torso, legs, and the head slowly to the floor at the same time.**

4. **Repeat Steps 2 and 3 three times; then stay in Step 2 (the last raised position) for 6 to 8 breaths.**

In the beginning, for Step 2, try sweeping your arms only half way forward in a T position. The T position allows your back muscles to gradually become accustomed to the physical demands on the back.

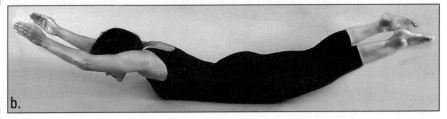
a.

Figure 12-6: Make sure you're ready for this "super" posture.

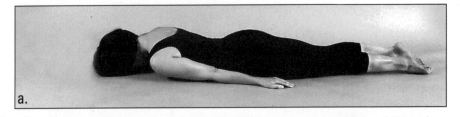
b.

Bending from Side to Side

The spinal column can move in four basic ways: It can bend forward *(flexion),* bend backward *(extension)*, bend sideways *(lateral flexion)*, and twist *(rotation)*. Of these four, the side bend is most often neglected in Yoga practice. This missed opportunity is unfortunate because side bends help to stretch and tone the muscles along the sides of the abdomen, rib cage, and spine, which keeps your waist trim, your breathing full, and your spine supple.

A true side bend fully contracts one side of the body while expanding the other. You can experience the effects of a side bend right now: Whether you're reading these words while sitting on a chair or the floor, simply lean over with an exhale to your right (or left) side and reach the same-side arm downward. To realize the full effect of the stretch, reach the opposite-side arm up toward the ceiling. In this section, we cover some safe, creative ways to use side bends on the floor.

Seated side bend

All the side bends have similar benefits. They stretch and tone the muscles along the sides of the torso and increase the flexibility of the spine.

1. **Sit comfortably in a simple cross-legged position (for the easy posture, or *sukhasana*, see Chapter 7).**

   Place your right palm on the floor, near your right hip.

2. **As you inhale, raise the left arm out to the side and up above your head beside your left ear.**

3. **As you exhale, slide your right hand across the floor out to the right.**

   Let your torso, head and left arm follow, bending sideways to the right (see Figure 12-7).

4. **As you inhale, return to the upright position (as you were at the start of Step 2).**

5. **Repeat Steps 2 through 4 three times; then stay in the bent position (Step 3) for 6 to 8 breaths.**

   Repeat the same sequence on the other side.

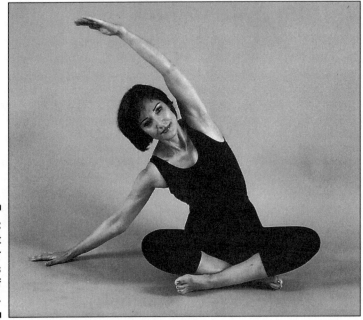

Figure 12-7:
Don't let
your
buttocks
come off
the floor.

All-fours side bend

The benefits of this side bend, which is a variation of *cakravakasana*, are the same as for the seated side bend. Many people with back or hip problems have a hard time sitting upright on the floor. The all fours position gives more freedom to the spine and is an easier side bend from the floor.

1. **Start on your hands and knees, with the your knees below the your hips and the your hands below the your shoulders, palms on the floor.**

   Straighten, but don't lock, your elbows. Look straight ahead.

2. **As you exhale, bend your head and torso sideways to the right and look toward your tailbone (see Figure 12-8).**

3. **As you inhale, return to the starting position in Step 1.**

4. **Repeat Steps 2 and 3 three times; then stay in Step 2 for 6 to 8 breaths.**

   Repeat the same sequence on the other side.

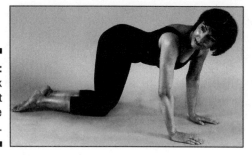

Figure 12-8:
Look back at what used to be a tail.

Folded side bend

The benefits of this side bend, which is a variation of *balasana,* the child's posture (see Chapter 6), are the same as for the seated side bend (see Figure 12-9). The Sanskrit word *bala* (pronounced *bah-lah*) means "child." This practice was inspired by a baby's folded position in the womb.

1. **Sit on your heels, toes pointing back, and fold forward by laying your abdomen on your thighs and your head on the floor.**

   Extend your arms forward with palms on the floor (see Figure 12-9a).

2. **As you exhale, stay in the folded position and slide your upper torso, head, arms, and hands to the right as far as possible, as shown in Figure 12-9b.**

   Wait for a few seconds and again, with another exhalation, slide further to the right, if you can without straining.

3. **Return to center (as in Step 1) and repeat the sequence to the left side.**

   Stay in Step 2 for 6 to 8 breaths on each side.

Figure 12-9:
Wait a few moments before you stretch further on each side.

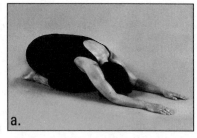

a.

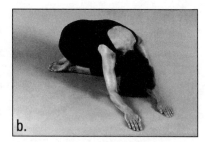

b.

Bending Forward

Of all the ways your torso (and spine) can move, bending forward is the maneuver most common to our species. People spend their first nine months growing in their mothers' wombs, folded in a forward bend; it's possible that because people instinctively associate this position with the peace and security of their prenatal lives, they often bend forward after strenuous or unfamiliar activities to calm and comfort themselves.

Forward bends are usually a good way to begin any movement routine (unless you're dealing with spinal disc injuries or certain other back problems). Although back bends are the lively extroverts of the *asana* family, forward bends are the retiring introverts; they are always performed with an exhalation — the passive, contracting phase of the breathing cycle.

In Sanskrit, the representative sitting forward bend is called *pashcimottanasana* (pronounced *pash-chee-moh-tah-nah-sah-nah*) which translates to the "extension of the West posture." In yogic jargon, the West refers to the back, while the East stands for the front. The symbolism refers to both the physical and psychological effects of this posture: It stretches the back of the body, especially the back of the spine and legs, and just as the sun sets in the West, so does the "light" of our consciousness draw inward as we fold upon ourselves.

Our constant bending forward *from the waist* tends to put stress on the lower back and neck. Yogic forward bends call for movement *from the hip joints,* which can help you maintain a healthy, stress-free spine as you correct poor forward-bending habits (see explanation in the beginning of this chapter).

Be very careful of all the seated forward bends if you have disc-related back problems.

Seated forward bend — pashcimottanasana

The seated forward bend intensely stretches the entire back side of the body, including the back of the spine and legs. It also tones the muscles and organs of the abdomen and creates a calming and quieting effect.

1. **Sit on the floor, with your legs at hip width and comfortably stretched out in front of you.**

   Bring your back up nice and tall and place your palms down on the floor near your thighs.

2. **As you inhale, raise your arms forward and up overhead until they are beside your ears (see Figure 12-10a).**

Keep your arms and legs soft and slightly bent in Forgiving Limbs, which we describe in Chapter 6.

3. **As you exhale, bend forward from the hips; bring your hands, chest, and head toward your legs.**

Rest your hands on the floor, your thighs, knees, shins, or feet. If your head is not close to your knees, bend your knees more until you feel your back stretching (see Figure 12-10b).

4. **Repeat Steps 2 and 3 three times, then stay folded (Step 3) for 6 to 8 breaths.**

Note: In the classic posture, the inner legs are joined, the knees are straight, and the ankles are extended (the toes point up). Also, the chin rests on the chest, the hands hold the sides of the feet, the back is extended forward and the forehead is pressed against the legs.

If you have a problem sitting upright on the floor in the seated forward bend or in any of the following forward bending postures, raise your hips with folded blankets or firm pillows, as shown in Figure 12-10c.

The Sanskrit word *pashcimottanasana* is composed of the words *pashcima* (pronounced *push-chee-mah*) meaning "Western," *uttana* (pronounced *oot-tah-nah*) meaning "extended," and *asana* or "posture."

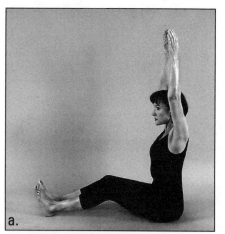
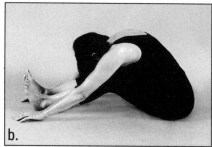
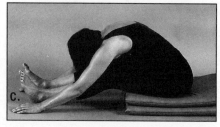

Figure 12-10: If your head is not close to your knees, bend your knees more.

Head-to-knee posture — janushirshasana

The head-to-knee posture keeps your spine supple, stimulates the abdominal organs, and activates the central channel (*sushumna-nadi*) (see Figure 12-11). As explained in Chapter 5, the central channel is the pathway for the awakened energy of pure consciousness (called *kundalini-shakti*), which leads to ecstasy and spiritual liberation.

1. **Sit on the floor, with your legs stretched out in front of you, bend your left knee and bring your left heel toward the right groin.**

2. **Rest the bent left knee on the floor (but do not force it down), and place the sole of your left foot on the inside of your right thigh.**

   The toes of the left foot point toward the right knee.

3. **Bring your back up nice and tall; as you inhale, raise your arms forward and up overhead until they are beside your ears (see Figure 12-11a).**

   Keep your arms and the right leg soft and slightly bent in Forgiving Limbs, which we describe in Chapter 6.

4. **As you exhale, bend forward from the hips.**

   Bring your hands, chest and head toward your right leg. Rest your hands on the floor, your thigh, knee, shin, or foot. If your head is not close to your right knee, bend your knee more until you feel your back stretching on the right side (see Figure 12-11b).

5. **Repeat Steps 3 and 4 three times; then stay in Step 4 (the final forward bend) for 6 to 8 breaths.**

   Repeat the same sequence on the opposite side.

Figure 12-11: This posture stretches the back more on the side of the extended leg.

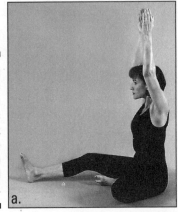

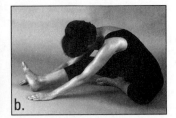

Keep your back muscles as relaxed as possible, which will help you achieve better extension.

The Sanskrit word *janu* (pronounced *jah-noo*) means "knee," and *shirsha* (pronounced *sheer-shah*) means "head."

Volcano — mahamudra

Ancient Hatha Yoga texts give high praise to the volcano posture. It strengthens the back, stretches the legs, and opens the hips and chest. This posture is unique in that has qualities of both a forward bend and a back bend.

When used with special "locks" (*bandhas*) that contain and channel energy in the torso, this technique has both cleansing and healing effects.

1. **Sitting on the floor, with your legs stretched out in front of you, bend your left knee and bring your left foot toward the right groin.**

2. **Rest your bent left knee on the floor to the left (but do not force it down), and place the sole of your left foot on the inside of your right thigh, with the heel in the groin.**

   The toes of left foot point toward the right knee. Bring your back up nice and tall.

3. **As you inhale, raise the arms forward and up overhead until they are beside your ears (refer to Figure 12-11a).**

   Keep your arms and the right leg soft and slightly bent in Forgiving Limbs, as we describe in Chapter 6.

4. **As you exhale, bend forward from the hips, lift your chest forward, and extend your back, but don't let your back round.**

   Place your hands on the right knee, shin, or toes and look straight ahead (see Figure 12-12).

5. **Repeat Steps 3 and 4 three times; then stay in Step 4 for 6 to 8 breaths.**

   Repeat the same sequence on the opposite side.

Note: In the classic posture, the front leg and the arms are straight, and the hands are holding the toes of the front leg. The back is extended and the chin is pressed on the chest. The abdominal muscles are pulled up into the abdominal cavity and the anal sphincter is tightened.

The Sanskrit term *mahamudra* (pronounced *mah-hah-mood-rah*) means literally "great seal."

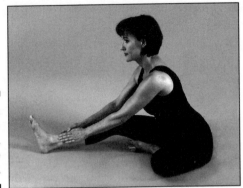

Figure 12-12:
The volcano
is a great,
all-inclusive
posture.

Spread-leg forward bend — *upavishta konasana*

The spread-leg forward bend stretches the backs and insides of the legs (hamstrings and adductors) and increases the flexibility of the spine and hip joints (see Figure 12-13). It improves circulation to the entire pelvic region, tones the abdomen, and has a calming effect on the nervous system.

Note: Muscle density may cause some men to find this posture more difficult.

1. **Sit on the floor, with your legs straight and spread wide apart (but not more than 90 degrees).**

   Because this posture is most challenging, give yourself an advantage by pulling the flesh of the buttocks (you may know them as "cheeks") out from under the sit bones (the ischium) and bending your knees slightly. Alternatively, sit on some folded blankets.

2. **As you inhale, raise the arms forward and up overhead until they are beside your ears.**

   Keep your arms soft and the legs slightly bent in Forgiving Limbs, as we describe in Chapter 6. Bring your back up nice and tall (see Figure 12-13a).

3. **As you exhale, bend forward from the hips and bring your hands, chest, and head toward the floor.**

   Rest your extended arms and hands, palms down, on the floor. If you have the flexibility, place your forehead on the floor as well (see Figure 12-13b).

4. **Repeat Steps 2 and 3 three times; then stay in Step 3 (the folded position) for 6 to 8 breaths.**

Note: In the classic posture, the legs are straight with the toes vertical, the chin and chest are on the floor, and the arms are extended forward with the palms joined.

The spread-leg forward bend is also called the *lifetime posture,* because it can take a whole lifetime to master. But don't despair if mastery eludes you. According to Yoga's outlook, if you do not master the pose in this lifetime, you can try again in the next lifetime.

The Sanskrit term *upavishta* (pronounced *oopah-vish-tah*) means "seated" and *kona* (pronounced *koh-nah*) means "triangle."

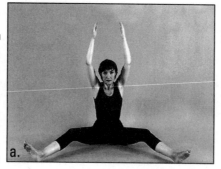 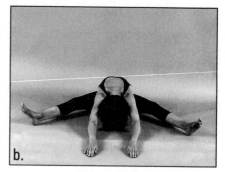

Figure 12-13:
Muscle density may make this posture difficult for most men.

a.

b.

Chapter 13

Twist But Don't Shout

. . . .

In This Chapter

▶ Enjoying spinal fitness — with a yogic twist

▶ Introducing six simple twists

. . . .

*I*magine that you're cleaning up the kitchen with a wet sponge. After mopping up some spills and a few stray crumbs, the sponge gets dirty — so you hold it under the kitchen faucet and turn on the water. You squeeze out the dirty water and, as you release the pressure on the sponge, it sucks up some clean water. You're ready for your next swipes across the countertops and floor.

This analogy of the sponge is often used to describe how yogic twists work on the spine. Of course, you don't have little sponges in your spine, but you do have pulpy pads that are like sponges, called the *intervertebral discs*, between the individual bones. These discs have no direct blood supply of their own, so they depend on your everyday movements to help them "wring out" the accumulated wastes and, in turn, soak up a fresh supply of blood and other revivifying fluids. Over time, if your discs aren't continually squeezed and soaked, they tend to harden and dry out, like a sponge left unused for a few days, and so your spine stiffens up and shrinks.

The yogic twists have multiple benefits:

✔ They "clean out" the discs and help keep them firm and supple.

✔ They "massage" the internal organs, such as your intestines and kidneys.

✔ They stoke the inner "fire" of digestion.

✔ They stretch and strengthen the muscles of your back and abdomen.

This chapter features sitting twists, which emphasize the upper spine, and reclining twists, which emphasize the lower spine. For standing twists, consult Chapter 8.

Putting a Positive Spin on Twisting

When it comes to the human body and mind, people often associate the word *twist* with pain or something undesirable. For example, people say things like:

✔ "She twisted her ankle."

✔ "He twisted his face in a wry smile."

✔ "He has a twisted mind."

✔ "You don't need to twist my arm."

✔ "He accused her of twisting his comments."

But twisting isn't all bad. Ropes get their strength from the twisted strands that compose them. Yogic twisting postures have the same positive effect. When done properly, they bring strength to your body, especially the weak spots (notably the lower back). True enough, twisting is part of your every-day movements. But unless your muscles are well-trained, you can easily injure yourself. The exercises in the following section can help you get your back in tip-top shape as you look forward to enjoyment and enlightenment along the way.

Starting Out with Simple Twists for Gnarly Spines

Approach all twists with caution if you're suffering from disc problems anywhere in your spine. Consult your physician or work with a reputable Yoga therapist.

Easy chair twist

If you're like most people, you probably sit most of the day. So why, you may wonder, do we ask you to sit on a chair for this exercise? Trust us — this is an excellent way for a beginner to achieve a good twist safely. Your spine will be grateful to you!

1. **Sit sideways on a chair with the chair back to your right, feet flat on the floor and heels directly below the knees.**

2. **Exhale, turn to the right, and hold the sides of the chair back with your hands.**

3. **As you inhale, extend or lift your spine upward.**

4. **As you exhale, twist your torso and head further to the right (see Figure 13-1).**

5. **Repeat Steps 1–4, gradually twisting further with each exhalation for 3 breaths (don't force it); then hold the twist for 6 to 8 breaths.**

   Repeat the same sequence on the opposite side.

If your feet are not comfortably on the floor for the easy chair twist, place a folded blanket or a phone book under your feet for elevation.

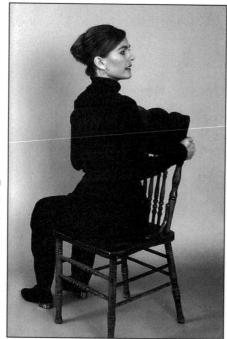

Figure 13-1:
Twist
mainly from
your
shoulders —
the head
and neck
come along
for the ride.

Easy sitting twist

Once you can twist comfortably while seated on a chair, you can transfer your newly gained skill to the floor and try the following exercise. Its effect is similar to that of the easy chair twist described in the previous section. The easy sitting twist is usually more convenient during regular Yoga practice because you do most yogic exercises on the floor. Of course, if you're at the office and want to liberate your spine with a yogic twist — without drawing too much attention to yourself — you may opt to stay seated instead.

1. Sit on the floor with your legs in a simple, cross-legged position and extend your spine upward nice and tall.

2. Place your left hand, palm down, on top of the right knee.

3. Place your right hand, palm down, on the floor behind your right hip to prop yourself up.

4. As you inhale, extend your spine upward.

5. As you exhale, twist your torso and head to the right (see Figure 13-2).

6. Repeat Steps 4 and 5, gradually twisting further with each exhalation for 3 breaths (don't force it); then hold the twist for 6 to 8 breaths.

Repeat the same sequence on the opposite side.

If you have difficulty sitting upright in this seated twist, use blankets or pillows to make your hips even with your knees.

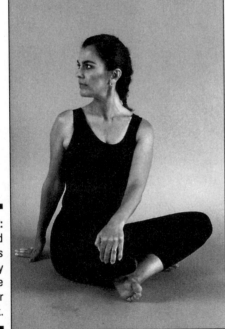

Figure 13-2:
Seated
twists
usually
emphasize
the upper
back.

The sage twist

The easy chair twist and the easy sitting twist are the simplest yogic twists. By changing the position of your legs, you can alter the level of difficulty and also enhance the overall benefit. The sage twist gives you extra rewards for your investment.

1. **Sit on the floor with both legs extended forward; bend your right knee and place your right foot on the floor just inside your left thigh, with toes facing forward.**

2. **Place your right hand, palm down, on the floor behind you; wrap the palm of your left hand around the side of your right knee.**

3. **As you inhale, extend or lift your spine upward.**

4. **As you exhale, twist your torso and head to the right (see Figure 13-3).**

5. **Repeat Steps 3 and 4, gradually twisting further with each exhalation for 3 breaths (don't force it), and then hold the twist for 6 to 8 breaths.**

   Repeat the same sequence on the opposite side.

If you have difficulty sitting upright in this seated twist, use blankets or pillows to sit on until your hips are even with your knees.

This posture is a variation of the classic posture called *maricyasana*. The Sanskrit word *marici* (pronounced *mah-ree-chee*) means "ray of light" and is the name of an ancient sage.

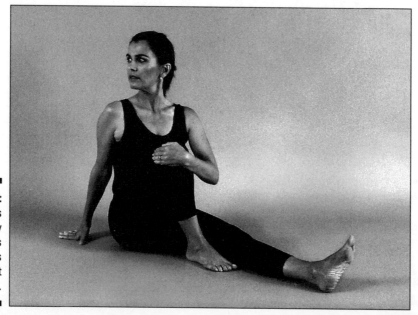

Figure 13-3: Beginners can enjoy benefits from this sage twist variation.

Bent leg supine twist

The previously described twists all require you to sit upright. The remaining exercises in this chapter call for you to lie down, which sounds easy enough — but there's a twist to this stipulation, literally. And it's in the twist that you harvest all kinds of benefits, including a delicious feeling of energy being released in your spine. The bent supine twist is a variation of the classic posture known as *parivartanasana*. The Sanskrit word *parivartana* (pronounced *pah-ree-vahr-tah-nah*) means "turning." We describe this standing posture in Chapter 8.

1. **Lie on your back with your knees bent and feet on the floor at hip width, extend your arms out from your sides like a "T," palms down, in line with the top of your shoulders.**

2. **As you exhale, slowly lower the bent legs to the right side, while turning your head to the left (see Figure 13-4).**

   Keep your head on the floor.

3. **As you inhale, bring the bent knees back to the middle.**

4. **As you exhale, slowly lower the bent knees to the left while turning your head to the right.**

5. **Follow Steps 1–4 alternating three times slowly on each side, and then hold one last twist on each side for 6 to 8 breaths.**

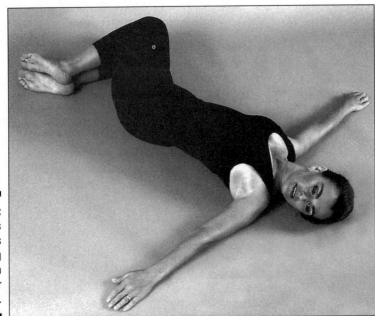

Figure 13-4:
This posture has a calming effect on the lower back.

The Swiss Army Knife

This posture, a variation of the classic *jathara parivritti,* tones the abdominal organs and intestines and stretches the lower back and hips. *Jathara parivritti* (pronounced *jat-hah-rah pah-ree-vree-tee*) means "belly twisting."

1. **Lie flat on the floor with your legs straight down, extend your arms out from your sides like a "T," palms up, in line with the top of your shoulders.**

2. **Bend your right knee and draw your thigh into the abdomen.**

3. **As you exhale, slowly lower the bent right leg to the left side and extend it out to a comfortable distance.**

4. **Extend your left arm overhead on the floor along the left side of your head (palm up), and then turn your head to the right (see Figure 13-5).**

   Keep your head on the floor.

5. **Follow Steps 1–4, and then relax and stay in Step 4 for 6 to 8 breaths.**

   Repeat the same sequence on the opposite side.

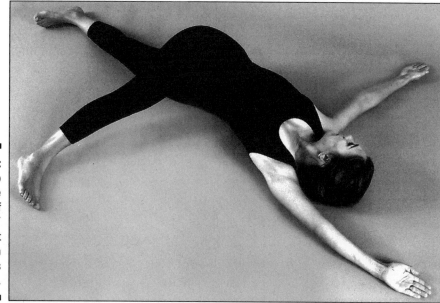

Figure 13-5: Try to visualize "lines of energy" going out through your arms and legs.

Extended legs supine twist — jathara parivritti

If you enjoy practicing the Swiss Army Knife, you are likely to enjoy the following, slightly more demanding exercise. This variation of *jathara parivritti* gives you the same benefits as the Swiss Army Knife, but affects an even more pronounced stretch of the lower back and hips. And, of course, stretching is good for your muscles and your spine.

1. **Lie on your back with your knees bent and feet on the floor at hip width, extend your arms out from your sides like a "T," palms down, in line with the top of your shoulders.**

2. **Bend your knees and draw both your thighs into your abdomen.**

3. **As you exhale, slowly lower your bent legs to the right side.**

4. **Extend both legs out to a comfortable distance, and then turn your head to the left (see Figure 13-6).**

   Keep your head on the floor.

5. **Follow Steps 1–4, and then relax and stay in Step 4 for 6 to 8 breaths.**

   Repeat the same sequence on the opposite side.

Note: In the classic version of this posture, the knees are straight and the joined legs are resting on the floor. The arms are straight and extended to the sides at right angles to the torso. The hand on the same side of the extended legs holds the top foot.

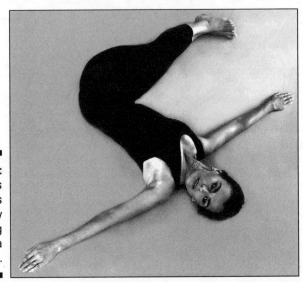

Figure 13-6: If this posture is difficult, try bending both legs a little more.

Chapter 14

Dynamic Posture: The Sun Salutation

. . . .

In This Chapter

▶ Discovering what the sun salutation can do for you

▶ Trying the 7-step sun salutation

▶ Experiencing the 12-step sun salutation

. . . .

The sun has long captured humanity's attention for its life-giving power. Sun worship is one of humankind's first and most natural forms of spiritual expression: Just think of the Sumerians, Egyptians, and Mayans. But nowhere has this homage to the solar spirit been as well preserved as in India's 10,000-year-old civilization, where to this day millions of people pay respects to the sun as a part of their daily rituals.

You don't have to be a sun worshiper, though, to benefit from Yoga's sun salutation (*surya namaskara,* pronounced *soor-yah nah-mahs-kah-rah*). This exercise — a special sequence of postures — is considered so profound that it is often used on its own.

The actual technique and number of steps in the sun salutation vary somewhat among the different Yoga schools and organizations. Of course, each school claims to practice the original sun salutation.

In this chapter, we focus on the best-known form of sun salutation — a 12-step sequence introduced to America in the early 1950s by the late Swami Vishnu Devananda, a disciple of the great Swami Shivananda of Rishikesh, India. We also introduce a modified 7-step version that is done from a kneeling position and is ideally suited for those who have yet to develop enough flexibility, muscle strength, and fitness for the 12-step version.

Shedding Light on the Benefits of Sun Saluting

Respected for its excellent effects, the sun salutation is reputed to provide an array of benefits, including:

- Stretching your spine and strengthening the muscles that support it
- Strengthening and stretching your arms and legs
- Improving your posture, coordination, and endurance
- Complementing the delicate balance between muscle tension and muscle relaxation
- Linking body, breath, and mind
- Granting (in most of its forms) aerobic benefits
- Improving the functioning of your lungs and the delivery of oxygen to your muscles (including the heart)
- Working well (with modifications) for people of all ages, from children to seniors

The Yoga masters also claim that the sun salutation has deeper psychological and spiritual implications, because it stimulates subtle vital energies leading to states of higher awareness. It's no wonder that so many Yoga videos on the market today include the sun salutation.

Exercising Your Yogic Solar Power

When doing the sun salutation, remember that your body is condensed sunlight! The saluting gesture, called *namaskara mudra* in Sanskrit (pronounced *nah-mahs-kah-rah mood-rah*), is a salute to the highest aspect within yourself — the spirit.

The dawn of the sun salutation

No one knows how old the sun salutation is, but at the beginning of the twentieth century, the Raja of Oudh, representing a small state in Northern India, encouraged all his subjects to learn and practice this exercise sequence. He personally practiced the sun salutation for health and happiness.

Traveling through the 7-step kneeling salutation

If you aren't quite ready to tackle the 12-step sun salutation, the following 7-step variation can give you many benefits and also help you get in shape for the standing variety of *surya namaskara*. Figure 14-1 shows you the various steps involved with this routine. Use any of the Yoga breathing techniques from Chapter 5.

1. **Sit on your heels in a bent-knee position, bring your back up nice and tall, and place your palms together in the prayer position, with the thumbs touching the sternum in the middle of your chest (see Figure 14-1a).**

2. **As you inhale, open your palms and slightly raise your arms forward, then up and overhead. Raise your buttocks away from your heels, arch your back, and look up at the ceiling (see Figure 14-1b).**

3. **As you exhale, bend forward slowly from the hips. Place your palms, forearms, and then your forehead on the floor and pause with your hips up (see Figure 14-1c).**

4. **Slide your hands forward on the floor until your arms are extended. Then slide your chest forward, bending your elbows slightly, and arch up into the cobra posture, as we describe in Chapter 13 (see Figure 14-1d).**

5. **As you exhale, turn your toes under, raise your hips up, extend your legs, and bring your chest down. Keep both hands on the floor (see Figure 14-1e).**

Figure 14-1:
Just follow your breath — inhale when you are opening, exhale when you are folding.

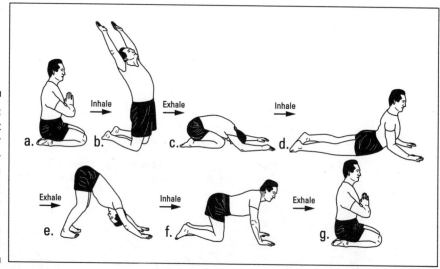

6. As you inhale, bend your knees to the floor and look straight ahead (see Figure 14-1f).

7. As you exhale, sit back on your heels and return your hands to the saluting position as in Step 1 (see Figure 14-1g).

8. Repeat the entire sequence 3 to 12 times. Move slowly, pausing after the inhalation and the exhalation.

Embarking on the 12-step sun salutation

To enjoy the greatest benefit from your Yoga postures, execute them with full participation of your mind. When you stand, really stand; plant your feet firmly on the ground. When you bend, bend with complete attention. When you stretch, stretch with full attention. Your mind not only makes your practice elegant, but also potent.

Use Figure 14-2 as a posture guide to help you through this routine. Use any of the Yoga breathing techniques from Chapter 5.

1. Start in a standing position with your feet at hip width. Place your palms together in the prayer position with your thumbs touching the sternum in the middle of your chest (see Figure 14-2a).

2. As you inhale, open your palms slightly and raise your arms forward, then up and overhead. Arch your back and look up at the ceiling (see Figure 14-2b).

3. As you exhale, bend forward from the hips, soften your knees (Forgiving Limbs posture; see Chapter 3), and place your hands on the floor. Bring your head as close as possible to your legs (see Figure 14-2c).

4. As you inhale, bend your left knee and step your right foot back into a lunge.

   Make sure that your left knee is directly over your ankle and your thigh is parallel to the floor, so that your knee makes a right angle. Look straight ahead (see Figure 14-2d).

5. As you exhale, step your left foot back beside the right and hold a push-up position. If your arms give out, bend your knees to the floor and pause on your hands and knees (see Figure 14-2e).

6. Inhale and then as you exhale, lower your knees (from the push-up), chest, and chin to the floor. Keep your buttocks up in the air (see Figure 14-2f).

7. As you inhale, slide your chest forward along the floor and then arch back into the cobra posture (see Figure 14-2g).

8. As you exhale, turn your toes under, raise your hips up, extend your legs, and bring your chest down. Keep both hands on the floor (see Figure 14-2h).

9. As you inhale, step your right foot forward between your hands and look straight ahead (see Figure 14-2i).

10. As you exhale, step your left foot forward, parallel to and even with the right. Soften your knees and fold into a forward bend, as in Step 3 (see Figure 14-2j).

11. As you inhale, raise your arms either forward and up overhead from the front, or out and up from the sides like wings, and then arch back and look up, as in Step 2 (see Figure 14-2k).

12. As you exhale, return your hands to the prayer position, as in Step 1 (see Figure 14-2l).

13. Repeat the entire sequence 3 to 12 times. First lead with the right foot, and then alternate with the left foot, for an equal number of times (each side counts as half a round).

Move slowly, pausing after the inhalation and the exhalation.

If you have back problems, lifting up from the forward bend (in Step 11) with your arms either to the front or sides may cause you some discomfort. If so, you can try the "roll up": Keep your chin on your chest and roll up, stacking the vertebrae one at a time, with your arms hanging at your sides. When you are fully upright, bring the arms forward, up, and overhead from the front, arch your back just a little, and look up.

If both the 7-step and the 12-step sun salutations are too difficult for you, repeat Steps 1–3 only of the 12-step version until you are ready to do more.

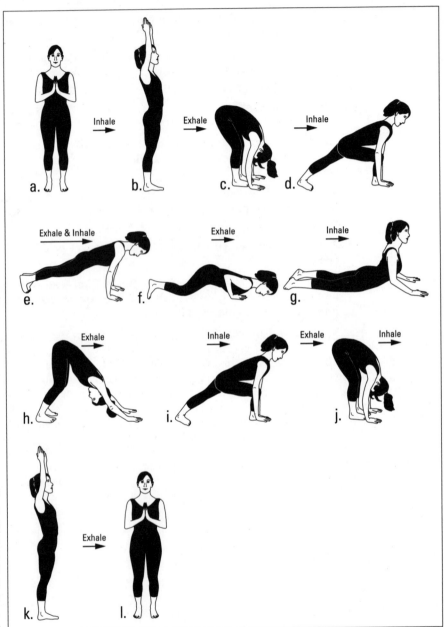

Chapter 15

Recommended Routines

• •

• •

The Yoga routines in this chapter are "tried and true" sequences from Larry Payne's User Friendly Yoga program. Taught around the world, these sequences have helped thousands of people — including the staff at the J. Paul Getty Museum in Los Angeles and, slightly further from home base, 100 members of the World Presidents Organization who convened all the way up at the North Pole. The WPO is a diverse and successful international organization of CEOs over age 50 who meet regularly for education and fun. The routines are safe and "do-able," and include segments that reduce stress and increase strength, flexibility, and overall pep and vitality.

Because this may be your first Yoga experience — and you may have turned directly to this chapter — we offer a quick trip through some basic principles. For an expanded picture of the basics and beyond, check out Parts I and II, plus the chapters we note in the following list.

✔ **Yoga is not competitive.** Be patient. If you follow the directions, you will improve over time no matter what your starting level. See Chapter 2.

✔ **Move slowly into and out of the postures.** Don't ever rush your Yoga session. Remember that coming out of a posture is an integral part of the posture itself.

✔ **Use yogic breathing throughout the routine.** See Chapter 5.

✔ **Pause briefly after each inhalation and exhalation.** See Chapter 5.

✔ **Challenge but don't strain yourself.** Yoga should never hurt or cause you pain. See Chapters 2 and 3.

✔ **Move smoothly into and out of a posture several times before holding the posture.** Doing so prepares your body for a deeper stretch and helps you concentrate on linking the body, breath, and mind (see Chapter 5). As another option, you can stay in a posture and breathe 6 to 8 times.

✔ **Don't change the order of the sequence and just randomly pick the postures that you want.** All the routines have a special order or sequence to give you the maximum benefits. (For details about how to put together your own routines, see Chapter 16.)

Starting at the Very Beginning

Most of this chapter outlines our 8-week course, which is designed to get you jump-started — painlessly but efficiently. If you follow the plan diligently, you can improve your flexibility, muscle tone and strength, and concentration. Very likely, you'll notice a number of other benefits as well, such as better stamina, digestion, and sleep. As the adage says, all beginnings are difficult. True enough, but we make your first steps in Hatha Yoga as simple as possible. Now you just need to take the first step — and then the next.

✔ **Weeks 1 and 2:** Use Beginner 1, Part I (about 15 minutes per session) a minimum of three times per week to a maximum of six times per week.

✔ **Weeks 3 and 4:** Use Beginner 1, Parts I and II (about 30 minutes) a minimum of three times per week to a maximum of six times per week.

✔ **Weeks 5 and 6:** Use Beginner 2, Part I, and Beginner 1, Part II (approximately 30 minutes) a minimum of three times per week to a maximum of six times per week.

✔ **Weeks 7 and 8:** Use Beginner 2, Parts I and II (about 30 minutes) a minimum of three times per week to a maximum of six times per week.

When practicing the various postures that we describe in the following sections, either follow the directions for breath and movement or simply stay in each posture for 6 to 8 breaths.

Beginner 1, Part I

You can use this routine as a 15-minute, stand-alone routine, or you can combine it with the Beginner 1, Part II routine for a 30-minute session. We include the necessary warm-up and compensation postures, as well as rest.

If you only have time for a 15-minute session, we advise you to practice the exercises of this part rather than Part II.

Corpse posture

1. **Lie flat on your back with your arms relaxed along the sides of your torso, palms up (see Figure 15-1).**

2. **Inhale and exhale through your nose slowly for 8 to 10 breaths.**

   Pause briefly after each inhalation and exhalation. Use focus breathing (see Chapter 5) in this posture and for the rest of this routine.

Figure 15-1:
First relax and then use focus breathing for the rest of this routine.

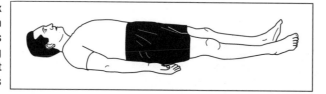

Lying arm raise

1. **Lie in the corpse posture, arms relaxed at your sides, palms down (see Figure 15-2a).**

2. **As you inhale, slowly raise your arms up overhead and touch the floor behind you (see Figure 15-2b).**

   Pause briefly.

3. **As you exhale, bring your arms back to your sides as in Step 3.**

4. **Repeat Steps 2 and 3 six to eight times.**

Figure 15-2:
Link the breath and movement from the very beginning.

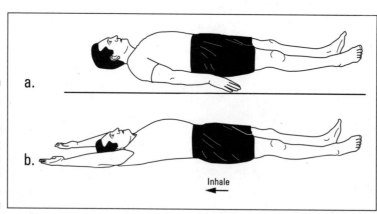

a.

b.

Inhale

Knee-to-chest posture

1. **Lie on your back, knees bent, feet flat on the floor.**

2. **As you exhale, bring your right knee into your chest and extend your left leg down.**

   Hold your shin just below your knee (see Figure 15-3). If you have knee problems, hold the back of your thigh instead.

3. **Stay in Step 2 for 6 to 8 breaths, and then repeat on the left side.**

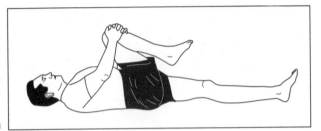

Figure 15-3: Prepare the lower body and tune each side of the back.

Downward facing dog

1. **Beginning on your hands and knees, place your hands directly under your shoulders, palms spread on the floor, with your knees directly under the your hips**

   Straighten your arms, but don't lock your elbows (see Figure 15-4a).

2. **As you exhale, lift and straighten (but don't lock) your knees.**

   As your hips lift, bring your head down to a neutral position so that your ears are between your arms (see Figure 15-4b). If possible, press your heels to the floor and your head toward your feet (stop if doing so strains your neck).

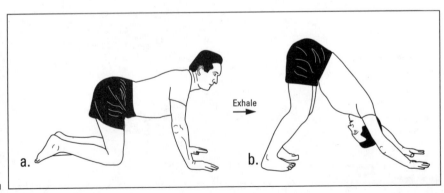

Figure 15-4: This first weight-bearing posture will prepare you for the main standing postures.

Exhale

a.

b.

3. As you inhale, come back down to your hands and knees as in Step 1.

4. Repeat Steps 1–3 three times; and then stay in Step 2 for 6 to 8 breaths.

Child's posture

1. **Starting on your hands and knees, place your knees about hip width apart, hands just below your shoulders.**

   Your elbows are straight but not locked.

2. **As you exhale, sit back on your heels; rest your torso on your thighs and your forehead on the floor. (You don't have to sit all the way back.)**

3. **Lay your arms back on the floor beside your torso, palms up, or reach your relaxed arms forward, palms on the floor.**

4. **Close your eyes and stay in the folded position for 6 to 8 breaths (see Figure 15-5).**

Figure 15-5:
A short rest before the most physical part of the routine.

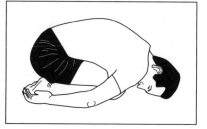

Warrior posture

1. **Stand in the mountain posture (see Figure 15-15, later in this chapter or refer to Chapter 6). As you exhale, step forward about 3 to 3¹/₂ feet (or the length of one leg) with your right foot.**

   Turn your left foot out (so the toes point to the left) if you need more stability.

2. **Place your hands on the top of your hips and square the front of your pelvis.**

   Then release your hands and hang your arms (see Figure 15-6a).

3. **As you inhale, raise your arms forward, overhead and bend your right knee to a right angle, so that your knee is directly over your ankle and your thigh is parallel to the floor (see Figure 15-6b).**

4. **Soften your arms (see Chapter 3 for a description of Forgiving Limbs) and face your palms toward each other.**

   If your lower back is uncomfortable, lean your torso slightly over the forward leg until your back releases any tension that may be present. Look straight ahead.

5. **Repeat Steps 3 and 4 three times, and then hold once on the right side for 6 to 8 breaths.**

6. **Repeat the same sequence on the other (left) side.**

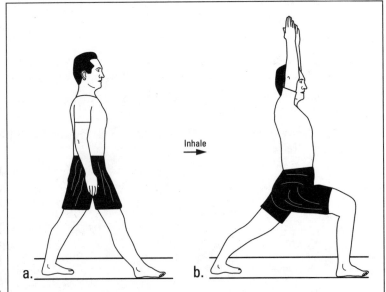

Figure 15-6: Imagine that you are a warrior — a symbol of power and strength.

Inhale →

a.   b.

Standing forward bend

1. **Start in the mountain posture (see Figure 15-15, later in this chapter). As you inhale, raise your arms forward, and then up overhead (see Figure 15-7a).**

2. **As you exhale, bend forward from the hips.**

   When you feel a pull in the back of your legs, soften your knees (see Chapter 3 for information about Forgiving Limbs) and hang your arms (see Figure 15-7b).

   If your head is not close to your knees, bend your knees more. If you have the flexibility, straighten your knees while keeping them soft. Relax your head and neck downward

3. **Exhaling, roll the body up like a rag doll stacking the vertebra one at a time. (See Chapter 8 for more advanced ways to come up from a forward bend.)**

4. **Repeat Steps 1–3 three times; and then stay down in Step 2 for 6 to 8 breaths.**

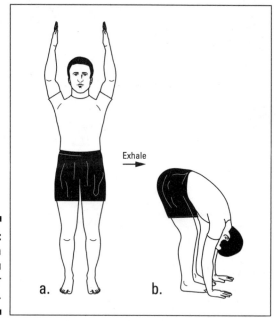

Exhale

a.   b.

Figure 15-7:
You're not a
wimp if you
soften your
knees.

Reverse triangle posture

1. **Stand in the mountain posture (see Figure 15-15, later in this chapter). As you exhale, step out to the right about 3 to 3$^1/_2$ feet (or the length of one leg) with the right foot.**

2. **As you inhale, raise your arms out to the sides parallel to the line of your shoulders (and the floor), so that your shoulders form a "T" with your torso (see Figure 15-8a).**

3. **As you exhale, bend forward from the hips and then place your right hand on the floor near the inside of your left foot.**

4. **Raise your left arm toward the ceiling and look up at your left hand.**

   Soften your knees and arms. Bend your left knee or move your right hand away from your left foot and more directly under your torso, if you experience strain or discomfort (see Figure 15-8b).

5. **Repeat Steps 2–4 to the same side three times; then stay down in Step 4 for 6 to 8 breaths.**

6. **Repeat the same sequence on the right side.**

You can strengthen or strain your neck in this posture. Turn your neck down if you're uncomfortable.

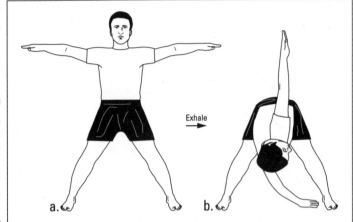

Figure 15-8:
This standing twist will rejuvenate your entire spine.

a. b.

Exhale →

Standing spread leg forward bend

1. **Stand in the mountain posture (see Figure 15-15 later in this chapter). As you exhale, step out to the right about 3 to 3¹/₂ feet (or the length of one leg) with your right foot.**

2. **As you inhale, raise your arms out to the sides parallel to the line of your shoulders (and the floor), so that your shoulders form a "T" with the torso (see Figure 15-9a).**

3. **As you exhale, bend forward from the hips and soften your knees.**

4. **Hold your bent elbows with the opposite-side hands and hang your torso and arms.**

5. **Stay folded in this posture for 6 to 8 breaths (see Figure 15-9b).**

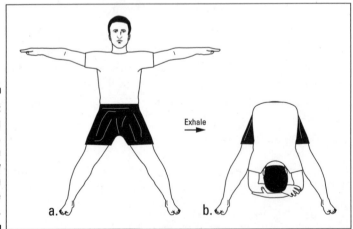

Figure 15-9:
Just hang comfortably. Notice each time how close you get to the floor.

a. b.

Exhale →

The karate kid

1. **Stand in the mountain posture (see Figure 15-15, later in this chapter). As you inhale, raise your arms out to the sides parallel to the line of your shoulders (and the floor), so that your shoulders form a "T" with the torso.**

2. **Steady yourself and focus on a spot on the floor 10 to 12 feet in front of you.**

3. **As you exhale, bend and raise your left knee toward the chest, keeping your right leg straight (see Figure 15-10).**

4. **Stay in Step 3 for 6 to 8 breaths.**

5. **Repeat with your legs reversed.**

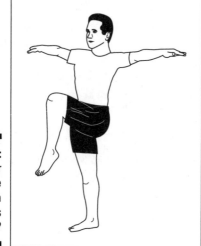

Figure 15-10:
Remember this posture from a famous movie?

After you become stable in the karate kid posture, extend your left leg down toward the floor, keeping your foot slightly off the floor. Then gradually, over time, raise your left leg higher and higher until it's parallel with the floor. Try this added step on both sides.

Corpse posture

Repeat the corpse posture exercise, as described at the beginning of this routine (refer to Figure 15-1). Stay for 6 to 8 breaths.

TIP

You're now at the halfway point, or approximately 15 minutes, of your routine. You may stop here or continue for the next 15 minutes to complete a 30-minute session.

Beginner 1, Part II

This routine expands on the exercise sequence of "Beginner 1, Part I." The sequences have the same level of difficulty. If you only have time for a 15-minute session rather than a full 30 minutes, we recommend that you use the exercises of Beginner 1 (Part I) rather than the following exercises.

Yogi sit-up

EXERCISE

1. **Lie on your back, knees bent, feet on the floor at hip width.**

2. **Turn your toes in "pigeon-toed" and touch your inner knees together.**

3. **Spread your palms on the back of your head, fingers interlocked, and hook your thumbs under the angle of the jaw bone, just below the ears (see Figure 15-11a).**

4. **As you exhale, press your knees firmly (but without causing yourself discomfort), tilt the front of your pelvis toward your navel and, with the hips on the floor, slowly sit up halfway.**

   Keep your elbows out to the sides in line with the tops of your shoulders. Look toward the ceiling (see Figure 15-11b). Don't pull your head up with your arms; rather, support your head with your hands and come up by contracting the abdominal muscles.

5. **As you inhale, slowly roll back down.**

6. **Repeat Steps 4–6 six to eight times.**

Figure 15-11:
Exhale as you sit up. Keep your eyes on the ceiling.

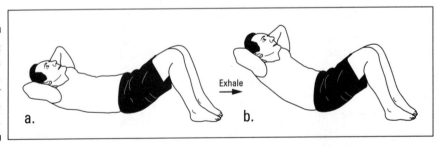

a.　　　Exhale →　　　b.

Cobra 2

1. **Lie flat on your belly, separate your legs to hip width and point your toes back with the tops of your feet on the floor.**

2. **Bend your elbows and place your palms on the floor with your thumbs near your armpits.**

   Put your forehead on the floor and relax your shoulders (see Figure 15-12a).

3. **As you inhale, begin to raise your chest and head. When you feel the muscles of your lower back engaging, press your hands down and arch your spine until you're looking straight ahead (see Figure 15-12b).**

   Keep the top front hip bones on the floor and your shoulders dropped away from your ears. Unless you are very flexible, keep your elbows slightly bent.

4. **As you exhale, lower your torso and head slowly back to the floor.**

5. **Repeat Steps 3 and 4 three times; then hold in the up position for 6 to 8 breaths.**

If cobra 2 is too strenuous, use cobra 1 (see Chapter 12).

Figure 15-12: Lift your chest only as high as you feel comfortable.

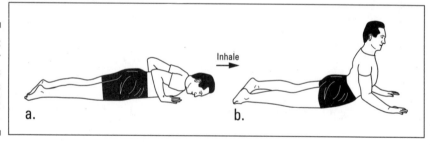

Inhale

a.

b.

Child's posture

Refer to Figure 15-5. Close your eyes and stay in the folded position for 6 to 8 breaths.

Hamstring stretch

1. **Lie on your back, legs straight, place your arms along your sides, palms down.**

2. **Bend just your left knee and put your left foot on the floor (see Figure 15-13a).**

3. **As you exhale, bring your right leg up as straight as possible (see Figure 15-13b).**

4. **As you inhale, return your leg to the floor, keeping your head and the back of your pelvis on the floor.**

5. **Repeat Steps 3 and 4 three times; then hold the right leg with your hands interlocked on the back of your raised thigh, just above your knee, for 6 to 8 breaths (see Figure 15-13c).**

6. **Repeat on the left side.**

Lift your head on a pillow or folded blanket if the back of your neck or your throat tenses while raising or lowering the leg.

Figure 15-13:
Stretching
your
hamstrings
will help you
to improve
a lot of
postures.

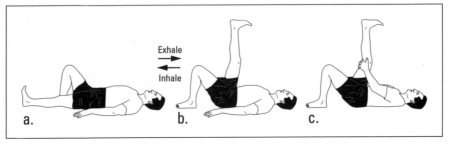

Head-to-knee posture

1. **Sitting on the floor with your legs stretched out in front of you, bend your left knee and bring your left foot toward your right groin.**

2. **Bring your bent left knee down to the floor on the left side (but don't force it) and place the sole of your left foot on the inside of the right thigh, heel in the groin.**

The toes of your left foot point toward the right knee.

3. **Bring your back up nice and tall and, as you inhale, raise your arms forward and up overhead until they are beside your ears.**

Keep your arms and the right leg soft and slightly bent in Forgiving Limbs, as we describe in Chapter 5 (see Figure 15-14a).

4. **As you exhale, bend forward from your hips, bringing your hands, chest, and head toward your right leg.**

Rest your hands on your leg, knee or foot. If your head is not close to your right knee, bend your knee more until you feel your back stretching on the right side (see Figure 15-14b).

5. **Repeat Steps 3 and 4 three times, then stay folded in Step 4 for 6 to 8 breaths.**

6. **Repeat the same sequence on the opposite side.**

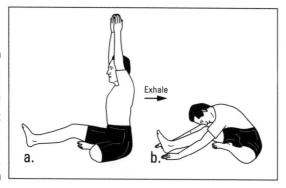

Figure 15-14:
Avoid pulling yourself down. Just relax in the posture and breathe.

Corpse posture

To perform this posture, refer to Figure 15-1 in the "Corpse posture" section. Stay for 8 to 10 breaths.

Beginner 2, Part I

After four weeks of practicing the exercises that we describe in Parts I and II of the Beginner 1 series, you're probably ready to move on to the slightly more challenging postures of Beginner 2. If you don't feel quite ready yet, however, continue to practice the Beginner 1 exercises for a few more weeks or for as long as necessary to achieve competence in the postures. Take your time. No one is rushing you.

This routine is either a 15-minute stand-alone routine, or you can combine it with the Beginner 1, Part II routine for a 30-minute session (in weeks 5 and 6 of our 8-week program) or the Beginner 2, Part II routine for a 30-minute session (in weeks 7 and 8 of our 8-week program).

Mountain posture

1. **Stand tall but relaxed with your feet at hip width.**

2. **Hang your arms at your sides, palms turned toward your legs.**

3. **Visualize a vertical line connecting the hole in your ear, your shoulder joint, and the sides of your hip, knee, and ankle.**

4. **Look straight ahead, eyes open or closed (see Figure 15-15).**

5. Use the three-part yogic breathing or chest-to-belly breathing (see Chapter 5) for 8 to10 breaths, and then continue with that breathing pattern for the entire routine.

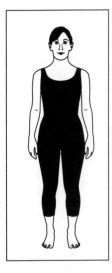

Figure 15-15: Starting with this first pose, keep a union with your body, breath, and mind.

Rejuvenation sequence

1. Stand in the mountain posture) with your feet at hip width and arms at your sides (see Figure 15-16a).

2. As you inhale, slowly raise your arms out from the sides and up overhead (see Figure 15-16b), then pause.

3. As you exhale, bend forward from the waist and bring your head toward your knees and your hands forward and down toward the floor in the standing forward bend (see Figure 15-16c).

   Keep your arms and legs soft (see Chapter 3 for an explanation of forgiving limbs). Then pause.

4. Bend your knees quite a bit and as you inhale, sweep your arms out from the sides, but only come halfway up with your arms in a "T" (half forward bend), as shown in Figure 15-16d.

   Then pause briefly.

5. As you exhale, fold all the way down again and hang your arms in the standing forward bend (see Figure 15-16e).

6. As you inhale, sweep your arms from the sides like wings and bring your torso all the way up again, standing with your arms overhead in the standing arm raise (see Figure 15-16f).

7. As you exhale again, bring your arms back to your sides as in Step 1 (see Figure 15-16g).

8. Repeat the entire sequence 6 to 8 times slowly.

   On the last round, stay for 6 to 8 breaths in the half forward bend (Step 4) and 6 to 8 breaths in the standing forward bend (Step 5).

For variation, you can replace the rejuvenation series with either the kneeling or standing sun salutation for 6 to 8 rounds (see Chapter 14).

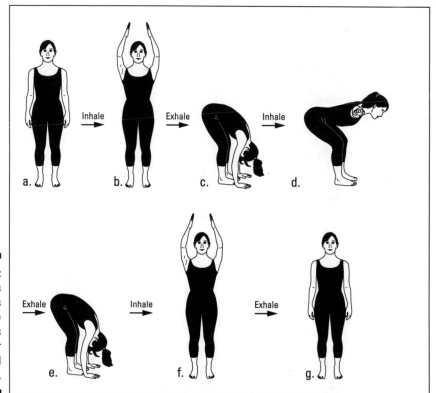

Figure 15-16: This series invigorates your entire torso, as well as your arms and legs.

Half chair

1. **Start in the mountain posture (refer to Figure 15-15). As you inhale, raise your arms forward, up and overhead, palms facing (see Figure 15-17a).**

2. **As you exhale, bend your knees and squat halfway to the floor.**

3. **Soften your arms but keep them overhead; look straight ahead (see Figure 15-17b).**

4. **Repeat Steps 1 through 3 three times, and then stay in the half chair posture (Step 3) for 6 to 8 breaths.**

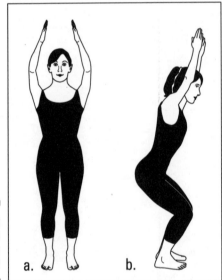

Figure 15-17:
Anyone in
favor of firm
thighs?

a.   b.

Standing forward bend

Repeat the posture shown in Figure 15-7 in the "Beginner 1, Part I" section. Remain folded for 6 to 8 breaths.

Balancing cat

1. **Begin on your hands and knees, place your hands directly under your shoulders, palms spread on the floor, with your knees directly under your hips.**

   Straighten your arms, but don't lock your elbows.

2. **As you exhale, slide your right hand forward and your left leg back, keeping your hand and toes on the floor.**

3. **As you inhale, raise your right arm and left leg as high as is comfortably possible for you (see Figure 15-18).**

   Stay for 6 to 8 breaths.

4. **Repeat with opposite pairs (left arm and right leg).**

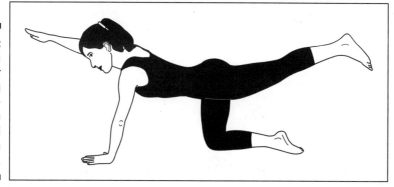

Figure 15-18:
A classic posture for balancing the para-spinals, the small muscles in your back.

Corpse posture

Refer to Figure 15-1 in the "Beginner 1, Part I" section. Relax in this posture for 8 to 10 breaths.

Beginner 2, Part II

You're probably in week 7 of our 8-week program, and you're now reasonably competent in the exercises of Beginner 1 (Parts I and II) and Beginner 2 (Part I). Beginner 2, Part II, offers you more of a cardiovascular workout than Beginner 1. Don't become concerned if you find that you're perspiring when doing these exercises. As your body cleans out from applying Yoga as a lifestyle, your perspiration becomes odorless anyway.

Extended leg slide-ups

1. **Lie on your back, knees bent, feet flat on the floor at hip width.**

2. **Bend your left elbow and place your left hand on the back of your head, just behind your left ear.**

3. **Raise your left leg toward the vertical, but keep your knee slightly bent.**

   Draw the top of your foot toward the shin (to flex the ankle) and place your right palm on your right thigh near your pelvis (see Figure 15-19a).

4. **As you exhale, slowly sit up halfway and slide your right hand toward your knee.**

   Keep your left elbow back in line with your shoulder and look at the ceiling. Don't push your head forward (see Figure 15-19b).

5. **As you inhale, roll back slowly and return to Step 1.**

6. **Repeat Steps 4 and 5 six to eight times.**

7. **Repeat the same sequence on the opposite side.**

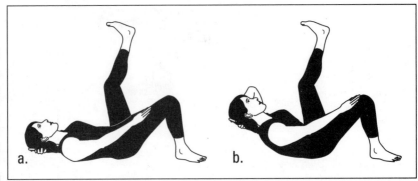

Figure 15-19: This posture works the abs and the hamstrings. A great combination!

a.　　b.

If this posture bothers your neck, support your head with both hands behind your head. If the problem persists, stop the exercise.

Dynamic bridge

1. **Lie on your back, knees bent, feet flat on the floor at hip width.**

2. **Place your arms at your sides, palms turned down (see Figure 15-20a).**

3. **As you inhale, raise your hips to a comfortable height (see Figure 15-20b).**

4. **As you exhale, return your hips to the floor.**

5. **Repeat Steps 3 and 4 six to eight times.**

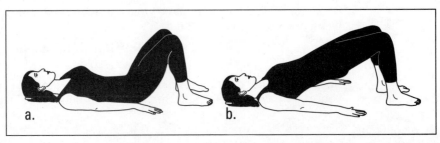

Figure 15-20: The bridge compensates or neutralizes the muscles you used in the slide-ups.

a.　　b.

Locust 2

1. **Lie on your belly, and separate your legs to hip width, extend your toes, and lay the tops of your feet on the floor.**

   Place your forehead on the floor.

2. **Extend your right arm forward, palm resting on the floor; extend your left arm back behind you and let it rest on the floor near your left side, palm up (see Figure 15-21a).**

3. **As you inhale, slowly raise your chest, head, right arm, and left leg up and away from the floor, as high as you feel comfortable.**

   Try to keep your right arm and ear in alignment and your left foot as high as your right hand (see Figure 15-21b).

4. **As you exhale, slowly lower your right arm, chest, head, and left leg to the floor at the same time.**

5. **Repeat Steps 3 and 4 three times, and then hold in the up position (Step 3) for 6 to 8 breaths.**

6. **Repeat with your left arm and right leg.**

Be careful of locust variations that lift just the legs, which increases chest pressure, heart rate, and tension in the neck. Definitely avoid these variations if you have heart problems or hypertension.

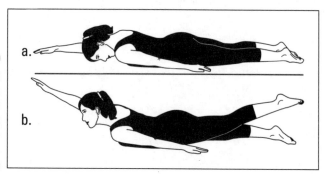

Figure 15-21:
Try to bring the raised arm and foot to the same height.

Child's posture

Refer to Figure 15-5 in the "Beginner 1, Part I" section to perform this pose. Close your eyes and stay in the folded position for 6 to 8 breaths.

Hamstring stretch

1. **Lie on your back, legs straight. Place your arms along your sides, palms down.**

2. **Bend your left knee and put your foot flat on the floor (refer to Figure 15-13a).**

3. **As you exhale, bring your right leg up as straight as possible (refer to Figure 15-13b).**

4. **As you inhale, return your leg to the floor.**

   Keep your head and the top of your hips on the floor.

5. **Repeat 6 to 8 times, and then hold your leg up with your hands interlocked on the back of your raised thigh, just above the knee, for 6 to 8 breaths (refer to Figure 15-13c).**

6. **Repeat Steps 1 through 5 with the legs reversed.**

Lift your head on a pillow or folded blanket if the back of your neck or your throat tenses when you raise or lower your leg.

Be very careful of all seated forward bends if you have disc-related back problems. Avoid these movements completely if you have pain or numbness in the back, buttocks, or legs.

Seated forward bend

1. **Sit on the floor with your legs at hip width and comfortably stretched out in front of you.**

   Bring your back up nice and tall and place your palms down on the floor near your thighs.

2. **As you inhale, raise your arms forward and up overhead until they are beside your ears.**

   Keep your arms and legs soft and slightly bent in forgiving limbs, as discussed in Chapter 3 (see Figure 15-22a).

3. **As you exhale, bend forward from the hips and bring your hands, chest, and head toward your legs.**

   Rest your hands on your thighs, knees, shins, or feet. If your head isn't close to your knees, bend your knees more until you feel your back stretching (see Figure 15-22b).

4. **Repeat Steps 2 and 3 three to four times, and then stay folded for 6 to 8 breaths.**

If you have a problem sitting upright on the floor in the seated forward bend or any of the following forward bending postures, raise your hips on a folded blanket or firm pillow (see Figure 15-22c).

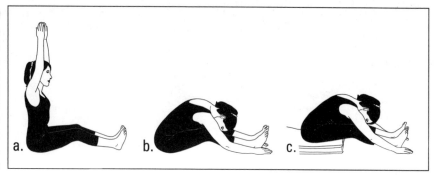

Figure 15-22:
Forward bends are calming and quieting and often used toward the end of a routine.

a.   b.   c.

Corpse posture

To perform the corpse posture, refer to Figure 15-1 in the "Beginner 1, Part I" section. Relax in this posture for 15 to 30 breaths.

Reaching Beyond the Beginning

After you complete the 8-week course, we recommend the following possibilities:

✔ Continue the recommended programs, using Beginner 1 (Parts I and II) and Beginner 2 (Parts I and II) on alternate days.

✔ Use Beginner 2 (Parts I and II) and substitute six rounds of the kneeling sun salutation or six rounds of the sun salutation (see Chapter 14) for the rejuvenation sequence.

✔ Turn to Chapter 16 to discover how to create your own Yoga program.

Of course, now that you have a taste of Hatha Yoga, you may want to take private lessons or go to a group class for feedback, to boost your morale, or simply to practice — with new confidence — in the company of others. If you have practiced on your own up to this point, we recommend that you ask a Yoga teacher to check for any bad postural habits and, if you like, to give you some suggestions for taking the next step.

Part IV
Creative Yoga

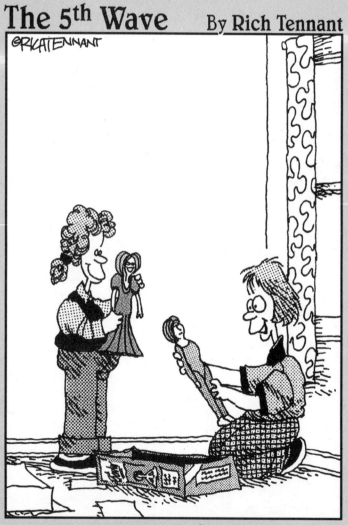

The 5th Wave   By Rich Tennant

"...and this one's Yogini Barbie. She doesn't come with a lot of stuff, but you can bend her into 13 different positions without anything breaking."

In this part . . .

Since routines can become boring rather quickly, it is important to add the spice of variety to your practice of Yoga. In Part III, we gave you a wide range of postures in all categories, such as sitting, bending, twisting, and so on and also offered you several routines. In this part, we go one step further and put you in control of your own Yoga practice by giving you the principles of designing an efficient routine for yourself. Here we also introduce some of the most widely used props, which can help increase the efficiency, safety, and enjoyment of your practice of Yoga postures.

Chapter 16

Designing Your Own Yoga Program

....

In This Chapter

▶ Introducing the classic formula

▶ Outlining 30- to 60-minute routines

▶ Presenting 15-minute routines

▶ Refreshing with 5-minute routines

....

*I*f you're like most people, you can't wait to cook up your own exercise routines. Opinions are plentiful about how to create an efficient Hatha Yoga program. In this chapter, we give you some practical guidelines, including a classic formula, that you can use to put together a variety of routines — exercises for different occasions throughout your life.

We don't intend for our advice to be a universal remedy. Some situations call for highly personalized attention. We're not offering a panacea for readers with serious muscular or skeletal problems, such as acute back pain, or those who have a serious illness. In Chapter 21, we address two *manageable* special situations — back problems and pregnancy. Providing a formula that fits every conceivable ailment or special circumstance is, however, beyond the scope of this book — or any book.

If you're dealing with a specific health challenge, you need to work one-on-one, under the guidance of your doctor, with a Yoga therapist or other health professional. This chapter focuses on "do-it-yourself" Hatha Yoga for general conditioning and stress reduction. Our emphasis is on prevention rather than therapy.

In Chapter 6, we consider a number of practice elements, which include:

✔ Determining your goals for each session

✔ The rules of sequencing, including warm-up or preparation, compensation, and rest

> ✔ Your starting point
>
> ✔ Your next activity
>
> ✔ How much time you have available

Then in Chapters 7 to 15, we describe step-by-step procedures for using the main postures. Although all the chapters in this book are designed to be self-contained, you can get more out of this chapter if you read or reread Chapters 5 and 6 and use the remaining chapters of Part III for reference.

Cooking Up a Creative Course of Exercise with the Classic Formula

Creating your own Yoga program is not unlike figuring out how to create your own fabulous meals. You determine how much time you have and which cuisine you're likely to enjoy the most. You consult your cookbook about the principles of combining main and side dishes and preparing each one properly. When the food is cooked, you sit down and relish each bite. You eat slowly to savor every single morsel. When you finish, you don't jump up right away, instead you sit back and relax for a while and let your stomach begin its digestive work.

When you create your own Yoga program with our classic formula, you

> ✔ Determine how long you want the routine to be.
>
> ✔ Select the main postures from the range of postures covered in Chapters 7 to 14 (or, of course, from any source you consider reliable).
>
> ✔ Decide how you want to prepare and/or compensate for each main category of postures.
>
> ✔ Allocate time for rest and for relaxation at the end in order to digest the nutritious meal of Yoga exercises that you prepared for yourself.

What we call the Classic Formula consists of the following 12 categories:

1. Attunement (integrating body, mind, and breath)

2. Preparation or warm-up (also used between main exercises wherever necessary)

3. Standing postures

4. Balance postures (optional)

5. Abdominals

6. Inversions (optional)

7. Back bends

8. Forward bends

9. Twists

10. Rest (to be inserted between main exercises whenever you feel the need)

11. Compensation (to be inserted after main exercises)

12. Final relaxation

You don't have to use all these categories as long as you follow the proper sequence (from 1 to 9 and always concluding with 12). The categories of *rest, preparation/warm-up,* and *compensation* are repeated where appropriate. Balancing postures, and inversions are marked *optional,* because their inclusion depends on your available time.

The Classic Formula is optimal for 30- to 60-minute general conditioning programs, but we also refer to it in the 15- and 5-minute programs. The beauty of our formula is that, as your Yoga practice grows over the years, you can explore safe postures from any book or system and then insert them into their appropriate slots within our 12-category module.

Enjoying a Postural Feast: The 30- to 60-Minute General Conditioning Routine

An old saying proposes that you can give someone a fish or you can hand that person a fishing pole and teach him or her how to fish. In a similar way, we can just offer you some precooked Yoga routines like we did in Chapter 15, or we can teach you how to cook up your own postural feasts. Most beginning Yoga students find it difficult to sustain more than a 30- minute practice on their own; however, if your appetite increases, we want you to have the tools to be a 60-minute gourmet. Simply follow the recipes in each of the categories to create your own great, custom routine.

If you live 70 years, you spend 23 years asleep and about 6 years preparing meals and eating. If you watch only one hour of television a day (and most people watch a lot more), this adds up to an amazing three years in your lifetime. How much time do we spend shopping, commuting, reading advertisements, and so on? Scary, isn't it? In light of this, even 30 to 60 minutes of Yoga practice 5 times a week seems more than reasonable, especially considering Yoga may well extend your life span.

An average of about two minutes for each posture you select is a good general yardstick for planning your practice time. Some postures take more time, some take less. An asymmetrical or two-sided (right and left) posture like the warrior (see Chapter 8) is counted as one exercise or posture. If you choose our sun salutation or a similar dynamic series (see Chapters 14 and 15) from another source, double or triple the time allotted, depending on the series and the number of rounds.

Note: Many of these postures are versatile: You can often use some of the same postures in more than one category when developing a general conditioning routine.

Attunement

To help you understand *attunement* — your personal connectedness — think of it this way: Attunement is like logging on to the Internet. Your "password" is the type of breathing you select for your attunement and the rest of your program. After you log on and establish the conscious link between your body, breath, and mind, all the benefits of the Yoga universe are yours. If you forget about the attunement stage, you'll be logged off the cosmic Internet before you have a chance to receive all the benefits of your Hatha Yoga session.

First, for routines of any length, select a style of breathing from Chapter 5. If you're a beginner, choose something simple like focus breathing or belly breathing. Later you can try either the classic three-part breathing or chest-to-belly breathing, or adopt the *ujjayi* technique.

Be sure not to confuse these styles of breathing with the traditional techniques of breath control *(pranayama)* that we also describe in Chapter 5.

Next, select one of the resting postures from Chapter 6, or a sitting posture from Chapter 7, depending on your frame of mind, physical condition, or what you have planned for the rest of your routine. The corpse posture (lying flat on your back) is always a good starting point for beginners. With our hectic lifestyles, we usually need to shift gears and slow things down before we can begin our postural exercises. Lying flat on your back definitely shifts your mood toward relaxation. However, sitting in the easy posture or standing in the mountain posture also makes a great starting point. Figure 16-1 shows some examples of rest postures that you can use to help achieve attunement.

Use 8 to 12 breaths to achieve attunement. The more you "remember" (pay attention to) the breath and your attunement, the more benefit you can expect to derive from your program.

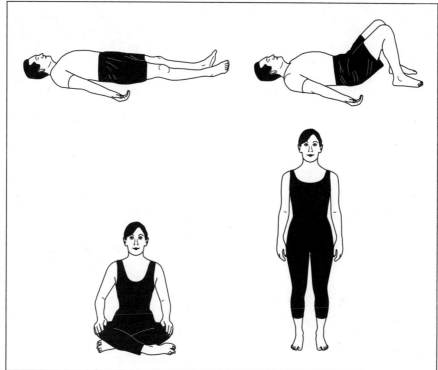

Figure 16-1:
These rest
postures
are great
starting
points when
working
toward
attunement.

Warm-up

You may notice that almost all the warm-ups in Chapter 6 are folding and opening motions (flexion and extension). Either motion provides the easiest way for your body to prepare for breath and movement. Select a warm-up posture or sequence from Chapter 6 that is a *similar* position to your attunement posture.

Make your Yoga practice as smooth as possible. Flow like a gentle river. For example, your attunement and warm-up both can take place on the floor; then you can stand up for all the standing postures. Avoid getting up and down like a yo-yo. Economy of movement is one of the principles of good Hatha Yoga practice.

If you're composing a routine designed for 30 minutes or more, you usually have room for at least 2 warm-up postures. Because the neck is a frequent site of tension, we often suggest using a warm-up posture that incorporates moving the arms. In addition to stretching the spine, arm movement prepares your neck and shoulders and helps you release tension. Also, warm-ups that move the legs and prepare the lower back are helpful for the standing postures that usually follow. Check out Figure 16-2 for some examples of common warm-ups in the lying, sitting, and standing positions. Chapter 6 provides full descriptions of all our recommended warm-ups.

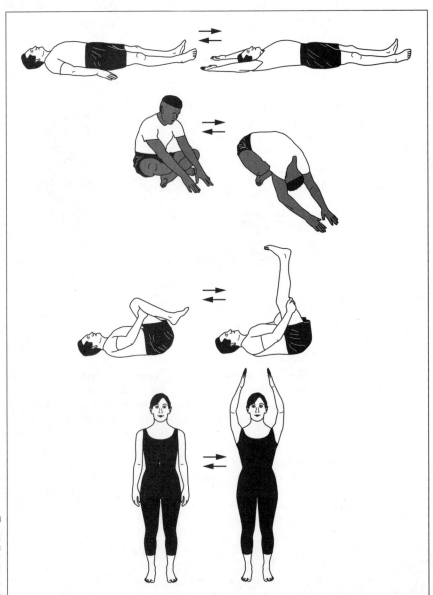

Figure 16-2:
Examples of
warm-up
postures.

Standing postures

The standing postures tend to be the most "physical" part of a program. If you're doing a 30-minute routine, you usually have time for 3 or 4 standing postures. In a 60-minute program, you may have as many as 6 or 7 main *asanas*. You can choose any of the standing postures from Chapter 8 for this portion of your routine.

Before you begin picking your postures, run through a simple rule of sequencing: *back bends, twists, and side bends are usually followed by forward bends.* Therefore, you want to include standing forward bends after most of the standing postures you choose. Figure 16-3 shows you examples of standing postures for a 30-minute or 60-minute program. As an alternative, you can also choose the dynamic kneeling or standing sequence (sun salutation) from Chapter 14 or the standing rejuvenation sequence for beginners from Chapter 15. In terms of time, the dynamic postures take the place of three to six standing postures, depending on which sequence you choose and how many rounds you do. When you select a dynamic sequence, try to allow time at the end for one twist and one compensating forward bend. We mention this because all our dynamic sequences are forward and backward bends only.

If you want your routine to be more physically challenging, simply do two sets of the standing postures.

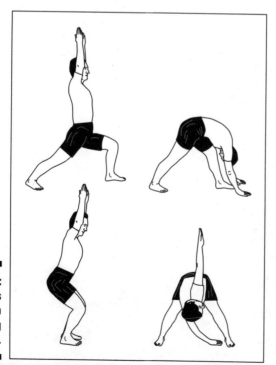

Figure 16-3: Examples of common standing postures.

The simplest way to expand a 30-minute routine into a 45-minute routine is to do 2 sets of your chosen standing postures and add 1 extra posture to the abdominal, back bend, and forward bend categories.

Balancing postures (optional)

Balancing postures are optional and depend on your time and stamina. They are often the most athletic postures and require overall coordination. Balancing postures are very rewarding, because you can see your progress immediately. They fit nicely after the standing postures because at this point in your routine, you're fully warmed up. Also, all our recommended balancing postures are either standing or kneeling, which means they fit smoothly into the sequence. Choose one balancing posture from Chapter 9 for a 30-minute to 60-minute routine (see Figure 16-4).

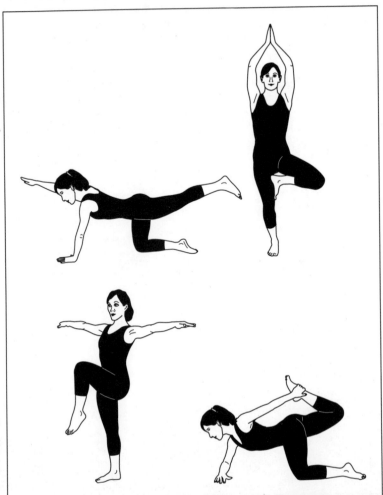

Figure 16-4:
Examples of balancing postures.

Rest

Most people usually welcome a rest at this point, and rest works nicely after any strenuous portion of your routine. Resting is usually done lying, sitting, or kneeling. We emphasize the importance of not feeling rushed during your Yoga session. At least for the short duration of your routine, believe that you have all the time in the world. In a 30- or 60-minute routine, the first rest usually comes at the halfway point. This resting period gives you the opportunity for inward observation of any physical, mental, or emotional feedback resulting from your Yoga practice so far.

Remember that you need to rest until you feel ready to move on. If you're really pinched for time, this first major rest is also a logical place to stop a session. Choose from any of our recommended resting postures in Chapter 6, or any of the sitting postures that you're comfortable with from Chapter 7, or select a posture from Figure 16-1.

Abdominals

As we say in Chapter 10, the belly is a focal point for exercise-conscious Americans. We recommend that you include at least 1, but not more than 2, abdominal postures in any program lasting 30 minutes or more. Think of your abdomen as "the front of your back" — a very important place. Choose 1 of the abdominal postures that we describe in Chapter 10 for a 30-minute routine or 1 or 2 for a 60-minute routine, or check out Figure 16-5.

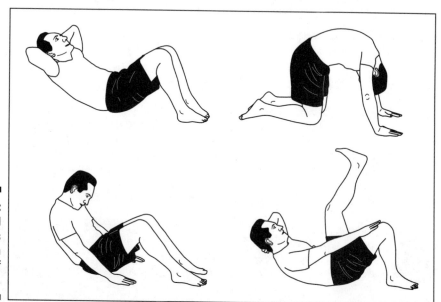

Figure 16-5:
Abdominal postures strengthen the front of your back.

Compensation and preparation

Take a short rest when you finish the abdominal exercises and then use the dynamic bridge, the dynamic bridge with arm variation, or the lying arm raise 6 to 8 times (see Chapter 6 and Figure 16-6). The action of the dynamic bridge plays a dual function here, because it *compensates* the abdomen, returning it to neutral. The bridge also warms up or *prepares* the back and the neck, if you choose to include an inversion posture or move on to back bends next.

Note: Compensation and preparation are normally done dynamically (moving).

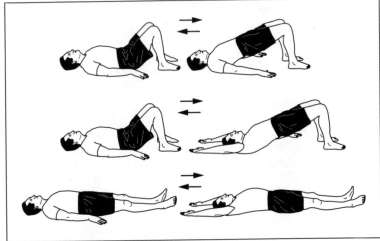

Figure 16-6: Compensation for abdominals can also be preparation for inversions.

Inversion (optional)

Indian Yoga teachers often teach inverted postures toward the beginning or at the end of a class. For Westerners, we prefer inverted postures closer to the middle of the program, when they've properly prepared their backs and necks and they have plenty of time for adequate compensation. Inverted postures, like those shown in Figure 16-7, are optional, and we recommend that beginners avoid the half shoulder stand and the half shoulder stand at the wall until they've practiced Yoga for 6 to 8 weeks.

TIP

Even after you're comfortable with your yogic practice, attempt inversions only if you have no neck problems. Inverted postures are worthy of a healthy respect rather than fear. They're powerful postures, but they demand a sense of balance and strong muscles. We offer you several easy and safe inversion postures in Chapter 11. Select just 1 for your 30- to 60-minute routine, assuming you are ready and want to include an inversion in your practice.

We advise against practicing the half shoulder stand or the half shoulder stand at the wall if any of the following conditions applies to you: glaucoma, high blood pressure, a history of heart attacks or stroke, hiatal hernia, the first few days of menstruation, pregnancy, or you are currently 40 or more pounds overweight.

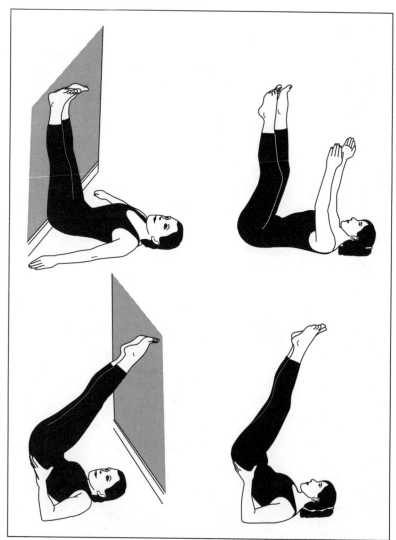

Figure 16-7:
Inversions
are
powerful
postures
that
deserve
respect.

Compensation for inversions and preparation for back bends

You should rest after the simpler inverted postures, normally in the corpse posture (see Chapter 4). After the half shoulder stand, rest and then compensate further with any one of the cobra postures (see Chapter 12) or the thunderbolt posture (see Chapter 7). The cobra and thunderbolt posture also prepare you for further back bends. Figure 16-8 shows these examples.

Back bends

Check for yourself how well back bends work after an inverted posture, and also how the cobra is an excellent compensation for the shoulder stand. The cobra also is a gentle back bend that serves as good preparation for more physical back bends, such as the locust posture. As Westerners, we bend forward far too much — that fact makes back bends a vital part of your Hatha Yoga practice. Whenever possible in general conditioning Yoga

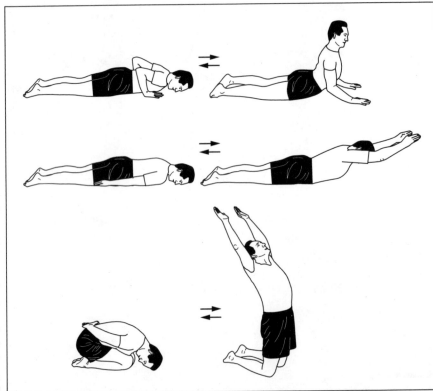

Figure 16-8:
These postures help you either compensate for an inversion or prepare for deeper back bends.

routines, select 1 back bend from Chapter 12; in programs over 30 minutes, select 2 back bends. Figure 16-9 shows some common back bends you can try.

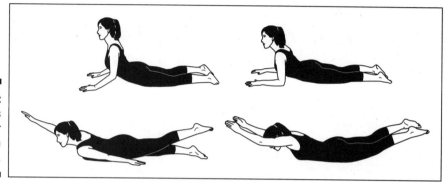

Figure 16-9:
Examples
of four
common
back bends.

Compensation for back bends

The compensation for prone back bends is usually some form of a bent knee forward bend (see Figure 16-10). We often recommend the knees-to-chest or the child's posture (see Chapter 6). After more strenuous back bends, such as any of the varieties of the locust postures, we suggest a short rest,

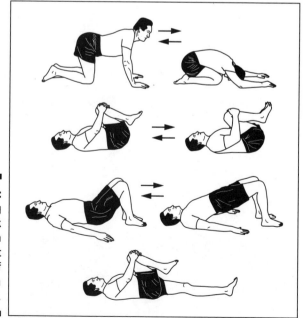

Figure 16-10:
Compensating
for back
bends is an
important
part of
your Yoga
program.

followed by one of the bent knee forward bends, and then the dynamic bridge posture as a second compensatory posture. This sequence helps neutralize the upper back and neck.

Preparation for forward bends

Preparation is particularly critical in the performance of extended leg forward bends. Stretching the hamstrings or the hips just before any of the recommended seated forward bends (see Chapter 12) not only improves the posture but also is safer for your back. Use the hamstring stretch, or the double leg stretch for a 30-minute routine. For a longer routine, use both and/or the rock the baby sequence, all of which we describe in Chapter 6 (see Figure 16-11).

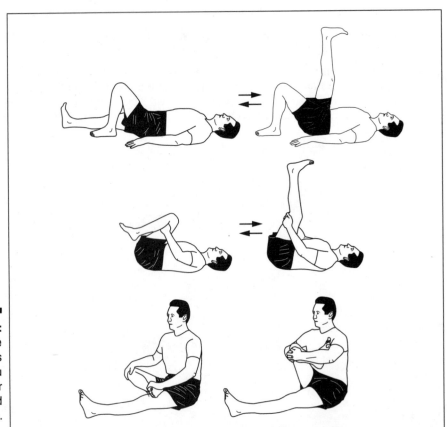

Figure 16-11:
These postures help you prepare for forward bends.

Forward bends

The seated forward bends are normally done toward the end of an exercise program because they have a calming effect. Of all the postures described in this book, the seated extended leg forward bends divide the sexes the most. Men have a higher muscle density, especially in the hip and groin area, and are usually tighter in the hamstrings. Preparation of the hamstrings is particularly important. If you have a hard time with this category, bend your knees more and, if necessary, place some blankets under your hips to give yourself a better angle for the forward bends (see Chapters 12 and 17). For a 30-minute routine, choose just 1 forward bend from Chapter 12. For a 60-minute routine, select 2 forward bends (see Figure 16-12). Alternately, you may substitute with one kneeling or sitting side bend from Chapter 12, and one sitting or kneeling forward bend from Chapter 6 for compensation.

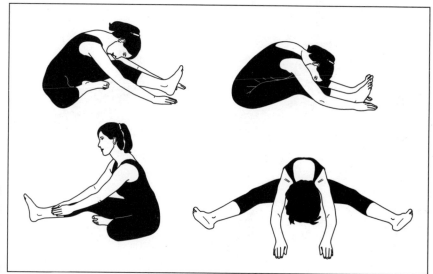

Figure 16-12: Examples of forward bends.

Compensation for forward bends

The forward bends are usually self-compensating. However, sometimes you may want to use a gentle back bend like the dynamic bridge as a counter pose (see Chapter 6).

Preparation for twists

The preparation for all twists is a forward bend. So, moving from the category of forward bends to twists is another grouping in the classic schema that flows naturally.

Twists

Twists, like forward bends, have an overall calming effect. The floor twists are the dessert in our program, because at the end of the routine they just feel so good. Choose 1 floor twist from Chapter 13 for a 30-minute routine and 1 or 2 for a 60-minute routine. Figure 16-13 shows some common twists.

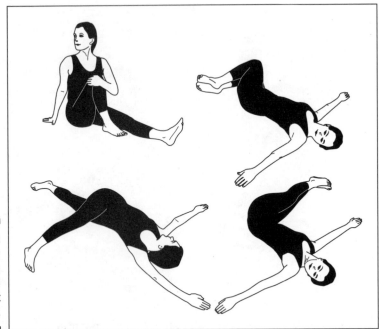

Figure 16-13:
Twists are calming postures and they just feel good.

Compensation for twists

Compensation for twists is always flexion, or a forward bend. After a floor twist, we usually recommend choosing one of the lying knees-to-chest or the knee-to-chest posture (see Chapter 6 and Figure 16-14).

Figure 16-14:
These postures help compensate for twists.

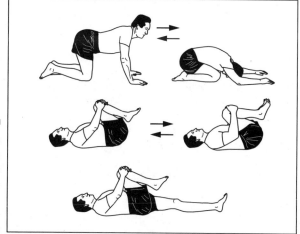

Relaxation

No matter how short your program, remember to include some form of relaxation. Rest provides a place where "absorption" can take place: You digest all the marvelous energies unleashed by your Yoga exercises.

This final category in our classic formula can take several forms: a relaxation technique (see Chapter 6), yogic breathing called *pranayama* (see Chapter 5), or meditation (see Chapter 20).

First, choose one of the rest postures from Chapter 6 or one of the sitting postures from Chapter 7. Next, select one of the breathing or *pranayama* techniques from Chapter 5, a relaxation technique from Chapter 4, and/or a meditation technique from Chapter 20. In a 60-minute routine you may choose both a breathing and a relaxation technique.

Whichever technique you choose, use it for at least 2 to 3 minutes and not more than 15 minutes.

Making the Most of Little: A 15-Minute Routine

Face it, available time is often limited. But rather than shelve your Yoga practice (and well-being), you can settle happily for a mini-routine. Even 15 minutes of Hatha Yoga can put you back on an even keel or remind your body and mind of how good stretching, moving, and breathing feel.

If we are honest with ourselves, most of us tend to spend a fair amount of time in idle motion — not really resting but not working either. Just picture revving your car engine when you're parked. We all have at least 15 minutes every day that we can put to good use to fortify our physical and mental health and/or put a dollar into our spiritual savings account.

When you opt for a 15-minute program, you need to be specific about your goals. Some of the more common uses for a short routine are

- ✔ A quick general conditioning program
- ✔ A stress-reduction and relaxation program
- ✔ A preparation program for Yoga breathing or meditation.

General conditioning

For the purposes of general conditioning, choose the following categories and do them in the order listed. You can also use the illustrations earlier in this chapter as a reference point.

The technique for each of the following postures as well as the recommended repetitions are listed in their corresponding chapters.

- ✔ Either a standing or sitting rest posture for attunement (see Chapters 7, 8, and Figure 16-1) and a Yoga breathing technique from Chapter 5.
- ✔ A dynamic series, such as either kneeling or standing sun salutation (see Chapter 14), the rejuvenation sequence, which counts as 3 or 4 postures (see Chapter 15), or 3 to 4 standing postures (see Chapter 8 and Figure 16-3) for 6 to 8 minutes.
- ✔ A lying twist (see Chapter 13 and Figure 16-13).
- ✔ Compensate with knees or knee-to-chest postures (see Chapter 6 and Figure 16-14).
- ✔ A lying or sitting rest posture (see Chapter 6 and Figure 16-1).
- ✔ A breathing exercise (see Chapter 5) and/or a relaxation technique (see Chapter 4).

Preparation for meditation and Yoga breathing

If you're looking for a routine to help you reduce stress, just plain relax, or prepare for meditation and Yoga breathing choose the following elements, and do them in the order listed:

- ✔ A lying or sitting posture for attunement (see Chapters 7, 8, and Figure 16-1) and a Yoga breathing technique from Chapter 5.

- ✔ Two lying warm-up postures, one that moves the arms and the other that moves the legs (see Chapter 6 and Figure 16-2).

- ✔ A supine (lying on your belly) back-bending posture such as the cobra or locust (see Chapter 12 and Figure 16-9) or a lying back bend such as the bridge (see Chapter 6 and Figure 16-6).

- ✔ A bent knee compensation exercise such as the child's pose or knees to chest (see Chapter 6 and Figure 16-10).

- ✔ A lying hamstring posture (see Chapter 6 and Figure 16-11).

- ✔ A lying twist (see Chapter 13 and Figure 16-13).

- ✔ A lying bent knee compensation exercise (see Chapter 6 and Figure 16-14).

- ✔ A lying or sitting rest posture (see Chapters 7, 8, and Figure 16-1) with a breathing exercise (see Chapter 5) and/or a relaxation technique (see Chapter 4).

Satisfying an Appetite for a Quick Pick-Me-Up: A 5-Minute Routine

A 5-minute program is the easiest to create. For a busy person, even 3 to 5 minutes once or twice a day can provide beneficial effects. Choose a rest posture from Chapter 6 or a sitting posture from Chapter 7 or Figure 16-1 and then select a yogic breathing or *pranayama* technique (see Chapter 5) for 3 to 5 minutes. You'll not only enjoy a quick, relaxing routine, but you'll also have at least 60 possible combinations to choose from.

Chapter 17

"Prop Art" — The Why and How of Simple Props

. . . .

In This Chapter

▶ Weighing the pros and cons of using props

▶ Relying on props you probably already own

▶ Investing in store-bought props for Yoga practice

▶ Unplugging any connection to gimmicks and gadgets

. . . .

The mainstay for any Yoga practice is, of course, the body-mind itself. However, props — physical means of support — may enhance your Yoga experience, especially if you're a beginner.

Traditionally, *yogis* and *yoginis* have relied on just a few basic props for their postural, breathing, and meditation practice — a bundle of grass or a tiger skin to sit on, a T-shaped arm rest (called *hamsa danda*) for prolonged meditation, and a *neti* pot. (A *neti* pot, which looks like an undersized pitcher, is a popular prop for cleansing the nasal cavities with lukewarm — often salted — water prior to the practice of breath control.)

Unfortunately, most Westerners' lifestyles and diet don't produce either a naturally balanced mind or well-trained body, so during Yoga practice special attention must be paid to conditions like chronic muscular contractions and skeletal misalignments A variety of props are now available to help make exercising safer and more comfortable in such cases.

Yoga's growing popularity in the Western world has spawned an industry of Yoga-related props — gear that can be complicated and costly. But as a beginner, you can find a few simple props around your house to help you exercise in spite of tight hamstrings, stiff hips, and an inflexible back.

Usually, a couple of blankets, a strap, a chair, or a wall for support is all that you need. Of course, using props has both pros and cons, but this chapter gives you enough information to make your own intelligent decisions about what you want to include in your Yoga practice, and in some of our other chapters we give you the option to use props for certain postures and also show you how to use them.

Deciphering the Pros and Cons of Props

In your Yoga practice, you can use props as extensively as you want or not at all. In any event, don't dismiss props as "silly" or "gimmicky." Determine on your own how props can help support your yogic practice. Rather than try to look like a magazine-cover or calendar Yoga model, listen to your own body's needs. A folded blanket under your hips can make all the difference when you want to sit cross-legged for more than a couple of minutes; or a wall can be a welcome support for your legs or back while doing particular postures.

Exploring the advantages of props

- They give you the added advantage of leverage in many postures.
- They help to improve your alignment, balance, and stability.
- Props like the *Invertebod* and the *Body Slant* provide the benefits of a classic inversion, such as a headstand, without compressing your neck.
- They allow you to participate more fully in a group class. With safe tools, you can perform some postures that would otherwise be inaccessible to you.
- They are, for the most part, relatively inexpensive and usually last for a long time.

Looking at drawbacks to props

- Some people, given the advantage of a prop, will go too far in a posture and injure themselves.
- You have to carry some props around with you when you go to a class.
- You can become too dependent on props, which inhibits your progress.

✔ Some props take time to set up and take down and can break the flow of a class, especially if you have to wait in line to get the prop and then put it away.

✔ Some props are expensive.

Going Prop Hunting at Home

Yoga has always favored an experimental approach. We suggest that you proceed in the same way. Find out for yourself what works and what doesn't work in your own case. Instead of giving up on a challenging posture, experiment with one or the other recommended prop. For instance, if you can't sit comfortably with your legs folded in the tailor's seat (*sukhasana*), then try placing a folded blanket or firm pillow under your hips. Remember, the human species prides itself on its use of tools. And usually, you have to look no further than your own address for a ready resource of handy props for your yogic practice.

Working with a wall

Walls are everywhere, they're free and, best of all, they're a versatile prop. You can use a wall in a great variety of postures, whether to support your buttocks and improve the angle of your forward bend, brace the back heel in the standing postures, or to support the backs of your legs in the reclining raised-legs relaxation position. Walls also can support you in the more advanced inverted postures, such as the half shoulder stand (see Chapter 11). The wall also works well as a frame of reference by which you can check your posture and alignment.

Using a blanket for more than bedding

Besides the obvious use of keeping you warm during relaxation, blankets can prop the hips in sitting postures, the head and neck in lying postures, and the waist in prone back bends like the locust posture. You also can use blankets as protective padding under the knees when kneeling. Always be sure to fold the blanket thickly, or use more than one blanket when the need arises to raise the hips (or head or shoulders). Also, always use firm, flat blankets for props.

Most blankets nowadays are made out of synthetic materials (or synthetic/wool blend), so don't worry about your allergy. The firmness of the blanket is important. You want something under your knees or neck that won't sink or collapse, as would a padded blanket or comforter.

Choosing a chair for comfort

A folding metal chair or a sturdy wooden chair without arms can have multiple uses as a prop in Yoga. Many, if not most, beginners have a hard time sitting on the floor for prolonged periods during meditation or breathing exercises, and sitting on a chair is a great alternative to sitting on the floor. Make sure, though, that your feet are not dangling; if they don't easily touch the floor, place your feet on a phone book. Students with back problems often use a chair during the relaxation phase at the end of a Yoga class. Lying on your back and placing your lower legs up on a chair, combined with guided relaxation techniques from the instructor can really help to release back tension or pain. You can find numerous books and magazine articles about doing your entire Yoga practice in a chair, with suggestions for ways to take Yoga chair breaks around the house, or in your office for a quick pick-me-up.

Stretching with a strap

You most frequently use a strap with postures that involve stretching the hamstrings, most commonly from a supine reclining (lying on your back) or sitting position. Someone's old karate belt or necktie works great, but so does a rolled-up towel or a bathrobe belt. You also can order an *official* Yoga strap from one of the mail-order companies (see the appendix).

Prop proliferation

Yoga props and accessories from around the world are now big business in the United States. Yoga Master BKS Iyengar of Pune (pronounced Poon-ah) more than any other teacher has influenced the development of props for Hatha Yoga in modern times. Americans, however, have made some of their own breakthroughs in the area of Yoga-inspired props.

Renowned sports medicine physician Leroy R. Perry Jr., D.C., founder of the International Sports Medicine Institute in Los Angeles, California, has sold over 10,000 units of his *Invertebod*, a spinal decompression-inversion device, to Yoga teachers and Yoga enthusiasts internationally. Yoga teacher Larry Jacobs of Newport Beach, California, inventor of the *Body Slant* (see the "Body Slant" section for more information), offers an entire line of safe and practical inversion furniture through mainstream mail-order catalogs nationally.

Searching Out Props You May Want to Purchase

As you gain comfort and confidence with your yogic exercises, you're sure to become curious about the array of props you either see being used in class or hear about from your association with fellow Yoga practitioners. Whether you plan to spend freely as you experiment with the best props for your personal situation, or you expect to approach buying a bit more conservatively, keep in mind that you're likely to find a sweeping range of merchandise and price tags out there in consumer land. By investing wisely — with product research, plus understanding of your own needs — you can enjoy greater rewards from your Yoga experience (see Figure 17-1).

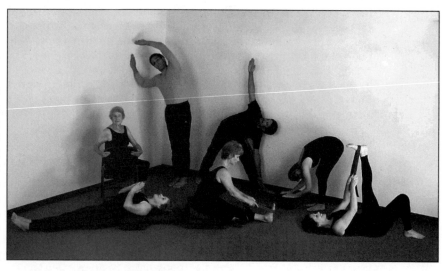

Figure 17-1: Just another day at a Malibu Yoga class: walls, straps, bolsters, blocks, and chairs.

Building better postures with the help of blocks

Some styles of Yoga incorporate wooden blocks (or sturdy foam blocks) for improving or facilitating certain postures. Either is fine, although wood is ten dollars higher. A block is especially helpful in standing twists, when your bottom hand cannot make it to the floor, or in standing forward bends, to support your hands. For beginners, put the block down on the floor horizontally or lying flat. Think of the block as a raised floor to support you. Try not to clutch the block with your hands, just use it to aid your balance. If you decide to make your own block, a good standard is nine inches high, six inches wide, and four inches deep. Be sure that the block is well-sanded and varnished to eliminate the possibility of splinters. Two blocks is plenty for your own personal use. Foam blocks are about $11, wood blocks about $20.

Students may prefer the more substantial feel and heft of a wooden block, or they may like the lightness of foam (especially if they drop the block on a floor or foot). Two blocks are ideal, but you can get by with one. You can also tightly wrap up an old hardback book or two in some masking tape and use that for support.

Bolstering support with pillows

Bolsters are large, firm, usually rectangular or oval pillows. You use them to support your knees in reclining postures, to help release the lower back and to raise the buttocks in forward bends, and to help soften tight hips and hamstrings. You can also place bolsters under your upper back so that when you lie over them you help open the chest. During the stress of pregnancy, bolsters are a great support for the side-lying posture (see Chapter 21). A good standard size for bolsters is 6 x 12 x 25 inches for the rectangular bolsters and 9 x 27 inches for the cylindrical shape. You can also buy a pranayama bolster (see Chapter 5) that is long and thin (about 8 x 30 inches). Bolsters cost from $35 to $50. One is usually plenty for your personal use. You can create your own bolsters by using thickly rolled blankets. In a pinch, sofa or bed pillows work, too — if they're not too soft. Bolsters are usually made of thick cotton batting with a removable canvas covering that you can wash.

Facing the many applications of eye bags

Eye bags — small bags filled with light materials (usually plastic pellets) — are used widely for various relaxation techniques. Although an eye bag may seem self-explanatory, there's actually more to an eye bag than, well, meets the eye. Eye bags, of course, block light (and visual stimuli), which helps to quiet the brain; they also put gentle pressure on the eyes, which slows the heart rate. You can just cover your eyes with a towel, but the effect is not quite the same. Eye bags are available in many shapes and sizes. Some eye bags are packed with herbal essences, which adds the in-scent-ive (no pun intended) of aroma therapy, but be sure the perfume isn't too strong so as to become bothersome. Eye bags are usually about 4 x 8 inches and cost from $10 to $20, depending on which type use choose (see the appendix). One eye bag is usually placed across the top of both eyes while you're in a lying position on your back. Some more expensive models tie down like a mask, which is usually unnecessary. If you decide to make your own eye bags, use materials such as cotton stuffed with rice to silk stuffed with flax seed. Be sure to do a good job on the seams, you don't want flax seed in your eyes!

If you are a do-it-yourselfer, you could make an eye bag out of an old sock and some rice or flax. Or you could fold up a thick towel and lay it across your eyes.

Turning to inversion props

We purposely omitted the headstand and the full shoulder stand from this book because we feel that these postures require the guidance of a competent Yoga teacher. Because our Western-world necks have become so weak and vulnerable, many physicians, and a large number of chiropractors, orthopedists, and osteopaths are not in favor of inverted Yoga postures, such as the headstand, the full shoulder stand, and the plow, because they can compress the neck. Because the benefits of inversion and reversing the pull of gravity are so great (see Chapter 11), many entrepreneurs have attempted over the last two decades to create safe and effective inversion devices.

You now have quite a selection of inversion apparatuses to suit various bodies and budgets. We feel that the following two are on the cutting edge of effectiveness, safety, and convenience.

Ask your physician before using the *Body Slant*, the *Invertebod*, or any new exercise device, to be sure that the prop is all right for your personal situation.

Avoid using the *Body Slant* or the *Invertebod* if you have the following conditions: glaucoma, hiatal hernia, high blood pressure, or heart disease, or if you have suffered a stroke.

Body Slant

The *Body Slant* (see Figure 17-2) created by yogi Larry Jacobs is the high-tech version of what used to be called Grandma's Slant Board. Three pieces of firm foam that fold and unfold easily make inversion safe and simple. Just lie back for 10 minutes to receive the rejuvenating effects of inversion (see the appendix).

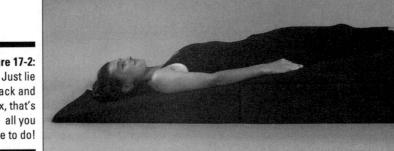

Figure 17-2:
Just lie
back and
relax, that's
all you
have to do!

Invertebod

Many health professionals consider Dr. Leroy R. Perry's *Invertebod* to be the top of the line in the Yoga inversion-decompression systems (see Figure 17-3).

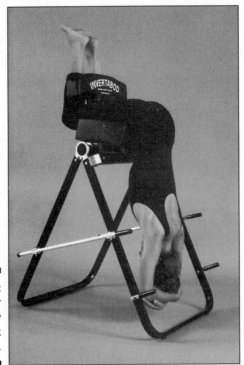

Figure 17-3:
A lifesaver
for many
back
problems.

The apparatus is known to be very effective in the treatment of back problems such as scoliosis, herniated and bulging discs, and muscle imbalance. Users hang forward comfortably from their thighs, which eliminates knee and ankle problems created by earlier inventions. You also can perform numerous additional therapeutic exercises while hanging on the Invertebod with the guidance of your health professional. Dr. Perry recommends that just hanging two and one-half minutes twice a day is all that's necessary to receive the benefits of the *Invertebod* (see the appendix for more information).

Relaxing with harmony screens

Of all the relaxation props on the market, we know of only one *nonelectronic* device that can actually help you relax. The apparatus uses your own body's energies to facilitate the relaxation response. Ernest Eeman invented the device, which goes by a variety of names (including *Eeman screens*, *polarity screens*, and *harmony screens*), in the 1920s. It consists of two small copper plates (or wire meshes), each of which attaches to a copper wire with a copper handle. You place one plate under your neck, the other under your lower back. You hold the handle of the neck plate in your left hand, the handle of the other plate in your right hand. With this device, you can balance and even strengthen the body's energy field. Even 15 minutes of rest on these plates can feel very rejuvenating. You also can use the plates or screens to combat insomnia, headaches, and jet lag. One of us (Georg Feuerstein) has used harmony screens on and off for the past 15 years and is so impressed with them that he makes them available through the Yoga Research Center (see the appendix for more information).

Avoiding Snake Oil Salesmen

In your travels over the Yoga path, you may encounter numerous electronic gadgets that promise to synchronize or harmonize your brain hemispheres or otherwise tune your nervous system to instantly give you the same benefits as yogic meditation — without the tedious discipline. Some of these gadgets are downright dangerous, others are useless, and very few may have at least some of the positive effects that they claim. Most Yoga masters and teachers look on such devices as mere gimmicks.

The fact is that no shortcut exists to the profound meditative states of Yoga; the only reliable route is direct control of your own mind. As Patanjali states at the beginning of his *Yoga-Sutra:* "Yoga is the control of the whirls of the mind." Yoga is about permanently changing your body-mind rather than merely temporarily altering your consciousness. Yogic practice isn't about having extraordinary experiences but rather making your most ordinary experiences significant by bringing full awareness to them.

Part V
Yoga as a Lifestyle

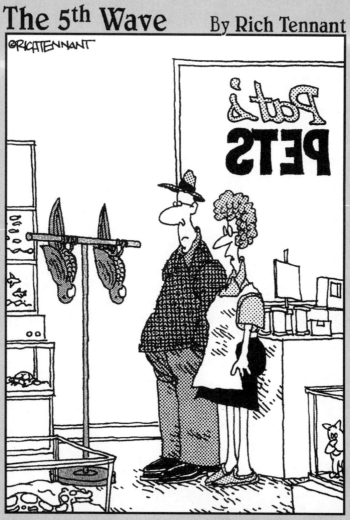

The 5th Wave   By Rich Tennant

"They belonged to someone who taught Yoga, and aside from hanging upside down from time to time, they're very quiet and well behaved."

In this part . . .

The focus in Parts II–IV was primarily on the physical exercises of Yoga. If practiced regularly, they can certainly improve your health and fitness and even positively affect your emotional and mental well-being. But, as we indicated in the Introduction and in Chapter 1, Yoga is a great deal more than physical exercise.

In this part, we show you how you can adopt Yoga as a lifestyle that will bring you inner peace and happiness, as well as the capacity to become a beacon of light for your family, friends, coworkers, and others. We specifically talk about the power of living with moral integrity, the deeper significance of sexuality, and your enormous spiritual potential. We also discuss how you can use Yoga for special situations.

Chapter 18

Yoga throughout the Day

- -

In This Chapter

▶ Applying Yoga throughout the day

▶ Looking inward for health and harmony

▶ Developing moral practices

▶ Rising above the ego's boundaries

▶ Reaping rewards from self-restraint

- -

*T*he postures and breathing exercises of Hatha Yoga — some of which we cover in preceding chapters — are merely a couple of tools from Yoga's well-stocked storehouse. When practiced correctly, they are extremely useful and potent in helping you regain or maintain your physical and mental health. Practicing postures and breathing can stabilize and boost your body's vitality and even harmonize your emotions and strengthen your mind.

But postures and breathing exercises are only a beginning; they are only two steps in the eightfold path of Raja Yoga (see Chapter 1 for more about the eightfold path). The real power of Yoga is unlocked when you approach it as a *lifestyle* or *spiritual path.* Yoga contains everything you need in order to transform your entire day — from rising in the morning, all the way through the night, and rising again. Just as a grand piano allows you to play music in eight octaves, Yoga gives you the means to tap into your full potential as a human being.

In this chapter, we show you how you can connect with your deeper potential and live your entire day the Yoga way. This approach includes paying proper attention to moral values, which are an important aspect of all branches and schools of Yoga but are often overlooked by Western practitioners.

Living Your Day the Yoga Way

When you decide to pursue Yoga as a lifestyle or spiritual discipline, you must be willing to practice it 24 hours a day, 7 days a week. You may think that this total commitment sounds difficult, and with good reason — living this way is truly a challenge! At least, staying on track is difficult while you're busy creating new habit patterns by laying down new pathways in your brain. After you change your thoughts and behavior, living the Yoga way is as easy as living any other routine, except the yogic lifestyle is far from routine.

Yoga is a *conscious* way of life. The power behind Yoga's extraordinary effectiveness is *awareness*.

Turning your face toward a Yoga morning

For thousands of years, Yoga practitioners have begun the day at sunrise, a time that's considered to be auspicious and especially potent for meditation, prayer, and tapping into your highest potential. Called *brahma-muhurta* in Sanskrit (pronounced *brah-mah moo-hoor-tah*), which means literally "hour of brahman" — brahman being the ultimate Reality — this time sets the right tone for the entire day.

Sunrise is not only a quiet and peaceful time, but also a time that's charged with symbolic significance for Yoga practitioners. Traditionally, the sun is celebrated as the first teacher, or *guru*, who brought the teachings of Yoga to humanity. According to Yoga, the sun is a symbol for the spirit, which shines with undiminished brightness forever. The sun salutation exercise described in Chapter 14 is one way in which yogis acknowledge their reverence for the inner sun.

Of course, India (Yoga's native home) is blessed with a lot of sunshine. Even if your climate doesn't offer much physical sun, you can still enjoy sunrise as a special, daily occasion — just ponder the sun's profound symbolism!

Too much of a good thing

Exposure to sunlight early in the morning is beneficial. Later on, the sun's ultraviolet rays become lethal, causing skin cancer from prolonged exposure. Yoga practitioners refrain from the widespread practice of baking in the sun (or under an artificial light source) to achieve a tan.

Here are some suggestions for transforming an otherwise mundane daily routine into a meaningful ritual that can energize and prepare you for the onslaught of the day:

- ✔ **Create a peaceful mood in your heart and remember your connection with everyone and everything.** Do this as soon as you wake up and before opening your eyes and getting out of bed. If you believe in a divine being (call it God, Goddess, or higher Self), this is a good moment for inwardly aligning yourself to it/him/her.

- ✔ **Write down any significant dreams.** When you live an active life of self-transformation, dreams often carry important messages. They may mirror and confirm your present inner development or stream of experiences, or they may provide you with a key for understanding what you are going through. If you don't write down your dreams shortly after waking, you're likely to forget them. If you find that they fade from your mind rapidly, you may want to consider jotting them down in your diary before making your daily resolution *samkalpa* (pronounced *sahm-kahl-pah*), which we cover next.

- ✔ **Affirm your highest resolve.** For example, repeat (aloud or in your mind) your resolution, such as "I intend to act all day long in accordance to the highest spiritual and moral principles," "I intend to be (more) compassionate today," "I intend to harm no one and benefit as many people as possible," "I intend to be kind and loving today," "I intend to speak only healing words today," "I intend to think only positive, benign thoughts today," "I intend to bless everyone today," "I intend to remember my true nature as often as possible throughout the day," and so on. Repeat your intention *(samkalpa)* with great conviction three or more times.

  Remembering an affirmation throughout the day is often difficult for beginning students. Try carrying something small around with you, such as a pebble, a button, or a ring, which will jog your memory whenever you see or touch it.

- ✔ **Before getting out of bed, consciously relax and take ten deep breaths.**

- ✔ **Stretch and thus fire up your muscles while you're still in bed.**

- ✔ **Use the bathroom, wash, and brush your teeth.**

- ✔ **Meditate.** If you meditate sitting on your bed, your mind will inevitably associate "bed" with "sleep." See Chapter 20 for more information on the art of meditation. Some authorities recommend that you do postures and breathing exercises before meditation, but we feel this preparation is only necessary when your mind tends to be sluggish in the early morning and you need to jumpstart it. If you wake up easily and happily in the morning, use that time for meditation or prayer.

- ✔ **Do your Hatha Yoga program to vitalize your body and fortify your mind.**

If you can't practice in the morning because, for example, you have to be at work when the rooster crows, make sure that you leave room in your schedule for Hatha Yoga and/or meditation at some other time during the day or in the evening. Even a few minutes of postures and breathing exercises are better than no exercises at all. But more importantly, always start your day right by making your resolution upon waking and centering yourself by breathing consciously.

If you have a family, make formal agreements with your partner and/or children so that you can practice Yoga as undisturbed as possible. Be sure that everyone is aware of and honors *your* private time. If need be, lock your door or put up a reminder sign on the outside. You may not always be able to get private time, especially when you have young children. In that case, try to do whatever practices you can while you're still in bed, and then include your children in your Yoga program. As a parent, you are the best role model for your children, and even toddlers can participate in your Yoga practice.

Some people are super-busy — going to bed late at night after they're exhausted and starting out the next morning still feeling tired. A regular Hatha Yoga routine can give you energy, making regular practice well worth the time it takes. Beyond the physical and mental benefits, Yoga provides much-needed quiet time, where you can be by yourself without distraction. If your situation permits, arrange to have 15 minutes a day that you can consider all yours. Make a creative deal with your partner and/or children that can benefit everyone.

Or, if you live alone and feel the pressures of time and attention to lots of details, just negotiate an agreement with the person who shows up in your mirror. You can be a better friend to that face if you set aside some time for inward glances.

Yoga with your youngsters

If you have young children and have no leisure time to practice Yoga on your own, don't despair! Make the most of the situation. As the saying goes, if you can't conquer them, join them. Your kids will love it — at least while the novelty lasts. Depending on their age and general disposition, the youngsters may get used to this little routine and happily participate in it or, if not, they may at least allow you to practice your own Yoga routine without too many interruptions. If you don't want them to get bored, you must make the session fun for the kids. As you well know, the universe revolves around children and their needs — until they learn otherwise. Your own peacefulness can definitely have a calming effect on them. Look at the section "Introducing Children to Yoga" in Chapter 21.

Practicing Yoga throughout the day

You have many opportunities to apply the wisdom of Yoga as activities and situations during the day. Whether you stay at home with your children or hold down a job outside the home, you have at your disposal an array of tools from Yoga's versatile toolbox for all circumstances. Here are only a few situations in which you can fruitfully apply yogic wisdom (remember that any situation can benefit from good Yoga practice):

- ✔ Running into heavy traffic during your daily commute to and from work
- ✔ Dealing with customers, a demanding boss, or fellow employees
- ✔ Enjoying breakfast, lunch, and dinner (see sidebar)
- ✔ Experiencing pregnancy and childbirth (see Chapter 21)
- ✔ Responding when your child's behavior leaves much to be desired
- ✔ Living through a health crisis
- ✔ Enjoying vacations and holidays
- ✔ Doing the daily shopping
- ✔ Grieving over the death of a loved one
- ✔ Watching television
- ✔ Having sex (see Chapter 19)

To all these situations you can bring awareness, which is the foundation for all other positive attitudes and practices. You can also bring understanding, patience, calmness, forgiveness, kindness, compassion, love, good humor, and a host of other virtues. By practicing various Yoga techniques, you can also calm your mind and raise your energy level or bring energy to others.

Don't think of the world as "out there" and your Yoga practice as "in here." Because Yoga connects inside and outside, such a distinction is artificial. Allow your practice to flow over into all situations. You're never so busy that you can't transform a few seconds of free time into meaningful time through Yoga: Exhale deeply, center yourself, silently recite a *mantra*, or bless someone.

The yogic art of conscious eating

What you eat forms your body. In turn, the condition of your body and especially the nervous system affects your mind. Your state of mind affects your entire life. Thus the traditional maxim "You are what you eat" holds true to a certain degree. Hence Yoga masters, typically, have been vegetarians, favoring grains, legumes, and fruit. In your diet, stick as close to Mother Nature as possible.

(continued)

(continued)

As important as *what* you eat, is *how* you eat. Of all the recommendations made by Yoga masters, the single most important is to *practice moderation*. This is called *mitahara* (from *mita* or "moderate" and *ahara* or "food" in Sanskrit, pronounced *mee-tah-hah-rah*). It implies:

✔ Don't overeat.

✔ Don't starve yourself.

Overeating not only puts pounds on you but also multiplies toxins in your body and makes you feel emotionally weighed down. Similarly, if you don't feed your body adequately, you will weaken it and also run the risk of causing disease. The best policy is to eat only when you are hungry (not merely a little peckish). The right amount to eat varies from person to person, and also according to climate and season. Find out for yourself by trial and error. Remember, though, that certain health conditions require frequent eating.

Another important yogic rule about diet is to eat with awareness. Here are some simple suggestions for changing unyogic or mechanical habits while you eat:

✔ Calm down first if you are agitated.

✔ Keep your attention on the task of eating.

✔ Eat slowly and chew your food well.

✔ Pay attention to all the wonderful taste sensations in your mouth.

✔ Breathe.

✔ Be grateful for your food.

Incorporating Yoga into nighttime routines

When you live Yoga as a spiritual discipline, the practice extends even to your sleep. In Chapter 6, we give you a relaxation technique that's better than any sleeping pill for preparing you for sleep. You can make this technique even more powerful by repeating the same intention *(samkalpa)* that you also use upon waking: "I intend to be more aware," "I intend to be more compassionate," "I intend to be a better listener," "I intend to be true to my innermost feelings," and so on. Repeat your intention when your relaxation is deepest and before emerging from it or falling asleep.

Sleeping peacefully with lucid dreaming

You can benefit from taking note of your dreams, keeping a diary of at least the more significant ones. But dedicated yogis and yoginis seek to transform their dream life altogether by training themselves in *lucid dreaming,* a special state of consciousness in which you retain a degree of self-awareness while dreaming. In other words, you know that you're dreaming and, with practice, even are able to direct your dreams. Usually lucid dreaming occurs spontaneously, but by priming your mind before going to sleep you can increase the likelihood of becoming self-aware in the midst of a dream. If you're interested in exploring this art, we recommend that you study the resources listed in this book's appendix. In the meantime, here are some pointers for programming yourself to dream lucidly:

- ✔ Become generally more aware of your thoughts, feelings, and sensations.

- ✔ Take an interest in your dreams.

- ✔ Get up a couple of hours earlier than usual and go about your regular chores.

- ✔ Slip back into bed and for about 30 minutes think about lucid dreaming and what sort of dream you want to create.

- ✔ Allow yourself at least two hours for dreaming before finally getting up.

- ✔ Induce lucid dreaming by doing the kind of deep relaxation exercise ("Yoga Nidra") that we describe in Chapter 4.

- ✔ Clearly form the intention to dream lucidly.

You may not succeed the first or second time you try, but then again, pleasant surprises may be just a dream away!

Aiming toward awareness through lucid waking

More important than lucid dreaming is *lucid waking* — the art of being present in the moment, of living with mindfulness throughout the day. In a way, lucid dreaming is an extension of lucid waking. If you acquire the knack of becoming aware in the dream state, but continue to sleepwalk in your waking life, you can't expect to gain very much. If you're aware but lacking in understanding or wisdom in the waking state, you'll also lack understanding or wisdom in the dream state. Yoga is first and foremost about lucid waking, which means penetrating the illusions and delusions of ordinary life with the searchlight of full awareness. After you clear your mind of its inherent misconceptions and biases, you can bring the same clear mind to nonordinary states of consciousness, including dreaming and deep sleep.

Swami Rama baffles scientists

In 1969, Swami Rama volunteered to have his yogic abilities tested at the Menninger Foundation in Topeka, Kansas. Among other things, he demonstrated his ability to produce all types of brain waves at will. He remained fully aware even when producing slow delta waves characteristic of deep sleep. In fact, he was able to remember what happened during his supposed deep sleep much better than did the researchers themselves. Two years later, Swami Rama (1925–1996) founded the Himalayan Institute in Honesdale, Pennsylvania, which continues to spread his teachings. Check out the appendix for the Institute's address.

Approaching mindfulness in deep sleep

For the serious Yoga practitioner, even deep sleep is not a no-man's land. On the contrary, dreamless sleep is a great opportunity for breaking into higher levels of consciousness. After you are able to retain mindful awareness during the dream state, you can extend your awareness to those periods where the mind is devoid of contents. The great Yoga masters are continuously aware throughout the day and the night. They are never unconscious, because they have realized the spirit, or Self, which is pure consciousness.

If constant awareness sounds exhausting, consider the deep peacefulness that the Yoga masters are able to achieve. Pure consciousness is the simplest thing in the world. Hence, it's called the "natural state," or *sahaja-avastha*, which is pronounced *sah-hah-jah ah-vahst-hah*. By comparison, the mind is vastly complicated. Just remember how thinking (especially when you're obsessing over something) can be incredibly exhausting.

Seeking Your Higher Self by Discovering the True You

However they may conceive the ultimate goal, all schools of Yoga seek to open a door to your true nature, which we call the *spirit* or *higher Self*. There are as many approaches to Self-realization (or enlightenment) as there are human beings. Everyone's spiritual journey is unique, yet our inner evolution follows certain universal principles. The most significant principle is that in order to discover our essential nature, we must overcome the gravity pull of our ordinary habit patterns (laid down as neural pathways in our brain).

You can say that there are numerous approaches to Self-realization, such as Hatha Yoga or the eightfold path of Raja Yoga, but there is only one underlying process. That fundamental process is marked by progressive *self-observation, self-understanding, self-discipline,* and *self-transcendence,* which are all interconnected practices.

Observing yourself

In Yoga, you simply begin to observe yourself. Staying in tune with yourself is different from the neurotic self-watching that is merely a form of self-involvement. Self-observation means being consciously aware of how you think and behave without judging yourself in any way.

Self-observation includes noticing — in a nonjudgmental way — how you react to people and situations. For instance, you may discover that in many ways, you're often overly critical or too gullible and accommodating. Or you may determine that you tend to be rather inward and afraid of engaging life or that you never think before you leap. The natural calmness that you create through Yoga's physical exercises can help you start uncovering your tendencies — without collapsing into self-recrimination or exploding into anger with others.

Understanding yourself

Based on self-observation, self-understanding involves grasping the deeper reasons for your habit patterns. Ultimately, self-understanding is the realization that all your thoughts and behaviors revolve around the ego, an artificial psychological pole. Your ego allows you to identify yourself in a very specific way. For example:

"I am Frank, a 35-year-old, Caucasian male and a United States citizen. I am 5 foot 11 inches tall, of athletic build, weigh 165 pounds, and have blue eyes and brown hair. I am married, have two children, and am an electronic engineer who likes to go parachuting. I am a capitalist, reasonably ambitious, but not very religious."

These ego-identifications are useful in your daily life — as long as they don't cause you to feel separated from your spiritual core or to create barriers to other people.

You have to be very careful not to take the ego habit too seriously; the ego is nothing more than a way of quickly identifying yourself both verbally and psychologically. It is not your true nature, the spirit or Self. Most importantly, it is not an actual entity in its own right but merely something we habitually do. The ego is based on the process of self-contraction (*atma-samkoca*, pronounced *aht-mah sahm-koh-chah*). The symbol for the ego is a clenched fist. Yoga shows you how to release that fist and engage life from the viewpoint of the spirit or Self, which is in harmonious relationship with everyone and everything.

Practicing self-discipline

When a seed sprouts, it must first push through the soil before it can benefit from the sunlight. Similarly, before you can experience the higher levels of Yoga, you must overcome the built-in lethargy of your ego-driven personality, which doesn't want to change. Self-observation and self-understanding become increasingly effective through the practice of *self-discipline* — the steady cultivation of spiritual practices.

By exercising voluntary self-control over your thoughts, behaviors, and energies, you can gradually transform your body-mind into a finely tuned instrument for higher spiritual realizations and harmonious living. You can't practice self-discipline without frustrating the ego a little, because the ego always tends to move along the path of least resistance. Yogic practice creates the necessary resistance to spark further growth in you.

Transcending yourself

Self-transcendence is at the heart of the spiritual process. This impulse and practice of going beyond the ego-contraction in every moment — through self-observation, self-understanding, and self-discipline — comes to full blossom in the great event of enlightenment, when your entire being is transformed by the spirit, or Self (see Chapter 20).

Making Inroads into the Eightfold Path

The eightfold path of Yoga, as we outline it in Chapter 1, is a useful model for the stages of the yogic process. In the following, we explain the first two limbs of the eightfold path in more detail, because they give you the essential moral foundation for practicing Yoga successfully. We start with the five practices of moral discipline *(yama),* which Yoga insists that you must practice under all circumstances. They are the same moral virtues that you find in all the world's great religious traditions:

- Nonharming or *ahimsa* (pronounced *ah-heem-sah*)
- Truthfulness or *satya* (pronounced *saht-yah*)
- Nonstealing or *asteya* (pronounced *ahs-the-yah*)
- Chastity or *brahmacarya* (pronounced *brah-mah-chahr-yah*)
- Greedlessness or *aparigraha* (pronounced *ah-pah-ree-grah-hah*)

These five disciplines are meant to harmonize your interpersonal life and are especially important in today's enormously complex world. Much of the social chaos in today's world is due to the collapse of a common system of basic moral values. Yoga reminds you that you can't attain self-fulfillment in isolation from others. You cannot hope to realize your higher nature without fostering what is good and beautiful in your day-to-day life in interaction with your family, friends, coworkers, teachers, and students. Thus, universally recognized moral virtues are the rich soil in which you plant all your other efforts on the path of inner growth and ultimate Self-realization (or enlightenment).

Yoga understands these virtues to be all-comprehensive, extending not only to your *actions* but also to your *language* and even your *thoughts.* In other words, you are called to abstain from doing wrong to others, speaking wrong of them, as well as poisoning them with your thoughts.

Vowing to do no harm

The practice of nonharming comes — or should come — into play hundreds of times a day. The more sensitive you become toward the effect that you have on others, the more you are called to live with moral mindfulness. How do you practice the virtue of nonharming in your life? You may think of yourself as a fairly harmless individual, because you don't physically or verbally abuse anyone, but have you ever started or listened to gossip? And what about feeling negatively toward an annoying client or customer or feeling angry with an inconsiderate driver who just took your parking space?

Moreover, nonharming is not only merely abstaining from harmful actions, speech, and thoughts, but also actively doing what is appropriate in a given moment to avoid unnecessary pain to others. For example, even withholding a smile or kind word from someone when you sense that the gesture may benefit that person is a form of harming.

In order to live, we involuntarily harm and even kill other beings — just think of the billions of microorganisms in your food and even in your own body that give up their lives so that you can stay alive and be healthy. The ideal of nonharming is just that: an ideal to which you may aspire. The concept calls for abstaining from deliberately harming other beings. As a useful exercise, ask yourself these questions:

- ✔ How many times today have I spoken harshly?

- ✔ When did I last kill a harmless spider instead of leaving it alone or relocating it?

- ✔ Are my thoughts about things and people preponderantly pessimistic, overly optimistic, or simply realistic?

- ✔ When I have to correct someone's behavior do I merely criticize or also encourage?

Yoga definitely expects you to control your anger and murderous thoughts — not to be confused with merely suppressing your feelings (which never works anyway). Yoga also encourages you to cultivate, *step by step,* better habits and mental dispositions. As you become more peaceful and content, you won't react so strongly and irrationally to life's pressures, but become more and more able to go with the flow — with awareness, a smile, and a helping hand. According to Yoga, a person grounded in nonharming is surrounded by such an aura of peace that even wild beasts become tame.

If you become aware of the various ways in which you harm others through your thoughts, words, and actions, don't succumb to feeling overwhelmed with guilt. That negative response is just another way of perpetuating violence. Simply acknowledge the situation, feel remorse, resolve to behave differently, and then also actively change your mental, verbal, and physical behavior.

Telling the truth all the time

These days, we seem to believe that truth is relative. Yoga, however, insists that facts and perspectives are many, but truth is always one and that truthfulness *(satya)* is a supreme moral virtue. Truth is the cement that holds together good relationships and entire societies.

The sorry condition of our own modern society says something about our commitment to truth, or rather the lack of it. For instance, consider the following questions:

- ✔ Have you ever told a "little white lie" not because you wanted to protect someone but because you deemed it more convenient than to tell the truth?

- ✔ Have you ever prettified or omitted certain facts from your resumé to look more suitable to a prospective employer?

- ✔ Have you ever failed to declare taxable income (even that small negligible amount that no one could possibly care about)?

- ✔ Have you ever instructed your spouse to say you aren't at home when an unwanted caller is on the phone for you?

- ✔ Have you ever lied about your age?

- ✔ Do you ever fail to keep your promises? (This question is a must for politicians.)

Probably, few people can answer all these questions with a resounding "No," unless, of course, they are lying to themselves. Admittedly, lies appear to vary by degree of severity. You may consider these examples fairly insignificant, and from a conventional point of view, they are. But Yoga doesn't let you off the hook so easily. Yogic practice values simplicity and clarity, whereas lying usually ends up being more complicated and confusing. Yoga is also concerned about the pathways you build in your brain. If you become accustomed to not telling the truth in little matters, sooner or later you may not be able to distinguish truth from falsehood in big matters as well.

Truthfulness is a marvelous tool for keeping your energy pure and your will undiluted.

Of course, in your attempts to be truthful, you must bear the principal moral virtue of nonharming in mind. Life is not black and white; many gray areas exist. If speaking the truth may bring more harm than good to another person, you're wise to remain silent. As with nonharming, your *intention* is the key.

Stealing means more than material theft

Nonstealing (*asteya*), the third moral discipline, is trickier than it looks at casual glance. You need not be a pickpocket, shoplifter, bank robber, or embezzler to violate this virtue. From the perspective of Yoga, depriving someone of his or her due reward or good name is also theft. So is appropriating someone's ideas without due acknowledgment, stealing someone's boyfriend or girlfriend, or denying your child proper parental guidance.

Our highly competitive society is designed to promote self-centeredness to the point where we constantly infringe the virtues of nonharming, truthfulness, and nonstealing. The kind of aggressive competitiveness that is rampant in the business world is all about elbowing your way to the top, beating the other guy, using any means necessary to outsmart your opponent, and winning the game at all costs.

To ponder the ideal of nonstealing, you may want to answer these questions:

- ✔ What percentage of your income do you allocate for charitable causes?

- ✔ Have you ever used someone else's time left on a parking meter, knowing that this widespread practice is actually in violation of the law?

- ✔ Are any of your computer programs bootlegged copies (a criminal offense)?

- ✔ Did you ever withhold love from a family member or friend because you wanted to punish him or her?

Traditionally, those people who are well-established in the virtue of nonstealing are described as always being sustained by life; they never lack anything for their further growth. The greatest antidote to the vice of stealing is generosity. A fulfilling life is a life in which giving and taking are elegantly balanced.

Observing chastity in thought and deed

Chastity (*brahmacarya,* pronounced *brah-mah-chahr-yah*), which is a highly valued virtue in all traditional societies, means abstention from inappropriate sexual behavior. According to Yoga, only adults who are also married householders should be sexually active. All others should practice sexual abstinence. For many Westerners, this standard is very difficult.

Yogically speaking, you must extend the ideal of chastity to action, speech, and even thought. We leave it up to you to determine where, in your own case, you can change your behavior to bring it more in line with Yoga's moral orientation. Bear in mind that Yoga isn't asking you to go against human nature, which includes sexuality. Rather, Yoga invites you to consider your higher spiritual potential. The Yoga masters recommend chastity not for prudish reasons but because it's an effective way of harnessing your body's vital energy. The practitioner who is firmly grounded in chastity is said to obtain vigor or vitality.

If you engage Yoga as a lifestyle or spiritual discipline, periodically taking stock of your virtues and vices can help you build toward achievement of your higher Self. When considering your sexuality, ask yourself:

- ✔ Do I tend to use sexually suggestive or explicit language?
- ✔ Do I use sex for emotional security or for personal power?
- ✔ Am I flirtatious and, if so, why?
- ✔ Do I know the distinction between sex and love?
- ✔ Am I capable of true intimacy, or do I treat my partner as a sex object?

Acquiring more by living with less

Greed — the habit of needing more and more, especially money — is a vice that underlies much of modern consumerism. From a yogic point of view, greed is a failed search for happiness, because whatever possessions you may acquire cannot fulfill you. On the contrary, the more you are surrounded by "stuff," the more likely you are to experience a big gaping hole in your soul. Intrinsically, money and possessions aren't "wrong," but few people ever master the art of relating to them properly. Instead of owning things, they are owned (controlled) by them.

Yoga holds high the ideal of voluntary simplicity — to choose to live simply. How do you measure up to it? Try to answer these questions honestly:

- ✔ Have you ever been called a miser?
- ✔ Do you have too much "stuff"?
- ✔ Do you expect to be pampered?
- ✔ Do you tend to overeat?
- ✔ Do you accumulate money and possessions because you worry about the future?
- ✔ Are you overly attached to your partner or child?
- ✔ Do you like to be the center of attention?
- ✔ Are you envious of your neighbors?

Yoga encourages you to cultivate the virtue of greedlessness in all matters. The Sanskrit word for this is *aparigraha,* which means literally "not grasping all round." The Yoga practitioner who is well-trained in the art of greedlessness is said to understand the deeper reason for his or her life. Behind this traditional wisdom lies a profound experience: As you loosen your grip on material possessions, you also let go of the ego, which is doing the gripping or grasping. As the ego-contraction relaxes, you increasingly become in touch with the abiding happiness of your true self. Then you realize that you need nothing at all to be happy. You are unconcerned about the future and live fully in the present. You are not afraid to give freely to others and also share with them your inner abundance.

Adding other moral practices

In addition to the five moral virtues listed by Yoga master Patanjali in his *Yoga-Sutra,* other Yoga texts mention the following as belonging to the first limb of the eightfold path:

- Sympathy or *daya* (pronounced *dah-yah*)
- Compassion or *karuna* (pronounced *kah-roo-nah*)
- Integrity or *arjava* (pronounced *ahr-jah-vah*)
- Patience or *kshama* (pronounced *kshah-mah*)
- Steadfastness or *dhriti* (pronounced *dhree-tee*)
- Nonattachment or *vairagya* (pronounced *vie-rah-gyah*)
- Modesty or *hri* (pronounced *hree* — the initial letter *h* is sounded out loud)
- Humility or *amanitva* (pronounced *ah-mah-neet-vah*)

As you can see, Yoga has the highest expectations of a serious practitioner. But becoming a saint isn't the goal. Yoga is about freedom and happiness. The moral virtues are natural side effects of a life dedicated to Self-realization, or spiritual enlightenment.

Exercising Yogic Self-Discipline

The second category, or "limb," of the eightfold path is known as "restraint" *(niyama),* also translated as "self-restraint." We explain the second limb here because it is an integral part of the moral orientation of Yoga, which is frequently given short shrift by Western practitioners. According to Patanjali, restraint comprises five practices:

- Purity or *shauca* (pronounced *shau-chah* — the *au* sounds similar to *ow* in *cow*)
- Contentment or *samtosha* (pronounced *sahm-toh-shah*)
- Austerity or *tapas* (pronounced *tah-pahs*)
- Study or *svadhyaya* (pronounced *svahd-hyah-yah*)
- Dedication to a higher principle or *ishvara-pranidhana* (pronounced *eesh-vah-rah prah-need-hah-nah*)

Purifying mind and body

An old saying from the Puritan tradition suggests, "Cleanliness is next to godliness." Yoga goes further, stating that perfect purity and divinity are one and the same. All of Yoga is a process of self-purification. It begins with mental purification (through the practice of the moral disciplines described earlier) and proceeds to bodily cleansing (through various purification techniques, including postures and breath control), followed by more profound mental purification (through sensory inhibition, concentration, meditation, and the ecstatic state), and ends with realizing the perfect purity of the spirit itself.

The Sanskrit word for "purity" is *shauca,* which has the root meaning of "being radiant." The ultimate reality, or spirit, is pure radiance. As you clean the windows of your body-mind, you invite in more of the spirit's light. Accomplished Yoga masters have a radiance about them.

Calming the quest through contentment

Contentment *(samtosha)* is traditionally defined as being satisfied with what life presents to you. When you are content, you have joy in your heart and you don't need anything else. You can face life with great calm. That doesn't mean, however, that you need to avoid improvements in your situation, such as finding a better job or studying for a diploma or degree. But your quest for improvement won't come from a place of neediness or gnawing dissatisfaction.

Focusing with austerity

Austerity *(tapas)* entails all kinds of practices designed to test your will-power and awaken the energy locked away in your body. Traditionally, these tests included strict dieting or prolonged fasting, staying awake for several days, or sitting completely still in meditation directly under the hot Indian sun. Few of these practices are possible for modern Westerners, but the basic principle behind *tapas* (literally meaning "heat") is as valid now as it was thousands of years ago: Whenever you want to make progress on the path of Yoga, you must avoid wasting your energy on things that are irrelevant to your inner development. By carefully regulating your mental and physical behavior, you generate more energy for yogic practice.

But progress calls for overcoming all kinds of inner resistances. *Tapas* makes a demand on you, which creates a certain amount of inner heat. Change is never easy, and for many people, self-discipline is a big stumbling block. They tend to give up too soon. Yet self-discipline — through the strength of your will — is within reach. Just persist and observe how your goals move closer. For instance, your effort to overcome laziness and practice Yoga regularly is a form of *tapas,* which gradually strengthens your willpower.

A good way to do *tapas* is by periodically going on retreat, where you have nothing to distract you from your inner work. Retreats provide an opportunity to clearly see all your tendencies in technicolor and also to start turning them around by creating better patterns of thought and behavior. Austerity is not about self-chastisement; it's an intelligent way of testing and strengthening your willpower. Remember, Yoga doesn't seek to increase pain and suffering but to remove it. Always be kind to yourself and, as your commitment to inner growth increases, don't hesitate to challenge yourself firmly.

Partnering research with self-study

Self-study *(svadhyaya)* is an important part of traditional Yoga, although contemporary Western practitioners who fail to understand its great value often neglect it. Self-study means both studying for oneself and studying oneself. Traditionally, this commitment involved pouring over the sacred scriptures, reciting them, and meditating on their meanings. In this way, practitioners stayed in touch with the tradition and also gained self-understanding, because study of the scriptures always confronts you with yourself. For basic study, we recommend the following Yoga texts, which are all available in good English translations:

- *Yoga-Sutra* of Patanjali, the standard text on Raja Yoga

- *Bhagavad-Gita,* the earliest available Sanskrit text on Jnana Yoga, Karma Yoga, and Bhakti Yoga

- *Hatha-Yoga-Pradipika,* one of the classical manuals of Hatha Yoga

> ✔ *Yoga-Vasishtha,* a marvelous work on Jnana Yoga; filled with traditional stories and beautiful poetic imagery
>
> ✔ *Bhakti-Sutra* of Narada, a classical work on Bhakti Yoga

You can find full or partial translations of numerous Yoga texts in Georg Feuerstein's *The Yoga Tradition* (see the appendix for more information).

Why study the Yoga scriptures? They are the distillations of several thousand years of experimentation and experience. If you are serious about Yoga, why not benefit from the wisdom of the accomplished adepts of this tradition?

Today, study can be usefully extended to include not only important Yoga scriptures but also contemporary knowledge that can further your self-understanding. Yoga practitioners who recognize the great ideas and forces that are shaping our modern civilization are better equipped to study themselves. To understand yourself, you must also understand the world you live in. You don't have to become an intellectual (unless you happen to be one), but studying of the various components of human nature is wonderful mental training, and it can help you to thoroughly comprehend the wisdom of Yoga.

Relating to a higher principle

The third element of self-restraint *(niyama)* is devotion to a higher principle. The Sanskrit term is *ishvara-pranidhana,* where the word *ishvara* means literally "lord," referring to the divine. We translate it as "higher principle" to emphasize that you don't need to believe in a personal God to perform this practice. Devotion to a higher principle essentially means keeping your sight fixed on realizing your highest spiritual potential. If you happen to believe in a personal deity, you can use the traditional practice of repeating whatever name you have for the divine until your mind becomes absorbed in the state of contemplation. Or you can employ prayers and invocations to feel near to God or Goddess. But always remember that, according to Yoga, the divine is not a separate being but the essence of everything.

Chapter 19

Sex and Yoga Make Good Bedfellows

• •

In This Chapter

▶ Going with the flow: How habits express energy

▶ Seeing sexual libido as psychophysical energy

▶ Pairing attitude and awareness for sexual good health

▶ Including your mind and heart in lovemaking

▶ Fostering vitality with three helpful exercises

• •

*Y*oga affects your entire body and mind. Through Yoga, you can loosen up, strengthen and tone your muscles, and boost your metabolism, as well as hone your concentration, improve your memory, and even enhance your creativity. Above all, Yoga enables you to tap into the inexhaustible pool of energy from which all life arises. Throughout your yogic journey, you can look forward to greater harmony and balance as you enjoy increased vitality and joy.

Everyone has a certain level of vitality or psychosomatic energy, which is called *prana* in Sanskrit. Your individual vitality is partly an expression of your state of health and partly a sign of your interest in something. Sometimes, a person seems to continually bubble over with energy — perhaps from nervous excitement, which isn't backed by adequate energy resources. Usually such people become exhausted quite quickly, and they constantly ride an emotional seesaw. You want both energy and balance. Others have a hard time getting started on something, but once they are moving, they are as difficult to stop as a freight train. You want adaptability in addition to energy.

In this chapter, we explain the role of physical vitality and psychosomatic energy. In particular, we present Yoga's perspective on sexual energy (libido), which is a manifestation of the primary psychosomatic energy, and we also describe two exercises — called "locks" — that can help you maintain, recover, or even boost your vitality. In Chapter 18, we discuss chastity as one of the moral practices of Yoga, explaining how to behave spiritually in our oversexed contemporary world. Here we offer advice for sexually active individuals who want to bring their sex lives in consonance with yogic ideals.

Sharing Energy: A Bundle of You and the Universe

According to Yoga, life is energy, and energy exists in infinite abundance. You are a manifestation of the same energy that is also the foundation of flowers, mountains, rivers, stars, galaxies, and your pet dog or cat. Without it, nothing exists.

Binding your energy through habit patterns

Your personality, or character, is shaped by your habit patterns. Habits in turn represent what you typically do with the energy at your disposal. Here are four principal ways in which you can express the life force in you:

- ✔ **Repression:** You are afraid to cut loose and so you keep the lid on your energy. You believe that you have no energy and so feel disempowered. You deny yourself pleasure and joy, and others call you a "wet blanket" or a "downer." You have a hard time coming to terms with the present and worry about the future.

- ✔ **Digression:** You bubble over with energy but don't really know what to do with it. You can't sit still or are chronically lost in thoughts — a daydreamer. You start projects but never finish them because your mind wanders from one thing to the next. Your life is unfocused, and you always wonder why you can't seem to succeed.

- ✔ **Obsession:** You know how to access your energy but you run it on a single track. You are fixed on a single idea or ideal — be it a task or another person. In its pursuit, you ignore everyone and everything else and are even willing to sacrifice your own happiness.

- ✔ **Integration:** You are energetic and know how to deploy your energy appropriately. Your timing tends to be excellent, and you are neither timid nor reckless, neither frenzied nor sullen.

If you find that you fit into all four categories at one time or another, then examine which one best describes your behavior. Make this exercise a regular part of your self-study *(svadhyaya)*, as we describe in Chapter 18.

How you express the life energy determines what sort of experiences you can expect to have in the course of a lifetime. Your habit patterns are the various ways in which you restrict and channel the infinite flux of energy. They are your limitation, your bondage, your karma. Yoga helps you not only immerse yourself more fully into life's ocean of energy but also to use the resource wisely — which can, of course, set you free.

Telling the truth about sexual energy

One way in which people commonly express the infinite life energy is to channel it into sex — as one Yoga master described, "down and out." From a yogic perspective, *libido* is universal energy as it manifests at the genital level. Although this point is very important, even Western Yoga practitioners seldom understand it. Sexual energy is just a variation of the energy — *prana* — that animates the body-mind as a whole and that sustains all life processes. Consequently, there is no conflict between living a yogic lifestyle and having a sexual body.

Sex is only "dirty" if your mind is polluted. The misconception that spirit and sex are mutually exclusive causes this world a great deal of unhappiness. In the past, people chastised themselves for even a fleeting sexual thought or stirring. Despite the so-called sexual revolution of the 1960s and 1970s, many Westerners still feel guilt and shame about sexuality.

Yoga offers a more wholesome perspective: Sex is an integral aspect of human life. You don't need to feel guilty or ashamed about your sexual impulses and thoughts. Rather, you are called to *understand* them. When you understand why you express universal energy in specific sexual ways, you can begin to engage that energy with awareness and, if appropriate, redirect it.

Cultivating Healthy Sexual Attitudes

Yoga teaches that true happiness resides within you. Therefore, the widespread notion that someone or something can make you happy is profoundly mistaken. Sex can make you feel good, even momentarily ecstatic, but it cannot give you lasting happiness. Contentment must grow from inside you. Once you are basically happy, your happiness can flow through all your experiences, including sex.

What you may find, however, is that basic happiness inspires you to stop using sex for the wrong reasons. Here are six popular wrong reasons:

- ✔ You have a poor self-image and need sex for emotional reassurance either to prove yourself (the typical male version) or to feel loved and accepted (the typical female version).

✔ You are bored and have nothing better to do.

✔ You offer sexual favors in order to gain some benefit. For instance, some women only sleep with their husbands when they can expect a gift in return.

✔ You feel you are expected to keep up with some spoken or unspoken standard.

✔ You are promiscuous to take revenge on a partner who betrayed you.

✔ You lack the wisdom and willpower to invest your life energy into expanding your consciousness beyond the genital level.

By contrast, the right reasons for sex always involve the heart. Many traditional schools of Yoga have an ascetic orientation and consider sex appropriate only for marriage partners who want to procreate. The fact is, however, that human sexuality is not seasonal like other animals. Therefore, some Yoga authorities believe that engaging in sex for intimacy and enjoyment is perfectly all right. You certainly don't have to become a killjoy to adopt yogic principles. Sexual repression can be more damaging than sexual expression.

Actually, Yoga is against sexual *suppression* and *repression,* which only lead to frustration and sickness. But Yoga also is against sexual excess, which is merely a form of self-indulgence. Yoga favors wholeness and balance in all things. Its focus is on happiness.

Experiencing happiness beyond sexual pleasure

Regular Yoga practice not only fans the life force in your body, but it also gradually redirects it from merely genital expression. The process is associated with what's called *heart opening.* When the life force becomes more active at the level of the heart — the dimension of feeling — sexuality ceases to be a problem. No more crisis over having or not having sex. When you do have sex, it is fully integrated with your emotions. In practice, this means that the sexual energy doesn't stay localized in the genitals but spreads throughout your body — from your toes to the top of your head. Because you are already basically happy, you don't feel deprived of anything when this intense sensation of pleasure finally subsides — either with or without orgasm. And you won't obsess about repeating the experience as quickly as possible. Instead, you allow your body's inner wisdom to regulate your sex life.

Generating subtle energy

By harnessing your sexual energy properly, you increase what is known in the Sanskrit language as *ojas* (pronounced *oh-jahs*), which means "subtle vitality." *Ojas* is the high-octane fuel that not only nourishes all your organs but also enables you to experience deep meditation and even ecstatic states of consciousness. In other words, *ojas* allows you to complete the yogic journey. The most important means for harnessing this subtle energy, as we note in Chapter 18, is self-control relative to your sexual thoughts, feelings, sensations, and actions.

The Yoga masters recommend *brahmacarya* (pronounced *brah-mah-chahr-yah*), or chastity (see Chapter 18 for more information). They are great believers in recycling your sexual energy rather than spending it liberally. For householders, this belief means sexual economy rather than complete sexual abstinence. Mainly it means not obsessing about sex and approaching sexual activity, whenever it occurs, with your whole body and whole mind. All Yoga masters argue against *casual* sex. You don't have to switch "it" off, just make each sexual experience count. Involve awareness and the heart. Great sex begins with an open heart and blossoms through awareness.

From a yogic perspective, sexual energy is the lowest octave of the universal life energy. This energy is necessary for procreation, but if you are eager to explore your body's full potential, you must channel the life energy upward by the various means of Hatha Yoga, especially meditation. But build the foundations first: Strengthen your body, discipline your emotions, and train your mind.

Appreciating Sexual Expression — the Yoga Way

To make each sexual experience count, prepare your inner and outer environment properly. Look upon your partner not merely as a body but as an embodied being of consciousness and spiritual beauty. We recommend that you read Dana Goodwin's *The Little Book for Lovers* to prime your mind and heart. Treating your partner with respect doesn't rule out enjoyment and playfulness. There is, of course, a big difference between *making love* and *having sex*. We can wholeheartedly recommend the former.

As for external preparations, take care of your personal hygiene and make your bedroom into a miniature Garden of Eden. Here are some simple tips to get your own creativity flowing:

- Tidy up your bedroom if necessary.
- Keep distractions at bay.
- Burn incense that you and your partner find pleasing.

  ✔ Light some candles.

  ✔ Play soft music.

When you see your partner as a being who is composed of body, mind, and spirit rather than as a proverbial sex object, your lovemaking naturally becomes more trusting, relaxed, and less goal-oriented. At times, the moment can even turn into a meditation experience for both partners. Here are some basic guidelines for making love the Yoga way:

  ✔ Begin your love play with the intention of being together not only at the physical level, but also emotionally and spiritually.

  ✔ Begin by consciously relaxing and breathing deeply.

  ✔ Take your time with foreplay (the female body generally takes longer to become sexually aroused than the male body).

  ✔ Be sensitive to the needs and preferences of your partner; you must always remain in relationship to your partner (don't go off into your private La-La Land, shutting out your partner).

  ✔ Communicate (unless your partner is a master of Yoga, he or she won't be able to read your thoughts).

  ✔ Don't make orgasm your goal; enjoy your lovemaking and see what happens (but don't frustrate yourself either).

  ✔ Enjoy and freely share with your partner the energy released during lovemaking.

  ✔ Don't be afraid to laugh at yourself and each other.

  ✔ Don't end your lovemaking abruptly. Let the golden rule of harmony be your guide in this and other matters.

Tantra Yoga

Tantra Yoga is widely touted as Yoga's answer to the sexual revolution, which is misleading. A clear distinction exists between traditional Tantra and what we call contemporary Western "Neo-Tantrism." The former is a rigorous spiritual discipline involving much renunciation and ritual; the latter focuses on sexual fulfillment, seeking to combine it with spiritual ideas and aspirations.

Traditional Tantra comprises two major orientations. Left-hand Tantra (which has always been in the minority) includes sexual rituals. Right-hand Tantra involves no sexual practices but emphasizes inner union through meditation. But even left-hand Tantra is 99 percent ritual and 1 percent sex. All Tantra is first and foremost *inner sex,* the union of body and mind, as well as breath and spirit. Delicious stuff when you know how to do it! And it's not impossible to learn.

Emphasizing Vitality with Sexual-Specific Exercises

Your general hygiene and postural practice contribute to your sexual health. In addition, a number of special Hatha Yoga techniques are available to keep your anus and genitals in excellent condition, notably *ashvini mudra* and *mula bandha*.

Definitely do not practice any of these exercises if you have heart disease. Also, if you are suffering from urogenital problems, consult your physician first.

Ashvini mudra

The Sanskrit phrase *ashvini mudra* (pronounced *ah-shvee-nee mood-rah*) means "horse seal." This technique consists of contracting the rectum's two ringlike sphincter muscles. An observant Yoga master created this exercise after watching horses practice it spontaneously. It strengthens the sphincter muscles and contributes to good rectal health.

1. **Sit, stand, or lie down in any comfortable posture.**

2. **Take several deep, even breaths.**

   Check that your whole body is relaxed.

3. **Inhale and, as you exhale, contract your anal muscles.**

   Don't strain! Picture a lotus flower opening and closing.

4. **As you inhale again, release the contraction.**

5. **Repeat 5 to 6 times.**

Note: If this breathing pattern is too difficult for you, breathe normally, but check yourself to make sure that you don't hold your breath when contracting the anal muscles.

Before you perform *ashvini mudra,* empty your bladder and bowels, if you can.

Mula bandha

The Sanskrit phrase *mula bandha* (pronounced *moo-lah bund-ha*) means literally "root lock". This technique consists in contracting the perineum (called *yoni* in Sanskrit), which refers to the muscles of the vagina and the penis. The perineum is the small area between the rectum and the vagina or penis.

Mula bandha is designed to affect the pubococcygeus (pronounced *pew-boh-cox-eh-jee-es*), or PC muscle. Los Angeles physician Arnold Kegel rediscovered this technique in the 1950s. Many sex therapists recommend his Kegel exercises for both men and women. In women, the *mula bandha* causes a tightening of the vagina as well as revitalizes the female organs and can help regulate menstruation. In men, it contributes to the health of the prostate and also offers better control over ejaculation.

Some Yoga authorities distinguish between contraction of the perineum and the muscles associated with the urethra. The latter is said to be achieved through *vajroli mudra* (pronounced *vahj-roh-lee mood-rah*) means "adamantine seal." You can identify the muscle associated with the urethra by stopping your urine midstream. We don't recommend this as a regular practice, though.

If you have serious medical problems with your urogenital tract, consult your physician before doing this or the following exercises. Before you do this exercise, empty your bladder and bowels first, if you can.

1. **Sit, stand, or lie down in any comfortable posture.**

2. **Take several deep, even breaths.**

   Check that your whole body is relaxed.

3. **Inhale and, as you exhale, contract the muscles of your perineum (but not the anal muscles).**

   Don't strain! Picture a lotus flower opening and closing.

4. **As you inhale again, release the contraction.**

5. **Repeat 5 to 6 times.**

Note: If this breathing pattern is too difficult for you, breathe normally, but check yourself to be sure that you don't hold your breath when contracting the muscles of the perineum.

If you can sit comfortably in *siddhasana* (see Chapter 9), we recommend that you use that posture for this and the other lock. Also, if you decide to breathe normally instead of using the above breathing pattern, make sure that you don't simply hold your breath when performing the contraction.

Chapter 20

Meditation and the Higher Reaches of Yoga

. . . .

In This Chapter

▶ Concentrating on finding your focus

▶ Approaching meditation as an art

▶ Making the most of your meditation practice

▶ Sitting correctly during meditation

▶ Clearing obstacles away from the road to successful practice

▶ Repeating mantras as you meditate

▶ Checking out a few meditation exercises

▶ Exploring states of ecstasy and enlightenment

. . . .

You've probably heard the saying, "You give as good as you get." The same goes for Yoga. Doing a few postures now and then certainly gives you some benefits; however, to reap Yoga's full rewards, you need to live a yogic lifestyle — a lifestyle that encompasses the physical, mental, and spiritual.

Yogic postures are a great place to start. Combined with a decent diet, Yoga postures take care of 80 percent of your physical well-being, and also have a positive effect on your emotional health. (The other 20 percent comes from adequate sleep, meaningful work, and a reasonably happy family life.)

Beyond the basic benefits of a healthy body, the physical practice of Yoga can help you continue to explore your deeper mental and spiritual potential. In fact, a vital, healthy body is the best foundation for meditation (yogic concentration) and the higher reaches of Yoga. Try meditating when your nose is blocked from a cold, when you are running a fever, or when your back is killing you! Pain and discomfort may make you philosophical ("Why me?"), but they don't contribute to a basically relaxed mind. And that's exactly why you need to meditate.

Many chapters in this book deal specifically with Yoga postures, which are designed to relax your body and thus prepare your mind for the higher stages of Yoga. This chapter explains how to integrate meditation into your routine so that you can reach the top rung of the Yoga ladder.

Playing Concentration

How busy is your mind? Can you concentrate easily? The following little exercise gauges your CQ (Concentration Quotient):

Think of a beautiful white swan. It looks neither left nor right, but just slowly and majestically glides across the surface of a pond. It barely causes ripples in the water. Just keep thinking of that swan. Try to form a clear image and then hold it as steadily as possible in your mind, while slowly counting 100, 99, 98, 97, 96 . . .

How far did you manage to count before your mental image of the swan faded into thin air or another thought intruded? Was it 97 or 96? Perhaps you lost your concentration with the count of 99. You may have been able to continue your counting for several more numbers, but reaching much beyond 96 is most unusual for beginners. If you did, your power of concentration is good — only a yogi or yogini can count all the way to 0 *and* think of the swan.

If you think you didn't do well with this exercise because visualizing is not your strong suit, try this one for good measure:

Sit quietly. Take a few deep breaths. Then let your mind go totally blank. No thoughts, no images, no counting — no ripples in your mental pond at all. Just sit. Just be.

How did you do? Don't feel bad if your concentration exercise went something like this:

. . . Okay, I'm not thinking. Heck, that's a thought, isn't it? Let me try again. . . . That's much better. See? Having no images is not that difficult. And what was it about counting? I didn't do too well with the counting test, but I hate tests. Oh *darn, I'm thinking again. Okay, back to no thoughts.* . . .

Don't be discouraged if your mind is a veritable speed train and your concentration is too poor to slow it down. The forward charge merely means that you have room for improvement, and you *will* improve with practice. Distraction is not negative in itself. Instead, you can look at your lack of clear concentration as an opportunity to gently refocus your attention. As you refocus repeatedly, your mind can become more obedient. Think of your mind as a spirited foal that exuberantly gallops around the meadow. With a little training, that frisky colt can become an excellent race horse.

JARGON ALERT

The inner limbs of Yoga

According to Raja Yoga, as described in the *Yoga-Sutra* of Patanjali, the yogic path comprises eight "limbs" *(anga)*. The first five limbs — moral discipline, self-restraint, posture, breath control, and sensory inhibition — are called *outer limbs*. These practices belong to the entrance hall of Yoga's vast mansion. In the interior of the estate you find concentration, meditation, and ecstasy, known as the *inner limbs*. You can practice these inner limbs successfully only after you achieve a certain degree of mastery in the other five practices.

In fact, many people confuse meditation with stopping all thoughts, but that's only one — and rather advanced — type of meditation. In the beginning, meditation is simply noticing the endless stream of thoughts flickering on your mental screen; consider your observations an important part of your overall effort to be *mindful,* or attentive.

Unleashing your essence

The ability to concentrate is a boon to everything you do. Without focus, you'd constantly hammer your finger instead of a nail, you'd miscalculate your taxes, and you'd be unable to follow the razor-sharp logic of Sherlock Holmes.

Yogic concentration is far more demanding than the kind of concentration you use in daily life; but it's also much more rewarding. Yoga can help you unlock the hidden chambers of your own mind. When you are able to focus your attention like a laser beam upon your inner world, you can discover the most subtle aspects of your mind. Above all, yogic concentration ultimately enables you to discover your spiritual essence.

Concentration, which leads to meditation, brings you clarity and peace of mind — two qualities that stand you in good stead in any situation. They enable you to live your life more fully, more meaningfully, and more competently. Whether you are a busy mother and homemaker or a top executive, the mental tranquility you produce through regular concentration and meditation exercises can transform your entire day.

Whenever you concentrate, your mind naturally turns away from the outer world. Thus, concentration involves a degree of sense withdrawal *(pratyahara),* which is the fifth limb of the eightfold yogic path. For instance, when you're listening intently to the radio, you may not hear someone calling your name.

As yogic concentration and meditation develop, you become increasingly able to shut down your senses at will — a useful ability when you sit in the dentist chair.

Putting your body into it

Concentration and meditation are special moments in the same *mindfulness* that you're asked to bring to every aspect of your life. The Sanskrit word for *concentration* is *dharana,* which means literally "holding." You hold your attention by focusing on a specific bodily process (such as breathing), a thought, an image, or a sound (as in Mantra Yoga — see the section "Adding sounds to meditation"). Through *concentration* you seek to become *concentric,* that is, properly centered and harmonious with yourself. When you are out of center *(eccentric),* or out of touch with your spiritual core, all your thoughts and actions are out of sync; they don't flow from your innermost core and thus they make you feel alienated, uneasy, and unhappy.

You can determine whether you are currently *concentric* or *eccentric* by checking in with your body. How do you *feel?* How does a decision you are about to make *feel?* How does a relationship *feel?* What does your body tell you about your present activity or your job? How do you *feel* about your life as a whole? This kind of mindfulness is called *focusing,* which means paying careful attention to how your mind is registering in your body. Body and mind go together. Keeping mentally in touch with your body regularly is important and, in fact, even fundamental to good postural practice.

Through focusing, you can also become aware of your own "stuff" — old resentments, disappointments, fears, and expectations. People tend to store negative experiences in the body, which make them predisposed to sickness. Sooner or later, each person needs to work through these stored memories for their own good health and to share their liberated selves with the world around them.

One way to begin replaying and diffusing negative experiences that are recorded in your body is to ask yourself: *Is anything preventing me from feeling good and happy right now? What, if anything, is keeping me from experiencing bliss?* Your body contains the answer(s): a sensation of tightness in the chest, a hollow feeling around the heart, a contraction in the pit of your stomach, fearful pounding in the head. All these are physical expressions of corresponding emotional states.

When doing this kind of focusing work, don't settle for the first answer that comes to mind. Instead, ask yourself: *What else is there to prevent me from feeling good and happy?* If you encounter too much inner pain, you may want to consider doing this work in the company of a trusted friend or under the guidance of a competent counselor or therapist.

Practicing Meditation

Meditation is a mental process involving focused attention, or calm awareness, which is also called mindfulness.

Many forms or styles of meditation exist, but two basic approaches stand out: *meditation with a specific focus* and *objectless meditation*. The latter is pure mindfulness, without narrowing attention to any particular sensation, idea, or other phenomenon. Most beginners find this kind of meditation very difficult, although some are drawn to it. We recommend that you start out with meditation on a specific object. The following categories of objects are suitable for this exercise:

- ✔ A bodily sensation, such as breathing, which makes an excellent focus.
- ✔ A bodily location, such as one of the seven cakras or energy centers (see the next section).
- ✔ A process or action, such as eating, walking, or washing dishes.
- ✔ An external physical object, such as the flame of a candle.
- ✔ A *mantra* (be it a single sound, a phrase, or a chant).
- ✔ A thought, such as the idea of peace, joy, love, or compassion.
- ✔ Visualization — a special form of meditation involving your creative imagination to picture light, emptiness, your spiritual teacher, a saint, or one of the many deities of Hindu or Buddhist Yoga.

Experiment with all these various focal points for meditation until you find what appeals to you the most. Then stick with it. For instance, if you choose to visualize a particular saint or deity, you benefit by always using the same figure in your daily visualization practice.

Cakras: Your wheels of fortune

According to Yoga, the physical body has a more subtle energetic counterpart. It consists of a network of energy channels called *nadis* (pronounced *nah-dees*) through which the life force *(prana)* circulates. The most important channel runs along the axis of the body, from the base of the spine to the crown of the head. It is called *sushumna-nadi* or the "gracious channel" (see the description of Kundalini Yoga in Chapter 1). In the ordinary individual, this central conduit of subtle energy is said to be mostly inactive. The purpose of many Hatha Yoga exercises is to clear especially this channel of any obstructions, so that the life energy can flow freely in it, leading to better health and also higher states of consciousness.

When the central channel is thus activated, it also sets the six principal psychoenergetic centers of the body in motion. These are the *cakras* (often spelled *chakras* in English), which are aligned along the central channel. The word means simply "wheel" and refers to the fact that these are whirlpools of energy that keep the physical body alive and functioning properly. You may see the cakras pictured as lotuses. In ascending order, the six *cakras* are:

- *Muladhara* (literally "root prop," pronounced *moo-lahd-hah-rah*): Located at the base of the spine between the rectum and genitals, this center is the resting place of the dormant "serpent power" (see Chapter 1), the great psychospiritual energy that Hatha Yoga seeks to awaken. This center is connected with elimination as well as fear.

- *Svadhishthana* (literally "own place," pronounced *svahd-hisht-hah-nah*): Located at the genitals, this center is connected with the urogenital functions, but also with desire.

- *Manipura* (literally "jewel city," pronounced *mah-nee-poo-rah*): Located at the navel, this center distributes the life force to all parts of the body and is especially involved in the digestive process, as well as the willpower.

- *Anahata* ("unstruck," pronounced *ah-nah-hah-tah*): Located in the middle of the chest, this center, which is also called the "heart *cakra*," is the place where the "unstruck" or inner sound can be heard in meditation. It is also linked with love.

- *Vishuddha* ("pure," pronounced *vee-shood-hah*): Located at the throat, this center is associated with speech, but also greed.

- *Ajna* ("command," pronounced *ah-gyah*): Located in the middle of the head between the eyebrows, this center is the contact place for the *guru's* telepathic work with disciples. It is also associated with the experience of higher states of consciousness.

- *Sahasrara* (literally "thousand-spoked," pronounced *sah-hahs-rah-rah*): Located at the crown of the head, this special *cakra* is associated with higher states of consciousness, notably the ecstatic state.

Following a few guidelines for successful meditation

Think of your meditation as a tree that you must water every day — not too much and not too little. Trust that one day your nurturing will bring the tree to bear beautiful blossoms and delicious fruit.

Here are seven vital tips to make your meditation tree grow:

✔ **Practice regularly:** Try to meditate every day. If this isn't possible, meditate at least several times a week.

✔ **Cultivate the correct motivation:** People meditate for all kinds of reasons: health, wholeness, peace of mind, clarity, spiritual growth. Be clear in your own mind why you are sitting down to meditate. The best motivation for meditation (and Yoga practice in general) is to live to your full potential *and* to benefit others by your personal achievements.

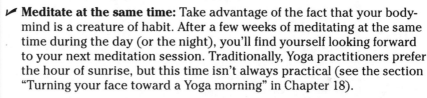

In Buddhism, this motivation is known as the *bodhisattva* ideal. The *bodhisattva* (literally "enlightenment being") seeks to realize enlightenment (the ultimate spiritual state) for the benefit of all other beings. As an enlightened being, you can be far more efficient in helping others in their own struggle for wholeness and happiness.

✔ **Meditate at the same time:** Take advantage of the fact that your body-mind is a creature of habit. After a few weeks of meditating at the same time during the day (or the night), you'll find yourself looking forward to your next meditation session. Traditionally, Yoga practitioners prefer the hour of sunrise, but this time isn't always practical (see the section "Turning your face toward a Yoga morning" in Chapter 18).

Inevitably, you'll have moments when meditation is the last thing you want to do. In that case, resolve to sit quietly for at least five minutes. Often, this break is enough to get you in the mood for full-fledged meditation. If not, don't beat yourself over the head; just go on to something else and try again later or the next day.

✔ **Meditate in the same place:** Choose the same time, same place for the same reason: Your body-mind enjoys what is familiar. Use this fact to your advantage by setting aside a room or a corner of a room that your mind can associate with meditation.

✔ **Select an appropriate posture for meditation and do it correctly:** Sit up straight, with your chest open, and your neck free (see the following section for instructions about posture). Don't recline while meditating — you fall asleep — and don't meditate on your bed, even in a sitting position. Your mind is likely to associate the experience with sleep. If you're not used to sitting on the floor, try sitting on a straight-backed chair or on a sofa with a cushion behind your back. If you can comfortably sit on the floor, you have a variety of yogic postures to choose from. We describe several of them in Chapter 7.

✔ **Select a meditation technique and stick with it:** In the beginning, you may want to try out various techniques to see which appeals to you the most. But after you find a good technique for your particular needs, don't abandon it until it bears fruit (in terms of increased peace of mind and happiness), a meditation teacher advises you to change to a different technique, or you feel really drawn to a different technique.

✔ **Begin with short sessions:** Meditate 10 to 20 minutes at a time at first. If your meditation naturally lasts longer, then simply rejoice in the fact. But don't ever force yourself if the timing creates conflict or unhappiness in you. Also, beware of overmeditating. Often, what beginners regard as a "nice long meditation" is just self-indulgent daydreaming. Make sure that your meditation contains an element of alertness. When you start drifting off into a comfortable space, you can be sure that you're no longer meditating. Like the practice of the Yoga postures, your meditation must have an *edge* (that is, you must push against the limitations of your mind but without frustrating yourself).

✔ **Be alert, yet relaxed:** Inner alertness, or mindfulness, is not the same as tension or stress. Make sure that your body is relaxed by regularly practicing some of the relaxation exercises we describe in Chapter 4. Cats are good examples of this alertness. Even when a cat is completely relaxed, its ears move around like radar dishes catching every little sound in the environment. The more relaxed you are, the more alert your mind can be.

✔ **Don't burden yourself with expectations:** Entering meditation with a desire to grow spiritually and to benefit from the experience is certainly acceptable. However, don't expect every meditation to be wonderful and pleasant.

✔ **Prepare properly for meditation:** As a beginner, don't expect to be able to jump from the fray of your daily activities straight into meditation. Allow your mind a little time to unwind before you sit for meditation. Have a relaxing bath or shower or at least wash your face and hands.

✔ **Be prepared to practice meditation for a lifetime:** You don't grow a tree overnight. On the yogic path, no effort is ever wasted. Therefore, don't give up if your meditation is not what you think it should be after a month or two. Don't conclude too hastily that meditation isn't working or that the technique you're using isn't effective. Instead, correct your understanding about the nature of meditation and then, persist. Your very effort to meditate counts.

Be wary of weekend workshops that promise immediate success, if not enlightenment itself. Meditation and enlightenment are lifelong processes.

✔ **Keep your meditation experiences to yourself:** In their enthusiasm, beginners understandably want to share their new discoveries with everyone. Resist the temptation to market your revelations to others, which turns most people off and won't do you any good either. Sharing your meditation experiences indiscriminately with others is like telling your friends (or anyone who will listen) about your intimate love life. It's in poor taste. Therefore, Yoga masters recommend silence on such matters.

Roses come with thorns

If you are a beginner and your meditations are consistently comfortable, you have every reason to be suspicious. The purpose of meditation is to clear the mind, and doing so entails clearing away the debris (or what one teacher has called "the frogs deep down in the well").

In the beginning, meditation consists largely of discovering just how unruly your mind is. If your meditation practice is successful, you will encounter your shadow side (all those aspects of your character you'd prefer not to think about). As you go on, more profound insights into your character can and will occur, which then require you to make the necessary changes in your attitudes and behaviors.

Few meditations are "spectacular," which is not at all what meditation is about. Even a "bad" meditation is a good meditation, because you are applying mindfulness. Don't be surprised to find that for no apparent reason, your meditation is calm and uplifting one day and turbulent and distracted the next. Until your mind reaches clarity and calmness, you can expect this fluctuation.

Graciously accept whatever happens in your meditation and don't hesitate to exercise your sense of humor.

✔ **At the end of your meditation, integrate the experience with the rest of your life:** Just as going straight from overdrive into a meditative gear is not prudent, you need to restrain from jumping up from meditation to return your other activities. Instead, make a conscious transition in and out of meditation. At the end of the session, briefly recall your reasons for meditating and your overall motivation. Be grateful for any energies and/or insights your meditation generates. Equally importantly, don't feel negative about a difficult meditation experience. Rather, be grateful for *any* experience. Sometimes important insights surface during meditation, and then your challenge is to translate these messages into daily life. When you continually perform this kind of integration, your meditation will deepen more quickly as well.

Maintaining right bodily posture

Correct posture is important for meditation. Here is a seven-point checklist that can help you develop good sitting habits:

✔ **Back:** The position of your back while sitting in meditation is the single most important physical feature. Your back should be straight but relaxed, with your chest open and your neck free. Correct posture enables your bodily energies to flow more freely, which prevents sleepiness. Most Westerners need a firm cushion under their sit bones to encourage good posture during meditation and to stop your legs from going to sleep. Make sure, however, that your pelvis does not tilt forward too much. Alternatively, sit on a chair. Any posture is acceptable as long as you can comfortably maintain it for the desired duration.

✔ **Head:** For the correct position of the head, picture an attached string pulling the back of your head upward so that your head is tilted *slightly* forward. Too much of a forward tilt invites drowsiness, not enough of a tilt can cause mental wandering.

✔ **Tongue:** Allow the front part of your tongue to touch the palate just behind the upper teeth. You will find that this position reduces the flow of saliva and the number of times you have to swallow, which many beginners find disturbing.

✔ **Teeth:** Don't clench your teeth, but keep your jaws relaxed. And be sure that your mouth doesn't hang open either.

✔ **Legs:** If you can sit cross-legged for an extended period of time without experiencing discomfort, we recommend especially the perfect posture *(siddhasana),* which we describe in Chapter 7. The folded legs form a closed circuit, which aids your concentration.

✔ **Arms:** Keep your cupped hands, palms up, in your lap, placing the right hand on top of the left. Relax your arms and shoulders. Leave a few inches between your arms and your trunk, which allows the air to circulate and prevents drowsiness.

✔ **Eyes:** Most beginners like to close their eyes, which is fine. As you develop your power of concentration, however, you may want to experiment with keeping your eyes slightly open while gazing downward in front of you. This again signals your brain that you aren't trying to go to sleep. Advanced practitioners are able to keep their eyes wide open without becoming distracted. In any event, make sure that your eye muscles are relaxed.

Overcoming obstacles to meditation

Whenever you deal with change, you also deal with resistance to change. Thus, the path of meditation is littered with various obstacles that can trip you up. Here are the most important potential hindrances:

✔ **Doubt:** The biggest boulder on the Yoga path: You either doubt the rightness or effectiveness of meditation (and the other methods) or you doubt yourself. You may, for example, wonder whether meditation is much too difficult for you (it isn't!); whether it will hypnotize you (it won't!); whether it's a form of escapism (it isn't!); whether you have to give up the things you enjoy to meditate (you don't!); whether it will clash with your religious beliefs (it won't!); or whether you first need to find a teacher (nope!). Everyone is worthy and capable of meditation, but don't expect fireworks from day one.

> *Remedy:* Take the time to write down all your doubts about meditation and Yoga and then analyze them — one by one. You may find that, on closer inspection, many of your concerns are unfounded, and some may be quite ridiculous. If, after this exercise, you have any serious doubts that prevent you from starting with your meditation practice, seek out a competent teacher who can help clarify your reservations.

✔ **Boredom:** Mindfulness (which consists of doing nothing other than paying attention) can quickly become "boring" for the overactive mind, which then invents various kinds of solutions to relieve itself of boredom, including dropping meditation altogether.

> *Remedy:* Accept that you are feeling bored and at least temporarily make boredom the focus of your mindfulness.

✔ **Sleep:** Many beginners succumb to sleep, because they subconsciously associate sleep with the slowing down of thoughts during meditation.

> *Remedy:* Check that your posture is good (see the preceding section). Keep your eyes slightly open. If necessary, stand up and do the walking meditation that we describe later in this section.

✔ **Physical discomfort:** Often, as soon as you settle down, your awareness of your body magnifies the least little sensation. Even a minor itch can become a major annoyance.

> *Remedy:* Notice the itch, breathe through it, and continue with your mindfulness. The itch can in fact provide you with additional energy to focus better. If the sensation gets out of control, just scratch yourself! Don't create a mountain out of a temporary rise in the road.

✔ **Negative thoughts:** Meditation tends to flush out the negative tendencies resident in your subconscious. Facing negativity can be very disturbing.

> *Remedy:* Don't dwell on any negative thoughts or moods that may arise. Remind yourself that you are not identical with the arising thoughts and feelings, and then choose to cultivate the exact opposite of whatever negative thoughts or moods are popping up on your mental screen. For instance, if you suddenly think dark, resentful thoughts about someone, simply dwell on the thought and feeling of loving kindness and project it everywhere.

✔ **Haste:** Nothing is more damaging on the Yoga path than "rushing to make it happen." You certainly can't hurry meditation.

> *Remedy:* Be patient! Give your body and mind enough time to change. Don't force anything.

✔ **Sanctimoniousness:** In Zen, which is the Japanese form of Yoga, this state of affected holiness is known as the *stink of Zen.* You let others know that you've *really* had a powerful meditation experience, that you're in the know — a kind of a master in your own right. This beginner's error is the same as bragging, or tooting your own horn, and we all know that pride comes before the fall.

> *Remedy:* Be realistic and modest about your attainments. Rejoice in progress along the path, but don't advertise it. If your inner growth is real, others will notice it sooner or later.

✔ **Phenomena hunting:** Some beginners relate to meditation as if it were a treasure hunt. They hope for all kinds of earth-shattering experiences — flashing lights, spectacular visions, extraordinary sounds, and so on. When these special effects aren't forthcoming, novice practitioners either become disenchanted with meditation or resort to fantasy.

> *Remedy:* Understand the nature and purpose of meditation, which is to train the mind in peace and insight to facilitate your inner growth. Keep it simple!

✔ **Illusionism:** Beware of the attitude that suggests that nothing really matters because everything is illusory anyway. Meditation does reveal just how much of your everyday reality is manufactured by the mind, but that doesn't mean that nothing is relevant. Often this attitude conceals a lack of grounding.

> *Remedy:* Understand that Yoga applies to all aspects of life. So, continue to do your work, care for your family and friends, and pay your bills as you enjoy the calming effects of yogic practice.

✔ **Kundalini symptoms:** Kundalini symptoms grew more popular and prevalent among meditators after publication of the fascinating spiritual autobiography of Gopi Krishna (see the appendix). These symptoms include psychosomatic phenomena such as energy streamings in the body, tremors of the limbs, involuntary body movements (called *kriyas*), hallucinations, and so on. In actual fact, genuine *kundalini* symptoms are very rare. Most of the reported cases are only precursors of an awakened *kundalini,* symptoms of mental illness, or pure imagination. (For a brief explanation of the *kundalini-shakti,* or serpent power, see Chapter 1.)

> *Remedy:* If your symptoms are light, you can deal with them through proper diet, a grounded lifestyle, and alternative medical therapies like homeopathy and acupuncture. If your symptoms are more severe, we advise you to find a competent healer familiar with the *kundalini* phenomenon (see the appendix).

Adding sounds to meditation

Using a sound or phrase to focus the mind is a popular approach in many spiritual traditions, including Hinduism, Buddhism, Christianity, Judaism, and Islamic Sufism. In Sanskrit, these special sounds are called *mantras.* They are thought to help better focus attention. Mantra Yoga made its debut in the Western world in the late 1960s with the Transcendental Meditation (TM) movement, founded by Maharshi Mahesh Yogi, whose most famous disciples were The Beatles.

Here are some well-known *mantras:*

- ✔ The syllable *om* is composed of the letters *a, u,* and *m,* and stands for the waking state, dream state, and deep sleep respectively. The long-drawn humming sound of *m* represents the ultimate reality. Hindus consider this syllable to be sacred and to symbolize the ultimate reality, or higher Self *(atman).* Begin the sound from the belly and move upward. The *m* sound is nasalized.

- ✔ The mantra *so'ham* (pronounced *so-hum*) means "I am He," that is, "I am the universal Self." It is repeated in sync with breathing; *so* on inhaling and *'ham* on exhaling.

- ✔ Buddhist Yoga widely uses the mantric phrase *om mani padme hum* (pronounced *om mah-nee pahd-meh hoom*). It means literally *"Om. Jewel in the Lotus. Hum,"* which is meant to convey that the searched-for higher reality is present here and now.

- ✔ The mantric utterance *om namah shivaya* (pronounced *om nah-mah shee-vah-yah*) is a favorite phrase among Hindu devotees of the Divine in the form of Shiva. It means *"Om. Salutation to Shiva."*

- ✔ The mantric utterance *hare krishna* (pronounced *hah-reh krish-nah*) was made famous in the West by the members of the Krishna Consciousness movement. It invokes the Divine in the form of Krishna, who is also called Hari.

According to the Yoga tradition, sounds are considered *mantras* only after a *guru* passes the sound to a worthy disciple. Thus, the syllable *om* on its own — without proper initiation — is not a *mantra.* Many Western Yoga teachers take a more relaxed approach and recommend both traditional and contemporary words for *mantra* practice. They relay the importance of finding a word (be it in Sanskrit or English) that appeals to you, because you will have to repeat it numerous times. That is to say, even words like the biblical *Amen* or the Hebrew *Shalom,* or the modern word *Peace* can serve as *mantras* — without official guru sanction.

Reciting your mantra

Whether you choose your own *mantra* or are given one, you must repeat it over and over again, either mentally or vocally (whispered or aloud), in order to make it effective.

This practice of recitation is called *japas,* (pronounced *jah-pah*) meaning literally "muttering." So, what happens after you recite a *mantra* a thousand, ten thousand, or a hundred thousand times? As you repeat the sound, your attention becomes more and more focused and your consciousness becomes absorbed into the sound. The *mantra* begins to recite itself, serving as an anchor for your mind whenever you don't need to engage your thoughts in specific tasks. This simplifies your inner life and gives you a sense of peace. Ultimately, your *mantra* can guide you to Self-realization, that is, enlightenment. Of course, to achieve enlightenment you must fulfill the other requirements of Yoga as well, notably honoring the moral disciplines, which we cover in detail in Chapter 18.

We recommend that beginners recite the *mantra* aloud, at a slow, steady pace. After you have some experience with this form of meditation, you can begin to whisper your *mantra,* so that only you can hear it. Traditionally, the most powerful form of mantric recitation is said to be silent or mental recitation. This, however, calls for a certain degree of skill in maintaining your concentration.

Using a rosary

Yoga practitioners often tell rosary beads while reciting their mantras — a practice that helps focus the mind The typical rosary *(mala)* consists of 108 beads plus an extra-large bead, which represents the cosmic mountain Meru. You tell the beads by using the thumb and middle finger. Your fingers should not cross the master or Meru bead. After 108 recitations (or beads), you simply turn the rosary around and start counting over again.

Breathing mindfully

Particularly taught in Buddhist circles, mindful observation of the breath is a meditation exercise that any beginner can try. As we note in Chapter 5, the breath is the link between body and mind. Since ancient times, the Yoga masters have made good use of this connection. Mindful breathing, or breathing meditation, is a simple and effective way of exploring the calming effect of conscious breathing.

1. **Sit up straight and relaxed.**

2. **Remind yourself of your purpose for meditation and resolve to sit in meditation for a given period of time.**

    We recommend at least 5 minutes for this exercise. Gradually extend the duration.

3. **Close your eyes or keep them half open while looking down in front of you.**

4. **Breathing normally and gently, focus your attention on the sensation created by the breath flowing in and out of your nostrils.**

   Carefully observe the entire process of inhalation and exhalation as it occurs at the opening of your nostrils.

5. **To prevent your mind from wandering, you can count in inhalation/exhalation breath cycles from 1 to 10.**

Note: Don't be concerned if you notice that your attention has wandered. Especially, don't be judgmental about any thoughts that may pop into your head. Instead, rededicate yourself to the process of observing your breath.

Walking meditation

Mindfulness is possible in any circumstance. You can eat, drive, wash dishes, have a conversation, watch television, or make love mindfully. For beginners, mindfulness while walking is an excellent form of meditation.

1. **Remind yourself of your purpose for meditation and resolve to meditate for a given period of time.**

   For a first try, we recommend at least 5 minutes for this exercise.

2. **Keep your eyes open but unfocused, looking down and a few steps ahead of you. Don't lower your head, but keep your neck relaxed.**

3. **Stand completely still and feel your entire body.**

4. **Focus your attention on your right foot, especially the toes and sole.**

5. **Slowly raise your right foot and take the first step.**

   Feel the sensation of the pressure lifting from your right foot and leg and shifting over to your left leg.

6. **As you slowly place the right foot back on the ground, become aware of the contact between your sole and the ground.**

   Also notice the rest of your body: your swinging arms that keep you balanced, your neck and head, your pelvis.

7. **Acknowledge any thoughts that arise without being judgmental; then return your attention to your whole body, not merely on one limb or movement.**

8. **At the end of your walking meditation, stand completely still for a few seconds, observing the clarity and calmness within you.**

Sharing love through meditation

We particularly recommend this meditation, because everyone can do with more love in his or her life. This exercise also provides a wonderful way of including others in your spiritual efforts and serves as a potent antidote for negative feelings toward others.

1. **Sit up straight but relaxed.**

2. **Remind yourself of your purpose for meditation and commit to sitting for a certain period of time.**

   We suggest 5 minutes for a first try.

3. **Observe your breath until you are calm.**

4. **Picture yourself surrounded by billions of living beings in ever-wider circles, with your parents and siblings closest to you, your other relatives forming the next circle, and so on.**

   Don't forget people who have hurt you or whom you dislike.

5. **Consider that, like you, all of them want to be happy and loved; even those who are angry and violent want and deserve love.**

6. **Generate the feeling of love in your heart, perhaps by thinking of the person you love the most.**

7. **As the feeling of universal love wells up in your heart, allow it to spread through your entire being, understanding that unless you can love yourself, you cannot love another.**

8. **Now let the warm loving feeling that pulsates in your body and mind flow out to all others in big embracing waves.**

   You can picture this process in the form of liquid light.

9. **As you allow your love to flow freely, mentally wish all beings well: "May you be happy; may your life flourish and be peaceful; may you be free from sickness, frustration, confusion, and negative emotions; may your lives be long and free from problems, and may you quickly attain enlightenment."**

10. **End the session by reaffirming your commitment to love all beings and to work on your limitations so that you become increasingly capable of benefiting others.**

Sparking wellness with a little "light" exercise

If you want to calm your mind or are in need of physical healing, you can benefit greatly from the following exercise.

1. **Sit up straight and relaxed.**

2. **Remind yourself of your purpose for meditation and resolve to sit in meditation for a given period of time.**

   We recommend at least 5 minutes for this exercise; gradually extend the duration.

3. **Close your eyes or keep them half open while looking down in front of you.**

4. **As you breathe normally and gently, picture pure white light coming from infinity and pouring into an opening at the crown of your head.**

5. **Allow the white light to fill your head and then flood your whole body, creating a feeling of calm and happiness in you.**

6. **Next, generate a feeling of love and compassion in your heart and visualize a deep blue color emanating from your heart and filling your chest; from there, picture the blue light radiating outward into all directions.**

7. **Strongly intend for this outward flow of deep blue energy to heal all the ills — physical, emotional, and mental — of all beings in the universe.**

   Feel a strong sense of kinship with everyone.

8. **Conclude this meditation by sitting still for a few moments.**

Although prayers can include a wide array of words and thoughts, most people know best what is called *petitionary prayer,* in which you ask for a favor or blessing. But in *meditative prayer,* you expect nothing and merely keep yourself open to divine influence. In recent times, the Trappist monk Thomas Merton did much to revive this kind of prayer within the Christian tradition. But meditative prayer also exists in non-Christian spiritual traditions, including Bhakti Yoga (see Chapter 1).

Associating prayer with meditation

A close relationship exists between meditation and prayer. In prayer, mindfulness is practiced in relationship to a being who is deemed "higher" than oneself — be it your own *guru,* a great master (dead or alive), a deity, or the ultimate spiritual reality itself. Prayer, like meditation, involves a feeling of reverence.

Working toward Ecstasy

When you start meditating, you are well aware that "you" — the subject — are quite different from the object of meditation. You experience the white or blue light or the visualized deity as distinct from yourself. But as meditation deepens, the boundary between subject and object — consciousness and its contents — becomes increasingly blurred. Then, at one point, the two merge completely. You *are* the light or deity. This is the celebrated state of ecstasy called *samadhi* in Sanskrit (pronounced *sah-mahd-hee*).

Yoga distinguishes two fundamental types or levels of ecstasy. At the lower level, the ecstatic state is associated with a certain form or mental content. The higher type of ecstasy is a state of formless consciousness.

Many Yoga practitioners won't experience the ecstatic state, but some will definitely encounter it in the course of their lives. If ecstasy occurs, count yourself fortunate, because the state is a wonderful spiritual opening. If you are practicing Yoga intensively and you still don't experience *samadhi,* count yourself fortunate as well, because your efforts are never wasted; just know that they may manifest differently for you: You may become serene, uncomplicated, basically happy. What matters is not how often or how long you enter into *samadhi,* but whether and how much you embody spiritual principles in your daily life. Are you compassionate and kind? Do you see others not as total strangers but fellow beings going through their own struggle of Self-realization? Can you love unconditionally? Are you forgiving and encouraging toward others?

Samadhi is not identical with enlightenment, which is the real goal of Yoga. You can attain enlightenment without ever experiencing *samadhi.* You can also have hundreds of *samadhi* experiences and still be far removed from enlightenment. The next section enlightens you about the state of enlightenment.

Reaching toward Enlightenment

People usually associate the word *enlightenment* with profound intellectual understanding. However, in Yoga, enlightenment means something completely different: It refers to the permanent realization of your true nature, which in Yoga is the ultimate or transcendental Self *(atman).* The Sanskrit word for enlightenment is *bodha* (pronounced *bohd-ha*), which means literally "illumination." The same realization also is referred to as *liberation,* because it liberates you from the misunderstanding that you are a separate self, referred to as ("I") in a unique body and gifted with a mind that is disconnected from everything else. Liberation is actually Self-realization, in which your journey of self-discovery meets with ultimate success.

Liberation is also called *open-eyed ecstasy* because, unlike other forms of ecstasy, it does not exclude awareness of the world. In order to achieve conventional forms of *samadhi* (see the preceding section), you typically focus your attention deep within yourself through concentration and meditation, losing awareness of the body and your surroundings. In the enlightened state, you simply are your true Self regardless of whether your eyes are open or closed, whether your body is awake or asleep, and whether your mind is active or still. Once you attain liberation, you cannot lose it. You are forever established in perfect ease.

Wherever you go, there you are

Sri Ramana Maharshi was one of the great Yoga masters of the twentieth century. When, on his deathbed, his disciples expressed their sorrow at losing him, he calmly said, "They say that I am dying, but I am not going away. Where could I go? I am here." He had realized the eternal Self, which is everywhere. To this day, his spiritual presence can be felt in the hermitage that disciples built for him long ago.

Chapter 21

Yoga for Special Situations

· ·

In This Chapter

▶ Using Yoga for a testy back

▶ Benefiting from Yoga during pregnancy

▶ Practicing Yoga during menstruation and menopause

▶ Sharing Yoga with children

· ·

*L*ife is a series of ordinary events punctuated by extraordinary situations. In this chapter, we address some of these extraordinary situations, which include physical limitations through ill health and pregnancy, and to a lesser degree, menstruation and menopause. Special situations also include a magic word: children. In all cases, you can bring Yoga into play, because it is a premium tool for making the most of any circumstance.

Unless you face medical complications, pregnancy, menstruation, and menopause are all perfectly normal processes. Although Westerners have the custom of giving birth in hospitals, pregnancy is, of course, not a sickness. Likewise, menstruation and menopause are ordinary physiological processes, which may require special attention but are certainly not afflictions. With Yoga, you can help prevent complications by harmonizing your body's physiological functions.

Should you find yourself in poor health — possibly even in a hospital bed — you can still benefit from Yoga. Yogic practice can help restore your physical vitality and emotional balance. In this chapter, we single out back problems, which are incredibly widespread in our sedentary culture. But Yoga's repertoire includes practices for all kinds of other health challenges, and if you are suffering from any health problems, we recommend that you seek out a competent Yoga therapist in conjunction with your physician of choice (see the appendix).

Befriend Your Back with Yoga

The number of people who have back problems in the United States is staggering. At least 85 percent of all Americans will seek professional help for a back problem sometime in their lives, and over 80 million people suffer from chronic back ailments. Seven million people miss work every day because of back-related problems, and over 250,000 men and women undergo back surgeries each year — with only a 50/50 recovery rate.

If you have a serious back problem or are currently in a great deal of pain, you need to first work one-on-one with a medical specialist, osteopath, or a chiropractor. Get a diagnosis from a competent health professional so that you can fully understand what you're dealing with. Then enlist the services of a qualified Yoga teacher/therapist or a competent physical therapist or exercise physiologist.

When you browse through the literature on lower back problems, you're likely to notice that many of the recommended exercises are very similar. On further investigation, you may discover that almost all systems of movement interface with Yoga somehow, simply because Yoga has explored human movement for a very long time. When it comes to back exercises, you can safely say that there's nothing new under the sun. The key is knowing what exercises fit an individual situation. Every case is a little different. Prescribing a particular Yoga posture or routine for a specific back problem is beyond the scope of this book — the variables are just too numerous.

In general, however, the most common cause of back problems is poor posture or poor lifestyle biomechanics (especially sitting) that begin to add up after days, weeks, and years of repetition. In addition, many people have weak abdominal muscles (see Chapter 10), tight hamstrings (see Chapter 6), and strained or sprained ligaments and muscles supporting the curvature of the spine. Additionally, many people have built-up scar tissue, either from injury or from operations, which they need to stretch out in order for the injured area to become functional again.

Five-step plan for a healthy back

After your healthcare professional tells you that you are ready for Yoga, the best way to prevent back problems or to keep them from becoming chronic is to use Yoga as part of a five-step plan. The key components of a five-step plan are as follows:

✔ **Biomechanical re-education:** Rebuilding your back is like fitting the pieces of a puzzle together. Re-education about biomechanics — how you sit, stand, walk, lift, sleep, and work — involves rethinking your entire lifestyle, a subject that could fill an entire chapter in this book.

✔ **Yoga or back exercise program:** All back problems are a little different, therefore, it is imperative that you have the guidance of a qualified Yoga therapist or health professional. One of the key issues is the length of your program. It has to fit your lifestyle. Most people new to a personal practice cannot commit to more than 15 to 20 minutes per day.

✔ **Back journal:** Keeping a journal is a simple way to discover more about how your lifestyle affects your back. It usually helps to first write down everything you can think of that agitates your back. Then go through the list with your health professional and see how many things you can eliminate from your daily activities. In addition, use a calendar to check off when you do your routine and rate the condition of your back each day on a scale of 1 to10 so you can chart your progress. Also keep track of your water intake. Hydrating, or drinking 6 to 8 glasses of water per day, is helpful to almost any muscular-skeletal rehabilitation program.

✔ **Proper food choices:** Dietary needs, just like back program designs, are different for every individual and require the direction of a health professional. However, we all do have a couple of things in common: We need to slow down when we eat and chew our food properly. And, with the exception of those who suffer from food disorders, we need to eat less as we age.

✔ **Rest and relaxation:** Just because we get into a bed and close our eyes does not mean that we are getting proper rest and relaxation. The last thing we see or listen to before bed has an effect on the subconscious mind and can affect your sleep pattern, which suggests that the local news coverage of crimes and disasters is not a good lullaby. Try reading something spiritual or listening to beautiful music and notice the difference.

For more information about the five steps, check out the original *Five-Step Healthy Back Plan with Larry Payne*. It first appeared in audio and booklet form in 1986 *(Healthy Back Exercises for High Stress Professionals)* and has helped thousands of back sufferers. The program offers guidelines for improving your entire lifestyle (see the appendix at the back of this book).

Yoga back class

The following exercises are not meant for acute back problems. If any part of this routine causes you back or neck pain, omit that part and check with your physician before you continue.

Yoga for athletes?

If you are in excellent health and fond of sports, well, don't think Yoga is only for the timid and sensitive. As many athletes already know, Yoga can be a marvelous ally in your sports ambitions. I (Georg Feuerstein) taught suitably adapted Hatha Yoga exercises to the British women's ski team for one season to help them get ready for the winter Olympics in the early '70s. Also, champion bodybuilder Frank Zane used Yoga meditation to focus his mind and win the coveted titles of Mr. Universe and Mr. Olympia several times. The Chicago Bulls basketball team used meditation to help them lead the NBA for many seasons. These athletes understand that the secret of Yoga lies in the control of the mind, be it through postures, breathing, or meditation.

A session or two of Yoga or back exercise during your week won't help much if you misuse or abuse your back the rest of the time.

No single Yoga routine is appropriate for all back problems. When your doctor feels that you're ready for a regular group class, the following routine can help you make the transition. Keep in mind that the Yoga breathing we recommend in this routine is just as important as the Yoga postures. Please note the options for many of the postures and remember that the proper sequence is very important.

Use Focus Breathing or Belly Breathing (see Chapter 5) for the entire routine. Inhale and exhale through the nose slowly, with a slight pause after the inhalation and the exhalation.

Corpse with bent legs (shavasana variation)

Relaxation and breathing are important ingredients for a healthy back. The corpse pose is a classic position to start the process.

1. **Lie flat on your back with your arms relaxed along the sides of your torso, palms up.**

2. **Bend your knees and place your feet on the floor at hip width.**

3. **Close your eyes and relax (see Figure 21-1).**

   Stay in the posture for 8 to 10 breaths.

Note: If your back feels uncomfortable, place a pillow or blanket roll under your knees. If your neck or throat is tense, place a folded blanket or small pillow under your head.

Figure 21-1: Think of this posture and your breathing as an oasis from the stressful world outside.

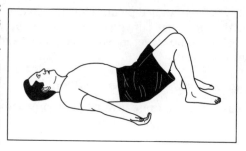

Lying arm raise with bent leg (shavasana variation)

Many back sufferers have problems on one side of the torso more than the other. The lying arm raise is a safe, classic way to gently stretch and prepare each side of the back and neck for the rest of the routine (see Figure 21-2).

1. **Lie in the corpse posture, arms relaxed at your sides and palms down.**

   Bend just your left knee, and put your left foot on the floor (see Figure 21-2a).

2. **As you inhale, slowly raise your arms overhead and touch the floor behind you, palms up (see Figure 21-2b).**

   Pause briefly.

3. **As you exhale, bring your arms back to your sides as in Step 1.**

4. **Repeat Steps 2 and 3 six to eight times, and then repeat with your right knee bent and your left leg straight.**

Figure 21-2: This sequence allows you to warm up each side of your back and also prepare your neck.

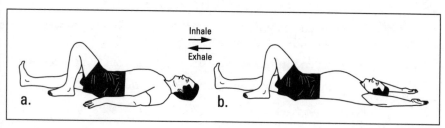

Knee to chest

Keeping your back healthy is like tuning a piano. The knee to chest posture helps to adjust and relax the lower back. If you hear a gentle pop when you bring your knee, consider the sound sweet music — you may have saved yourself a visit to the chiropractor.

1. **Lie on your back, knees bent, feet flat on the floor.**

2. **As you exhale, bring your right knee toward your chest, holding your shin just below your knee (see Figure 21-3).**

   If you have knee problems, hold the back of your thigh instead.

3. **Stay for 6 to 8 breaths, and then repeat on the left side.**

Figure 21-3:
Remember,
this is not a
biceps
exercise.
Just hold
the knee,
breathe,
and relax.

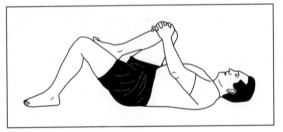

Push downs

The abdomen is considered the front of your back (see Chapter 10). This is a key area to keep strong and toned if you want to prevent back problems. The lower abdominals (see Chapter 10) are the focus of this exercise and a great place to start.

1. **Lying on your back, knees bent, feet on the floor at hip width, rest your arms near your sides, palms down.**

2. **As you exhale, push your lower back down to the floor for 3 to 5 seconds (see Figure 21-4).**

3. **As you inhale, your back releases from the push down.**

   Repeat Steps 2 and 3 six to eight times.

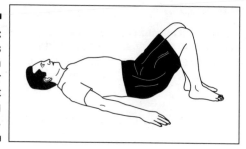

Figure 21-4:
Push downs
strengthen
your lower
abs without
involving
your neck.

Yogi sit-ups

Most exercises are traceable to Yoga, which has been around for thousands of years.

The yogi sit-ups are a contemporary variation of *navasana* (pronounced *nah-vah-sah-nah*), or the boat posture, and primarily work the upper abdomen (see Chapter 10).

1. **Lie on your back, knees bent, feet on the floor at hip width.**

2. **Turn your toes in pigeon-toed and touch your inner knees together.**

3. **Spread your palms on the back of your head, fingers interlocked, and hook your thumbs under the angle of the jawbone, just below your ears.**

4. **As you exhale, press your knees together firmly, tilt the front of your pelvis toward your navel and, with your hips on the ground, slowly sit up halfway.**

   Keep your elbows out to the sides in line with the tops of your shoulders. Look toward the ceiling (as shown in Figure 21-5). Don't pull your head up with your arms; rather, support your head with your hands and come up by contracting your abdominal muscles.

5. **As you inhale, slowly roll back down.**

   Repeat Steps 4 and 5 six to eight times.

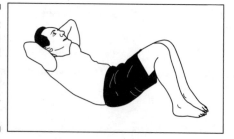

Figure 21-5:
Be careful
not to pull
your neck.
Just hold
the neck
and look up.

Dynamic bridge — dvipada pitha

The order or sequence in a back program is very important (see Chapter 6). The bridge posture lives up to its name by acting as a bridge from the abdominal postures to the back bending postures. The gentle action of the bridge compensates the abs and prepares the back for the next level of back bends.

1. **Lie on your back, knees bent, feet flat on the floor at hip width.**

2. **Place your arms at your sides, palms down.**

3. **As you inhale, raise your hips to a comfortable height (see Figure 21-6).**

4. **As you exhale, return your hips to the floor.**

   Repeat Steps 3 and 4 six to eight times.

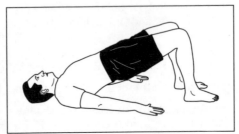

Figure 21-6: Only raise as high as you feel comfortable.

Cobra 2 — bhujangasana

Chapter 12 emphasizes that most of us simply bend forward too much. Finding a way to compensate (see Chapter 6) with some form of back bends is important. We offer three levels of back bends for this part of your routine.

Note: We recommend that you use either this posture or the Cobra 1 posture — not both.

1. **Lie on your abdomen, with your legs at hip width and the tops of your feet on the floor.**

2. **Bend your elbows and place your palms on the floor with your thumbs near your armpits.**

   Rest your forehead on the floor and relax your shoulders (see Figure 21-7a).

3. **As you inhale, engage your back muscles, press your palms against the floor, and raise your chest and head.**

4. **Look straight ahead (as shown in Figure 21-7b).**

   Keep the top front of your pelvis on the floor and your shoulders relaxed. Unless you are very flexible, keep your elbows slightly bent.

5. **As you exhale, lower your torso and head slowly back to the floor.**

   Repeat Steps 3–5 six to eight times.

Figure 21-7:
Unless
you're very
flexible,
keep your
arms a little
bent.

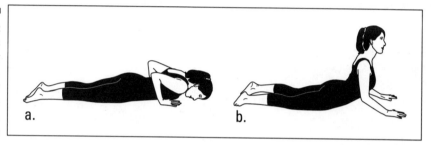

a.   b.

Move slowly and cautiously in all of the cobra-like postures. Avoid any of the postures that cause pain in your lower back, upper back, or neck. If Cobra 2 is too strenuous, use Cobra 1, which appears next in this section, or repeat the lying arm raise, which we cover earlier in this chapter (refer to Figure 21-2).

Cobra 1 — sphinx

Use cobra 1 only if you are not able to work with cobra 2 (don't use both). Listen carefully to your body and choose the right posture. Keep in mind that you are having a dialogue not a monologue.

1. **Lie on your abdomen, with your legs at hip width and the tops of the feet on the floor.**

2. **Rest your forehead on the floor and relax your shoulders (see Figure 21-8a).**

   Bend your elbows and place your forearms on the floor, palms turned down and positioned near the sides of your head.

3. **As you inhale, engage your back muscles, press your forearms against the floor, and raise your chest and head (see Figure 21-8b).**

   Looking straight ahead keep your forearms and the front of your pelvis on the floor. Continue to relax your shoulders.

4. **As you exhale, lower your torso and head slowly back to the floor.**

5. **Repeat Steps 2–4 six to eight times.**

If the cobra postures aggravate your lower back, separate your legs wider than your hips and turn your heels out. Also, if you move your hands further forward, cobra 1 or cobra 2 is less difficult. Then again, if you move your hands further back, to the sides of the navel, you increase the difficulty. However, we do not recommend increasing the difficulty level without guidance from your health professional

Figure 21-8:
Cobra 1
emphasizes
the upper
back until
your lower
back is
ready for
cobra 2.

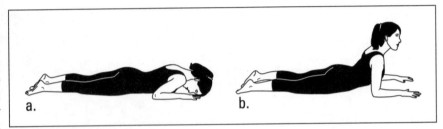

a.   b.

Prone resting posture

Back bends may be the most strenuous part of your back routine. Resting at the right times is an important part of the sequence. Remember, Yoga should never feel like you are in a hurry.

1. **Lie on your abdomen, with your legs at hip width and the tops of your feet on the floor.**

2. **Rest your forehead on the floor or turn your head to one side and relax your shoulders.**

   Bend your elbows and place the forearms on the floor, palms turned down and positioned near the sides of your head (see Figure 21-9).

   Stay for 6 to 8 breaths.

Note: If this resting position is uncomfortable for you, use the bent knee corpse posture.

Figure 21-9:
Just relax
and rest.

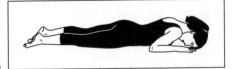

Locust 1 — *shalabhasana*

The cobra postures we recommend for this routine work primarily to stretch your back. The locust posture works more on strengthening your back. We need both.

1. **Lie on your abdomen, with your legs at hip width and the tops of your feet on the floor.**

   Rest your forehead on the floor.

2. **Extend your arms back along the sides of your torso, palms on the floor (see Figure 21-10a).**

3. **As you inhale, raise your chest, head, and your right leg (see Figure 21-10b).**

4. **As you exhale, lower your torso and your head slowly to the floor.**

   Repeat Steps 3 and 4 six to eight times, and then repeat with the left leg.

Note: If this posture is too strenuous for you, try it without lifting your leg. If you want to make the posture more challenging, raise both legs but again, let your health professional recommend the best time to make the posture more challenging.

Figure 21-10:
The locust posture helps to strengthen your back and neck.

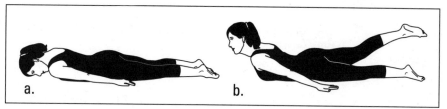

Child's posture — *balasana*

If you listen for feedback from your body after doing a number of back bends, you'll hear a clear desire to fold as compensation (see Chapter 6). The child's posture is a smooth and easy way to fold when you're concluding prone or front-lying back bends.

1. **Starting on your hands and knees, place your knees about hip width, hands just below your shoulders, elbows straight but not locked.**

2. **As you exhale, sit back on your heels, rest your torso on your thighs, and place your forehead on the floor.**

3. **Lay your arms on the floor beside your torso, palms up.**

   Close your eyes and breathe easily (see Figure 21-11). Stay for 6 to 8 breaths.

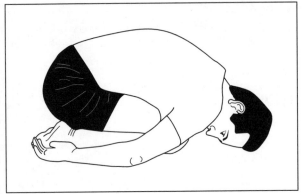

Figure 21-11:
Keep your arms at your sides or stretched out on the floor in front of you.

If you have knee or hip problems, lie on your back and do the knees to chest posture (see Chapter 6) instead of the child's posture.

Hamstring stretch

Tight hamstring muscles are a key factor in many cases of chronic back problems. A fine balance exists between stretching your hamstrings and not aggravating a chronic back condition. For this reason, we recommend keeping one leg bent with the foot on the floor to support your back (see Figure 21-12).

1. **Lying on your back, legs straight, place your arms along your sides, palms down.**

2. **Bend just your left knee, and put your foot on the floor (see Figure 21-12a).**

3. **As you exhale, raise your right leg until it's perpendicular to the floor — see Figure 21-12b — or as close as you can manage.**

4. **As you inhale, return your leg to the floor, all the while keeping your head and the top of your hips on the floor.**

   Repeat 3 to 4 times.

5. **After repeating 3 to 4 times, then hold the back of your raised thigh just above your knee, hold your leg in place for 6 to 8 breaths (see Figure 21-12c).**

If the back of your neck or your throat tenses when you raise or lower your leg, rest your head on a pillow or folded blanket.

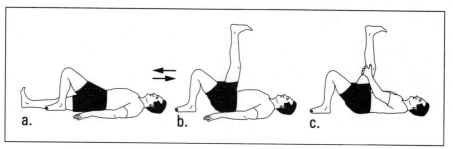

Figure 21-12:
Make sure you feel the stretch in your hamstrings not in your back.

a. b. c.

Head-to-knee posture — *janu shirshasana*

The head-to-knee posture allows you to stretch each side of your back separately (see Figure 21-13). Because so many back problems are asymmetrical or affect one side more than the other, this posture helps to bring balance back to your entire torso.

Be very careful of the head-to-knee posture or any extended leg forward bends if you are having a disc problem. Avoid it completely if you experience pain or numbness in your back.

1. **Sit on the floor with your legs stretched out in front of you.**

   Bend your left knee and bring your left heel toward your right groin.

2. **Rest the bent left knee on the floor (but do not force it down) and place the sole of your left foot on the inside of your right thigh.**

   Point the toes of your left foot toward your right knee.

3. **Bring your back up nice and tall, and as you inhale, raise your arms forward and up overhead until they're beside your ears.**

   Keep your arms and your right leg soft and slightly bent (see Figure 21-13a).

4. **As you exhale, bend forward from your hips, bringing your hands, chest, and head toward your right leg.**

   Rest your hands on the floor or on your thigh, knee, shin, or foot. If your head is not close to your right knee, bend your knee more until you feel your back stretching on the right side (see Figure 21-13b).

5. **Repeat Steps 3 and 4 three times, and then hold the final forward bend for 6 to 8 breaths.**

   Repeat the same sequence on the opposite side.

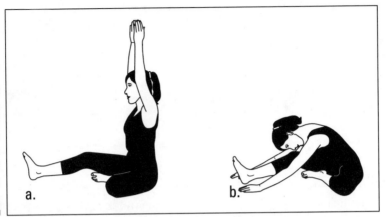

Figure 21-13:
If your head
is not close
to your
knee, bend
the knee a
little more.

Bent leg supine twist (parivartanasana variation)

A good back routine often includes a twist. The bent leg supine twist is appropriate here because of its ease of execution and the safeness of the movement. We offer you a number of other effective twists in Chapter 13.

If you are having a disc-related problem, be very careful of twists. If you have any negative symptoms, such as pain or numbness, leave the twist out. Speak to your physician before adding the twist back to your program.

1. **Lie on your back with your knees bent and feet on the floor at hip width.**

   Extend your arms out from your sides like a "T," palms down and in line with the top of your shoulders.

2. **As you exhale, slowly lower your bent legs to the right side, and then turn your head to the left.**

   Keep your head on the floor (see Figure 21-14).

3. **As you inhale, bring the bent knees back to the middle; as you exhale, slowly lower the bent knees to the left and turn your head to the right.**

   Follow Steps 1 to 3 and alternate three times slowly to each side; then hold one last twist to each side for 6 to 8 breaths.

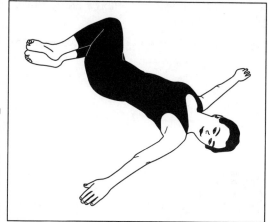

Figure 21-14:
Turn your
head in the
opposite
direction of
your knees.

Knees-to-chest posture— *apanasana*

One of the rules of sequencing (see Chapter 6) is to always follow a twist with some kind of forward bend. Knees-to-chest is a classic forward bend to use when the posture preceding it is a floor twist, as in this back routine.

1. **Lie on your back and bend your knees in toward your chest.**

2. **Hold your shins just below the knees (see Figure 21-15).**

   Stay for 6 to 8 breaths.

   If you have any knee problems, hold the backs of your thighs instead. Hold for 6 to 8 breaths.

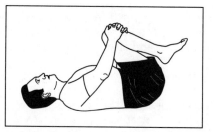

Figure 21-15:
Just hold
the legs,
breathe,
and relax.

Corpse with bent legs *(shavasana variation)*

When you come to the end of our back routine, the corpse with bent legs gives you a stable position to focus on your breathing and deeply relax your back. You don't want to skip this part.

EXERCISE

1. **Lie flat on your back with your arms relaxed along the sides of your torso, palms up.**

2. **Bend your knees and place your feet on the floor at hip width.**

   Close your eyes and relax (see Figure 21-16).

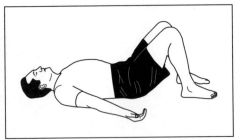

Figure 21-16:
Is it any wonder that the corpse postures are the most popular Yoga postures?

3. **Stay in this posture for 25 to 30 breaths, making your exhalation slightly longer than your inhalation.**

Note: If your back is uncomfortable, place a pillow or blanket roll under your knees. If your neck or throat is tense, place a folded blanket or small pillow under your head.

Partnering Yoga and Pregnancy

Experts disagree about the best way to approach Yoga or any other exercise during pregnancy. Of course, you need to involve your doctor in any decision about your health before, during, and after pregnancy.

TIP

If your doctor is not familiar with Yoga, show him or her a copy of this book.

We think that the best way to take full advantage of Yoga is to start your practice well before you are pregnant, or at least as soon as you receive the good news. Your Yoga practice can build a strong, healthy body and a stable mind, not only helping you conceive a child (by making you fit and relaxed) but also supporting you during the pregnancy, at birth, and thereafter. Many of our students continue their Yoga practice during their entire pregnancies, using the conservative principles that we outline in this book.

BEWARE

We don't recommend starting any new fitness regime, including Hatha Yoga, in the middle of a pregnancy. However, this caution does not exclude you from practicing conscious yogic relaxation and meditation. Your body and mind, as well as your baby will be grateful to you!

Womb with a (yogic) view

Dave and Adrian Lopez first attended Yoga classes in Southern California during the late 1980s. They later married, became heavily involved in their careers, and drifted away from Yoga for several years. In 1994, they decided they were ready for children and for three years tried unsuccessfully to get pregnant, despite resorting to all the latest medical methods. Adrian's doctor suggested that stress could be the problem and encouraged Dan and Adrian to return to Yoga together. Following their doctor's advice, they enrolled in a weekly class and used Larry Payne's User Friendly Yoga tapes (see the appendix) on two other days a week. Much to their joy, within 30 days, Adrian was pregnant. She continued her Yoga practice until the eighth month of her pregnancy and gave birth to a big beautiful baby boy.

Enjoying Yoga support as you — and the baby — grow on

Pregnancy involves major physiological and psychological changes. Apart from modifying your shape and weight, it also alters your body chemistry. All this, in turn, may lead to potentially unpleasant side effects, including the following:

- Back problems
- Emotional and physical instability
- Faster heartbeat
- Fatigue
- Lack of balance
- Morning sickness
- Physical pressure of extra weight
- Respiratory difficulties
- Swelling and leg cramps

Yoga can make a major difference in your pregnancy experience. Yogic practice provides the following benefits during that special time in your — and your baby's — life:

- Relaxes your whole body
- Helps with back problems
- Relieves nausea

✔ Reduces swelling and leg cramps

✔ Improves emotional and mental stability

✔ Provides focusing and breathing techniques for labor

✔ Offers camaraderie through prenatal and postnatal Yoga classes

The increasing self-awareness that comes with Yoga is very helpful during pregnancy. Each Yoga practice is like completing a self-examination — a valuable tool both during and after pregnancy.

You may want to call local Yoga schools to ask about prenatal classes, and always talk to the teacher before you go to class. Find out about her training and experience, and what kinds of things she teaches and stresses in class.

Exercising caution during pregnancy

Because pregnancy is a time when your actions directly and immediately affect more than your own person, we recommend that you keep the following cautions in mind as you exercise:

✔ Avoid extremes in all the postures, especially deep forward or back bends. Do not strain.

✔ Avoid sit-ups and postures that put pressure on the uterus.

✔ Avoid inverted postures other than putting your feet up on the wall or a chair.

✔ Avoid breathing exercises that are jarring, such as the shining skull (*kapalabhati*) or breath of fire (*bhastrika*).

✔ Do not jump or move quickly in and out of postures.

✔ Avoid lying on your stomach for any postures.

✔ Be careful not to overstretch, which you can easily do in pregnancy because of increased hormone levels that cause your joints to become very limber.

✔ Always do a little less than you're used to doing, and never hold your breath.

Most mothers-to-be have no problem resting on their backs. However, for about 15 to 20 percent of women, lying on their backs causes the weight of the uterus to compress the *vena cava,* the major vein that returns the blood from the lower body to the heart. If you experience this compression, you will most likely feel a tingling or numbing sensation in your lower or upper body. Importantly, lying on your back may be comfortable one day or one week and not the next. Speak to your doctor about this concern. The safest alternative to lying on your back is the side-lying variation of *shavasana* (refer to Figure 21-17).

Finding the right posture for pregnancy

Practicing Yoga during pregnancy calls for the same consideration as putting together a yogic plan to manage back problems — no single posture or routine works the same way for everyone. To make the most of your personal situation, rely on a qualified teacher for one-on-one instruction or join a good pre- or postnatal Yoga class. The following sections describe two of the more useful Yoga postures for you to use during and after pregnancy.

Side-lying posture

The side-lying posture relieves feelings of general fatigue or nausea during pregnancy, labor, and the postpartum period. Side-lying also is a good position for nursing. You need four blankets and two large pillows for this variation of the corpse posture, or *shavasana*.

1. **Lie on your side on a comfortable surface.**

2. **Place one of the pillows under your head and the other just in front of you on the floor between the top of your thighs and the bottom of your chest.**

   Hang your top arm over the large pillow in front of you.

3. **Bend your knees and place two blankets between your feet and two blankets between your knees (see Figure 21-17).**

   Stay and breathe naturally for as long as you feel comfortable. Repeat as often as you need to.

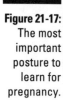

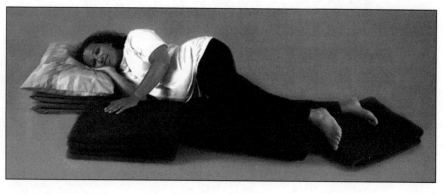

Figure 21-17: The most important posture to learn for pregnancy.

The cat and cow

This posture, a variation of *chakravakasana*, flexes and extends the lower back and helps relieve symptoms of general back pain caused by pregnancy.

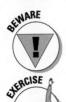

Do not exaggerate or force your lower back down in Step 4. Eliminate cat and cow if you experience any negative symptoms.

1. **Starting on your hands and knees, look straight ahead.**

2. **Place your knees at hip width, hands below your shoulders.**

   Straighten but don't lock your elbows.

3. **As you exhale, hump your back like a camel.**

   Turn your head down and look at the floor (see Figure 21-18a).

4. **As you inhale, slowly look up toward the ceiling and drop your lower back in the reverse camel posture (see Figure 21-18b).**

   Repeat Steps 3 and 4 six to eight times.

Figure 21-18:
Cat and cow can relieve back pain during pregnancy.

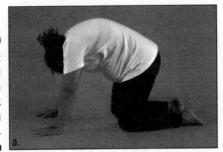
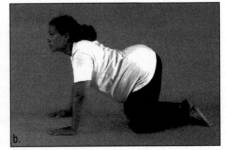

Practicing Yoga during labor

Yoga teaches you to connect your breathing with uterine contraction. Breathe into each contraction as though you're breathing through a difficult Yoga posture. Be patient: Breathing, relaxation, and concentration can get you through the labor process. If you have a *mantra,* labor is a good occasion to use it.

Continuing yogic exercise after pregnancy (postpartum)

Generally, you can resume a very gentle Hatha Yoga practice within two to three weeks after delivery or five to six weeks after a cesarean. Avoid all inverted postures for at least six weeks because of uterine blood flow (called *lochia*). Also, be careful with sit-ups, as the groin area is fragile from its recent stretch. A good way to get started is with short walks and the side-lying corpse posture (refer to Figure 21-17). Your hormone levels may make you feel emotional and a little unstable. Your Yoga practice will seem like an oasis. Don't feel guilty about taking time for yourself. You need to recharge. Nothing is more demanding than a new baby. Your child took nine months to grow inside your body, so give yourself nine months to get back into shape.

All women have postnatal bleeding for a few weeks after pregnancy. Watch your flow. Slow down your Yoga practice a little if the bleeding becomes heavier or turns bright red. In case of doubt, consult your physician.

Cycling Yoga into Your View of Menstruation and PMS

Menstruation is not normally a hindrance to Yoga practice. If your periods are irregular and painful, consistent Yoga practice, a nonstressful lifestyle, and good diet can often establish balance fairly quickly. Menstrual distress is unnecessary. Also, Yoga has a deep positive influence on your body's hormonal activity. You *can* overcome the mood swings that characterize premenstrual syndrome (PMS), also called premenstrual tension (PMT). Never think of yourself as a victim of biology. Instead, focus on your Yoga practice, especially relaxation (see Chapter 4) and breathing (see Chapter 5).

If you're bleeding heavily, go easy on yourself. We recommend that you avoid inversion exercises during menstruation and emphasize relaxation instead.

Inversions during menstruation can cause *endometriosis,* a condition in which the uterine lining tears loose and embeds itself in the abdominal organs.

Practicing Yoga through Midlife and Beyond

Yoga is a powerful tool for all seasons of life. Midlife, as the word suggests, refers to the middle of life. It's not, as some people think The End, but a new beginning. Yoga allows you to grow old gracefully, that is, healthily and actively.

Working through menopause

Menopause signals a major biochemical change, marked most obviously by the disappearance of a woman's monthly flow. Her body's sexual glands go into relative retirement, and she can no longer bear children. Most women would welcome this transition with open arms, if it weren't for the undesirable side effects: hot flushes, palpitations, dizzy spells, insomnia, vaginal dryness, urinary problems, and irritability. The most unwelcome and potentially damaging symptom, however, is the often-present sense of worthlessness, which can lead to depression.

Regular Yoga practice can help you alleviate the physiological side effects of menopause, especially if you start a few years before its onset. Inversions (see Chapter 11), which have a profound effect on the glands and inner organs, are particularly helpful. For soothing rest and whole-person recovery, we particularly recommend that you cultivate the corpse posture to perfection. Middle age is not *the end* but a new beginning! Just give your body a chance to rebalance its chemistry. Daily Yoga practice can do much to speed up this process.

Aging gracefully from the male perspective

What we call the *malopause* is very similar to the woman's menopause. Although changes in their sexual glands may lessen their sex drives, men can continue to sire children into old age. But when they see their vitality and hairline recede a little, men are often thrown into an existential crisis.

Midlife is a great opportunity to discover life's possibilities beyond sexual reproduction and raising children. Regular Yoga practice can buffer the unpleasant physiological side effects of the male version of menopause. Yoga also can stabilize the emotions that are triggered when you realize you are no longer quite so dashing — unless, of course, you have practiced Yoga all along. However, sooner or later midlife and old age catch up with everybody. The best idea is to prepare emotionally long before you realize how quickly the years are rolling past, by keeping the larger perspective in mind: Human life is not merely for reproduction, but also for moral, intellectual, and spiritual growth.

Bones of steel

With regular exercise, you can prevent the bone loss *(osteoporosis)* associated with midlife and old age. Bones want to be exercised, and they love relaxation. Regular weight-bearing exercises strengthen your bones, while stress causes acidity, which leaches the calcium from your bones. Many people don't realize that osteoporosis actually starts in your mid- to late 20s. Therefore, you can't begin Yoga too early — and it's never too late to take it up! Buns of steel ain't bad, but bones of steel are the better deal.

Keeping the pounds at bay

Midlife not only decreases bone mass but also increases fatty tissue. Yoga practice helps you step up a flagging metabolism and keep the rolls off your midriff. Of course, you still have to be wise about your diet.

Introducing Children to Yoga

Yoga for children really begins at birth. In both word and deed, parents right from the start can model yogic values like truthfulness, nonharming, and (though maybe not *all* the time) patience. Parents also serve as models for their children's postural and movement habits. We sometimes forget that children imitate not only *what* their parents do, but *how* they do it. Parents can stand and walk and sit in ways that promote proper biomechanics. Then, when these children become adults, they already have a leg up on Yoga practice.

Different people have different views on how early children should receive Yoga instruction. Traditionally in India, some children learn about Yoga while they are still toddlers, although regular instruction does not begin until the child is age 8. Simple lessons may include sun salutation and alternate nostril breathing, with more advanced Yoga instruction introduced after puberty.

In the United States, Yoga postures are taught at a growing number of private and public elementary schools, and many Yoga schools include classes for children. Classes are usually short, from 30 to 45 minutes, and fast-paced, moving quickly from one posture to the next. With the same guidelines as adults, children are asked not to eat for an hour or two before class, to be barefoot in class, and to appreciate a noncompetitive environment that focuses on body, breath, and mind. See the appendix for Yoga for kids videos.

Part VI
The Part of Tens

The 5th Wave   By Rich Tennant

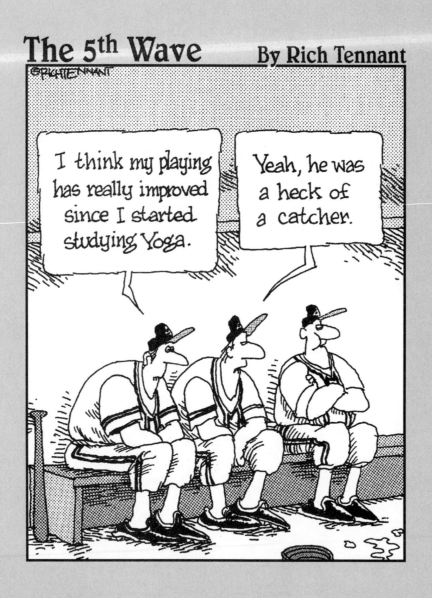

In this part . . .

This is the place to turn if you want to get clear about why you are practicing or ought to be practicing Yoga, or about how to approach Yoga correctly. This part is full of fun little snippets of information that remind you how wonderful Yoga practice is. Also, if you are thinking of enrolling in a Yoga class or workshop to get started or find out more about Yoga, we give you the top places in the United States to contact (with more addresses and other information in the appendix).

Chapter 22
Ten Tips for a Great Yoga Practice

*T*o succeed at anything, you must know two things: the ground rules and yourself. In this chapter, we give you ten hot tips for growing your Yoga practice into a sturdy, fruit-laden tree. If you bear these points in mind, you can expect to reap the benefits of your efforts surprisingly quickly. Although we don't promise overnight miracles, we are confident that regular, correct Yoga practice can bring you multiple advantages — physically, mentally, and also spiritually.

Understand Yoga

To engage Yoga successfully, you must first understand what it is and how it works. Sometimes people rush into Yoga practice without knowing anything about it, and then they have to work through a bunch of misconceptions before they can benefit from Yoga.

This book gives you a basic understanding of the nature and principles of this age-old discipline — enough for a solid start. But make time to read other books on Yoga to deepen your comprehension (see the appendix in the back of this book).

Traditional Yoga involves study, a key aspect of practice for thousands of years. We especially recommend that you acquaint yourself with the actual literature of Yoga — notably the *Yoga-Sutra* of Patanjali and the *Bhagavad-Gita* — through the many translations available today (see the appendix in the back of this book for more information). The Yoga tradition is vast and highly diverse. Discover which approach speaks to you the most.

Be Clear about Your Goals and Needs

If you want your Yoga practice to be successful, take the time to consider your personal situation carefully and then set your goals based on your abilities and needs. Ask yourself: How much free time do I have or want to make available for Yoga? What are my expectations? Do I want to stay or become fit and trim? Do I want to be able to relax more and discover the art of meditation? Do I want to adopt Yoga as a lifestyle or explore the spiritual dimension of life? When you're realistic, you're less likely to experience disappointment — or guilt, when your schedule seems overwhelming. If you're dealing with health issues or physical impediments, make sure that you consult your physician before you launch your Yoga practice.

Commit Yourself to Growth

Even if you don't choose to practice Yoga as a lifestyle, keep an open mind about Yoga's involvement in your life. Allow Yoga to transform not only your body but also your mind. Don't put a ceiling on your own development. Don't assume that you are incapable of ever achieving a certain Yoga posture or learning how to meditate. Let Yoga gently work with your physical and mental limitations and expand your abilities. Allow Yoga to help you outgrow useless attitudes and negative thoughts, and discover new horizons.

Stay for the Long Haul

Spoiled by our consumerist society, most people expect quick fixes. While Yoga can work miracles in a short span of time, it's not like instant coffee. To derive the full benefits from Yoga, you have to apply yourself diligently, which also nicely strengthens your character. The longer you practice Yoga, the more enjoyable and beneficial it becomes. Give Yoga at least a year to prove itself to you. We promise you won't be disappointed. In fact, you may very well come out of that year with a lifelong commitment to growing with Yoga!

Develop Good Habits from the Beginning

Bad habits die hard, so cultivate good Yoga habits from the outset. If possible, take two or three lessons from a qualified Yoga teacher, either in a group class or privately. At least read our book — and other practical Yoga books — carefully before trying out the postures and breathing exercises.

Wrong practice can do damage! Protect yourself by proceeding slowly and following the instructions step by step. Err on the cautious side. If in doubt, always consult a teacher or knowledgeable practitioner.

Vary Your Routine to Avoid Boredom

After you enjoy the initial wash of enthusiasm, your mind may start playing tricks on you. (Here are some favorite expressions of doubt: "Maybe Yoga doesn't work." "It doesn't work *for me*." "I really have other more important things to do." "I don't feel like practicing today.") If you're easily bored, vary your program periodically to keep your interest alive. Slugging through Yoga or any exercise program serves no purpose. Cultivate what the Zen Buddhists call "beginner's mind": Approach your Yoga sessions (and, in fact, everything else) with the same intensity and freshness that you brought to your very first session.

Yoga For Dummies gives you a well-tested formula for creating many efficient routines for a variety of situations. You can make your programs as diversified and challenging as you like. Anyway, if you focus on each exercise properly, your mind won't have time to feel bored. Also, the more you involve yourself in the spirit of Yoga, the more centered you become, lessening your likelihood of needing an exercise potpourri.

Make Awareness and Breath Your Allies

Yoga practice is so potent because, if practiced correctly, it combines physical movement with awareness and proper breathing. Awareness and breath are Yoga's secret weapons. The sooner you catch on to this concept, the more quickly you can enjoy really satisfying results. Bringing awareness to your exercise routine also automatically strengthens your overall capacity for concentration and mindfulness. You're able to work more efficiently and better appreciate your leisure time. In particular, conscious breathing during the exercises greatly enhances the effects of your practice on your body and mind, equipping you with the vitality you need to meet the challenges of a busy life.

Do Your Best and Don't Worry about the Rest

People often anxiously watch their progress. Progress isn't linear; sometimes you seem to take a step back, only to take a big leap forward in due course. Be diligent but relaxed about your Yoga practice. Perfectionism serves no purpose other than to frustrate you and irritate others. In aspiring to reach your goal, be kind to yourself (and others). Don't worry about what may or may not happen down the line. Focus on practicing now and leave the rest to the power of Yoga, providence, and your good karma (see Chapter 1).

Allow Your Body to Speak Up

Your body is your best friend and counselor. If something doesn't "feel" right, it probably isn't. Trust your bodily instincts and intuitions not only in your Yoga practice but also in daily life. All too frequently, your body tells you one thing and your mind another. Learn to go with your body.

When practicing Hatha Yoga, be especially careful about letting your desire to achieve quick results get in the way of common sense and bodily wisdom. For instance, if a forward or backward bend "feels" risky, don't test your luck. Or if your body tells you that you aren't ready for the headstand (which we don't recommend for beginners anyway), don't fall victim to your own ambition.

Listening to your body is an art — one well worth cultivating.

Share Yoga

In the beginning, plan to practice Yoga with others until you find your own momentum. Sometimes everyone needs a little encouragement, and a supportive environment is a great bonus. If you don't go to a regular Yoga class, take the initiative to enlist an interested family member or friend in your Yoga practice. Make sure, however, that you keep any missionary zeal under wraps. Yoga is a wonderful gift to give to anyone, and so offer it in an attractive way: with love and tempered enthusiasm.

Chapter 23

Ten Great Places in the U.S.A. to Discover Yoga

In This Chapter

▶ Great schools to practice Hatha Yoga

▶ Where to practice Yoga comprehensively

▶ Places that offer weekend courses and retreats

You can find literally thousands of Yoga centers — big and small — around the world. In this chapter, we highlight some of the long-established and more popular places in the United States. We focus on centers that include or focus on Hatha Yoga and cater to beginners. If you happen to be athletic and very flexible and want to try your hand at a more aerobic type of Yoga, you can easily find information and addresses in the summer issue of *Yoga Journal* or in *Yoga International's Guide to Yoga Teachers and Classes,* which is published annually. These publications also tell you where you can study forms of Yoga other than Hatha Yoga. The listings in either periodical are not exhaustive, but they do provide a good starting point.

Although we haven't visited all the places we list, we know that most of them have been in existence for many years, and we've had good reports about the more recently established organizations. In any case, we name the centers in the United States with the largest annual enrollments, which means that thousands of students take classes at each location every year. But feel free to make your own inquiries among Yoga-practicing friends and acquaintances. You may find an excellent small- to medium-size center or a wonderful private class near you. To avoid disappointment, use the guidelines we provide in Chapter 2 to check out all your prospects carefully before you sign up.

For more information on Yoga centers in the U.S. and overseas, see the appendix.

Kripalu

Kripalu is the largest center for Yoga and holistic healing in the United States. In its 300-room building on 300 acres in a beautiful rural environment, a staff of around 150 caters to more than 12,000 guests annually. Kripalu was founded on the yogic ideal that physical health is the best foundation for mental well-being and spiritual growth. Offering a wide variety of Yoga programs for more than 20 years, the center presents a curriculum that includes daily workshops, weekend, and weeklong programs, as well as monthlong training.

Kripalu, P.O. Box 793, Lenox, MA 01240; 413-448-3152 or 800-741-7353

Ananda

Ananda, an 800-acre retreat center, was established 30 years ago by Swami Kriyananda (Donald Walters), a disciple of the famous Paramahansa Yogananda and the author of many books. Ananda, which favors a spiritual orientation, offers daily classes, workshops on postures, breathing, meditation, and Ayurveda (India's naturopathic medicine), weekend and weeklong retreats, as well as personal retreats (without being required to participate in any of the programs). The center also offers a four-week teacher-training program.

Ananda, 14618 Tyler Foote Road, Nevada City, CA 95959; 800-346-5350

Himalayan International Institute

Himalayan International Institute, established in 1971 by the late Swami Rama, is situated on 420 acres of wooded land. The Institute offers many residential programs based on traditional yogic teachings, including the cleansing practices of Hatha Yoga, which Western instructors seldom teach. The Institute also has a ten-day teacher-training course.

Himalayan International Institute, RR1, Box 400, Honesdale, PA 18431; 800-822-4547

Sivananda Yoga Vedanta Center

Sivananda Yoga Vedanta Center in New York is one of many centers established by Swami Vishnudevananda, the author of *The Complete Illustrated Book of Yoga*. In addition to daily, public classes, the Center also offers an intensive four-week residential program several times a year, an advanced Yoga teacher's training course, and a *sadhana* (spiritual practice) intensive program.

Sivananda Yoga Vedanta Center, 243 West 24th Street, New York 10011; 212-255-4560

Satchidananda Ashram

Satchidananda Ashram, founded by Swami Satchidananda, has centers in New York City and San Francisco, and both locations offer daily public classes and a teacher-training program in Integral Yoga. At the ashram (retreat), *Yogaville* is available — a month-long program in Integral Hatha Yoga for beginners. This approach goes back to Swami Sivananda of Rishikesh and combines postures, breath control, and purification practices with meditation, chanting, and other more traditional practices. Swami Satchidananda, author of *Integral Hatha Yoga,* was one of the spiritual mentors of the Woodstock generation.

Satchidananda Ashram, Buckingham, VA 23921; 804-969-3121 and 800-858-YOGA

B. K. S. Iyengar Yoga Institute of San Francisco

B. K. S. Iyengar Yoga Institute of San Francisco, established in 1974, is one of the larger Iyengar Yoga centers in the United States. The Institute has daily public classes, weeklong summer intensives, retreats, workshops, and a teacher-training program. Iyengar Yoga, which emphasizes precision in the execution of postures and also makes extensive use of props (see Chapter 17), is the most popular approach to Hatha Yoga. For the various "dialects" of Hatha Yoga, see Chapter 1.

B. K. S. Iyengar Yoga Institute, 2404 27th Avenue, San Francisco, CA 94116; 415-753-0909

American Yoga Association

American Yoga Association, founded in 1968 by Alice Christensen, has centers in Ohio and Florida. The Association's varied curriculum includes free introductory classes, daily classes, continuing courses, three-day seminars, classes for practitioners with physical limitations, in-service training for health professionals, a stress management course, and on-site courses for nurses.

American Yoga Association, P.O. Box 19986, Sarasota, FL 34276; 941-927-4077

The Pierce Program

The Pierce Program was founded in 1975 by Margaret and Martin Pierce, authors of *Yoga for Your Life*. This organization uses the T. K. V. Desikachar approach of Viniyoga (see Chapter 1) and offers a whole range of classes on Hatha Yoga (including beginning level), Viryayoga (for advanced students), and meditation. The center has an active program for pregnant women and also offers a teacher-training course.

The Pierce Program, 1164 N. Highland Avenue NE, Atlanta, GA 30306; 404-875-7110

Yoga Works

Yoga Works, directed by Marty Ezraty and Chuck Miller since 1987, offers over 150 classes per week in the styles of Ashtanga, Iyengar, Viniyoga, and mixed approaches, including classes for children, seniors, as well as pre- and postnatal Hatha Yoga. Some of the country's finer instructors conduct workshops, and Yoga Works offers teacher-training twice a year.

Yoga Works, 1426 Montana Avenue, 2nd Floor, Santa Monica, CA 90403 and 2215 Main Street, Santa Monica, CA 90405; 310-393-5150

Unity Woods Yoga Center

Unity Woods Yoga Center, founded in 1979 by John Schumacher, is the largest Iyengar Yoga center in the United States, with three locations in the Washington, D.C. metropolitan area. The curriculum includes classes for beginners, pregnant women, teens, and people with special situations (such as breast cancer survivors and those people who have heart problems, arthritis, back pain, and chronic or acute injuries, and so on). Unity Woods also offers a teacher-training course.

Unity Woods Yoga Center, 4853 Cordell Avenue, Suite PH9, Bethesda, MD 20814-3036; 310-656-8992

Chapter 24

Ten Good Reasons to Practice Yoga

*Y*our journey of discovery in the world of Yoga is not only exciting but also immensely rewarding. In this chapter, we give you ten excellent reasons to begin that journey *now* and persist in it.

The effects of regular Yoga practice are pervasive and astonishing. You can see good results very quickly. If you practice Hatha Yoga (the form of Yoga that deals specifically with the body), you may first notice an improvement in your flexibility, muscle tone, and overall fitness. Certainly, expect to feel better. Other wonderful benefits manifest as you continue to practice regularly and go deeper into Yoga. You have every reason to proceed with confidence! Yoga is a savings bank that pays triple and quadruple interest.

Yoga Helps You Maintain, Recover, or Improve Your Health

Yoga is an amazing stress-buster. When you consider that 75 to 90 percent of all visits to the doctor are related to stress, Yoga's holistic approach is a prudent first choice for fostering well-being. Through its relaxation, postural, breathing, and meditation exercises, as well as dietary rules, Yoga can effectively lower your level of tension and anxiety. Thus, yogic practice boosts your immune system, which obviously keeps illness at bay and, if you are sick, facilitates the physical healing process. Research demonstrates that Yoga is a very effective way of dealing with a variety of health problems — from hypertension, adult-onset diabetes, and respiratory illnesses (such as asthma) to sleep disturbance, chronic headache, and lower back pain. Yoga can help improve your cardiovascular functions, digestion, and eyesight — even enable you to control pain. You can practice Yoga as both remedial and preventive medicine. You can't find a cheaper health and life insurance policy!

Yoga Makes You Fit and Energetic

Yoga relaxes your body and mind, thereby enabling you to mobilize all the energy you need in order to deal efficiently with the many challenges at home and at work. Yoga can greatly promote your body's flexibility, fitness, strength, and stamina. In addition, Yoga may even help you shed surplus pounds.

Yoga Balances Your Mind

Yoga not only assists you in maintaining or recovering your physical well-being, but it also has a profound influence on your mind via the hormonal system. The mind is the source of many of your troubles — sooner or later, the body reflects wrong attitudes, negative thoughts, and emotional imbalance that your mind holds. Yoga is a powerful tool for clearing your mind and freeing you from mood swings. Yogic practice supports greater results than any tranquilizer, and without the undesirable side effects of drugs. It balances you without dulling your mind. Through Yoga, you can stay alert but relaxed.

Yoga Is a Powerful Aid for Personal Growth

Yoga can help you discover the body's hidden potential. Your body is a marvelous instrument, but you need to play it properly to produce beautiful, harmonious melodies. Yoga also can guide you safely into the exploration of the hidden aspects of the mind, especially higher states of consciousness (such as ecstasy and enlightenment explained in Chapter 20). It progressively peels away misconceptions about yourself and about life in general and reveals your true nature, which is uncomplicated and blissful.

Yoga Is Truly Comprehensive and Integrative

Yoga offers you a sensible, growth-oriented lifestyle that covers all aspects of life — from cradle to grave. Its repertoire includes techniques for optimal physical and mental health, for dealing creatively with the challenges of modern life, for transforming your sexual life, and even for making creative use of your dream life through the art of lucid dreaming (see Chapter 18). Yoga makes you feel comfortable with your body, improves your self-image and self-esteem, and enhances your power of concentration and memory. Ultimately, Yoga empowers you to discover your spiritual essence and to live free from fear and other limiting emotions and thoughts.

Yoga Helps You Harmonize Your Social Relationships

By giving you a new outlook on life, Yoga can help you improve your relationships with family, friends, coworkers, and others. It gives you the means to develop patience, tolerance, compassion, and forgiveness. Through the techniques of Yoga, you can gain control of your mind and liberate yourself from obsessions and undesirable habits, which stand in the way of satisfying relationships. Yoga also shows you how to live at peace with the world and in attunement with your essential nature, the spirit or Self. It provides you with all that is necessary to harmonize and beautify your life.

Yoga Enhances Your Awareness

Yoga enables you to greatly intensify your awareness (see Chapter 1). Thus, yogic practice empowers you to approach all life situations, even crises, with clarity and serenity. In addition, Yoga makes you more sensitive to your bodily rhythms, heightens your five senses, and even develops your intuitive faculty (your sixth sense). Most significantly, Yoga puts you in touch with the spiritual reality that is the source of your everyday mind and awareness.

Yoga Can Be Combined with Other Disciplines

Although Yoga is complete in itself, you can easily combine it with any kind of sports or physical workout, including aerobics and weightlifting. You also can practice Yoga in conjunction with any existing mental discipline, including mnemonics (memorization) and chess. Not only is Yoga compatible in all cases, but it's also bound to improve your performance.

Yoga Is Easy and Convenient

Yoga doesn't require you to work up a sweat (unless you are practicing some modern aerobic-type Yoga). You can always look pretty cool! You can practice Yoga in the comfort of your own home. In fact, you can practice Yoga anywhere. Although you don't need to spend time traveling from place to place, beginners in particular should consider joining a Yoga class — even your trip there and back offers opportunities for a Yoga experience. Yoga creates rather than consumes time — a major benefit in the busy and stressed lives of Westerners! Moreover, Yoga is pain-free. In fact, Yoga helps overcome all forms of suffering (see Chapter 18).

Yoga Is Liberating

Yoga can put you more in touch with your true nature, giving you a sense of fulfillment, inner worth, and confidence. By assisting you in reducing egotism and negative thoughts and emotions, Yoga has the power to bring you closer to lasting happiness. It builds your willpower and puts you in charge of your own life.

Appendix

Additional Yoga Resources

· ·

Discovering Yoga Organizations

In Chapter 23, we give you our choice of the top ten Yoga places to check out. Here are additional names and addresses to help you with your explorations.

Yoga therapy and psychospiritual healing

Healing Buddha Foundation, directed by Lama Segyu Choepel Rinpoche, is a Tibetan Buddhist Yoga Center, which operates psychospiritual healing clinics that handle difficult cases of spiritual emergency, including *kundalini* problems (see Chapter 1).

> P.O. Box 87, Sebastopol, CA 95472;. phone 707-823-8700; fax 707-823-8787; e-mail buddhaheal@aol.com; Web site members.aol.com/buddhaheal/

International Association of Yoga Therapists, founded in 1979 by Larry Payne, Ph.D., and Richard Miller, Ph.D., has 1,000 members and publishes an annual journal (see the "Peeking into Periodicals" section later in this appendix).

> P.O. Box 1386, Lower Lake, CA 95457; phone 707-928-9898; fax 707-928-4738; e-mail mail@yogaresearchcenter.org (see the "Topnotch Web Sites" section, later in this appendix, for Web site address and details).

Maui School of Yoga Therapy, directed by Gary and Mirka Kraftsow, offers classes and personal sessions, as well as retreats and training programs in Yoga therapy in the Viniyoga style.

> P.O. Box 1662, Kahului, HI 96733; phone 808-572-1414; fax 808-572-5775; e-mail info@viniyoga.com; Web site www/viniyoga.com/

Phoenix Rising Yoga Therapy, founded and directed by Michael Lee, offers a range of classes and workshops, as well as teacher training.

> P.O. Box 819, Housatonic, MA 01236; phone 800-288-9642 or 413-274-6166; Web site www.pryt.com/

Stanford Yoga, directed by Yelena Fedotova, Ph.D. since 1997, offers Iyengar-style Yoga therapy classes in Stanford, California for chronic and acute ailments.

> Phone 650-329-0400; e-mail yelena@ionix.net; Web site www.stanfys.com

Yoga for Health Foundation, directed by Howard Kent, is internationally known as a residential Yoga center with a full program for the fit and the chronically disabled.

> Ickwell Bury, Biggleswade, Bedfordshire SG18 9EF, Great Britain; phone 01767-627271

Teacher training and academic programs

In addition to the teacher training programs listed in Chapter 23, we recommend that you check out the following organizations:

American Sanskrit Institute, directed by Vyaas Houston, offers extensive courses in the Sanskrit language, including immersion trainings, and also has audiotapes and CDs available.

> 73 Four Corners Road, Warwick, NY 10990; phone 914-986-8652; fax 914-987-7097

American Institute of Vedic Studies, directed by Dr. David Frawley (Vamadeva Shastri), offers in-depth correspondence courses on Yoga, Vedas, and Ayurveda.

> P.O. Box 8357, Santa Fe, NM 87504; phone 505-983-9385

International Yoga Studies, founded and directed by Sandra Summerfield Kozak, offers a well-rounded teacher training program based on the standards developed by the European Union of Yoga.

> 13833 South 31st Place, Phoenix, AZ 85048; phone 602-759-1972

Integrative Yoga Therapy, founded and directed by Joseph LePage, consists of a professional training program bridging the insights of Yoga and the latest advances in mind-body healing. IYT also offers advanced and continuing training for its graduates.

> 2975 Pacific Heights Drive, Aptos, CA 95003; phone 408-688-9642 or 800-750-9642; e-mail iyt@cruzio.com; Web site www.cruzio.com/~iyt

Corporate Yoga

Clarity Seminars, operated by David and Karen Gamow, offers corporate training in meditation and stress reduction. Their clients include NASA, IBM, and the U.S. Army.

> 240 Monroe Drive, Suite 215, Mountain View, CA 94040; phone 650-917-1186; e-mail: dkgamow@jps.net; Web site: http://www.jps.net/dkgamow/clarity.htm

Yoga research organizations

Guru Ram Das Center for Medicine and Humanology, directed by Shanti Shanti Kaur Khalsa, Ph.D., offers healing classes and courses in all aspects of Kundini Yoga and Humanology. Specializing in life-threatening illness, HIV, and cancer, the Center also serves as a resource for books, audios, and videos.

> P1114 N. Riverside Drive #184, Espanola, NM 87532; phone 505-995-2086 or 800-326-1322; e-mail Healthnow@grdcenter.org.

Kaivalyadhama, founded in 1925 by Swami Kuvalayananda and today directed by Dr. M. V. Bhole, is one of the more important Yoga research and educational organizations, which publishes Indology books and the quarterly research journal *Yoga Mimamsa.*

> 117 Valvan, Lonavla (Dist. Pune), Maharashtra 404 403, India

Yoga Biomedical Trust, directed by Robin Monro, Ph.D. since he founded the organization in 1983, explores the therapeutic applications of Yoga and publishes a quarterly newsletter and research reports. The Trust also offers Yoga and therapy classes, teacher training courses, and Yoga therapy diploma courses.

> 60 Great Ormand Street, London WC1N, Great Britain; phone 0171-419-7195; fax 0171-419-7196

Yoga Institute of Santacruz, founded in 1918 by Shri Yogendra, offers a rich program of practical and theoretical classes, Yoga camps for the chronically sick, and a teacher training course. The institute also publishes the monthly magazine *Yoga and Total Health* (see the "Peeking into Periodicals" section, later in this appendix).

Santacruz East, Shri Yogendra Marg, Prabhat Colony, Mumbai (Bombay) 400 055, India; phone 6110506 and 6122185; Web site www.geocities.com/athens/6709/

Yoga Research Center, directed by Georg Feuerstein, Ph.D., is dedicated to research and education on all branches and aspects of Hindu, Buddhist, and Jaina Yoga. Publishes a quarterly newsletter and other publications.

P.O. Box 1386, Lower Lake, CA 95457; phone 707-929-9898; fax 707-928-4738; e-mail mail@yogaresearchcenter.org (see the "Topnotch Web Sites" section, later in this appendix, for Web site address and details).

Other Significant Organizations in the United States and Canada

Astanga Yoga, directed by Beryl Bender Birch and Thom Birch, offers Power Yoga — an athletic and precision approach to Hatha Yoga.

325 East 41st Street, Suite 203, New York, NY 10017; phone 212-661-2895

Massachusetts New England Yoga Alliance, directed by Pat Burke, has a membership of 200 Yoga teachers. The Alliance publishes a newsletter for members and an annual Yoga Teacher Directory, and operates a referral service.

186 Main Street #14, Marlboro, MA 01752;.phone 508-480-8884; e-mail esyoga@aol.com; Web site www.newellness.com/neyoga/

Nityananda Institute, directed by Swami Chetanananda, operates a full service Yoga center and is one of the larger independent publishers of Yoga-related books, tapes, and videos in the United States.

P.O. Box 13390, Portland, OR 97213; phone 503-235-0175; fax 503-235-0909

White Lotus Foundation, established in 1967 and codirected by Ganga White and Tracey Rich, offers a synthesis of classical and contemporary styles of Yoga as well as teacher training programs and retreats.

2500 San Marcos Pass, Santa Barbara, CA 93105; phone 805-964-1944

Yasodhara Ashram Yoga Study and Retreat Centre, founded over 35 years ago by the late Swami Sivananda Radha, offers Yoga workshops and retreats aimed at personal and spiritual growth.

P.O. Box 9, Kootenay Bay, British Columbia V0B 1X0, Cananda; phone 800-661-8711 or 250-227-9224; fax: 250-227-9494; e-mail: yashram@netidea.com; Web site www.yasodhara.org/

Major overseas organizations

Here we bring you a selection of leading Yoga organizations outside the United States; these sources can refer you to teachers during your overseas travels.

Europe

The British Wheel of Yoga, founded in 1965, has around 4,000 Yoga teachers as members. It publishes *Spectrum* magazine (see the "Periodicals" section, later in this appendix).

> 1 Hamilton Place, Boston Road, Sleaford, Lincs NG34 7ES; phone 01529-306851; fax: 01529-303233; e-mail wheelyoga@aol.com.uk; Web site http://members.aol.com.wheelyoga

Life Foundation, a large, full-service Yoga and humanitarian organization dedicated to preserving the principles of Dru Yoga through international peace walks, a cancer center, and therapeutics; maintains a large selection of books, audios, and videos. Founder: Dr. Manushkh Patel.

> Maristow House, Dover Street, Bilston, W. Midlands, North Wales, WV145A; phone 01902-409164; fax 01902-497362; Web site www.nwl.co.uk/life

Weg Der Mitte, founded by Daya Mullins, Ph.D. Yoga teacher and holistic practioner certification courses. Located in Berlin with a retreat center in Gerode.

> Mill Str. 35 D-14169, Berlin, Germany; phone 011-49-30-813-1040; fax 011-49-30-813-8281; e-mail Berlin@wegdermitte.de; Web site www.wegdermitte.de

Latin America

Indra Devi Foundation, founded by David Lifar, is the largest Hatha Yoga center in South America, with over 2,000 students per week in 3 locations. It has a newsletter and teacher-training programs.

> Azuenaga 762, Buenos Aires, Argentina 1029; phone 54-1-962-3142

Latin American Union of Yoga, founded in 1985 and today directed by Liliana Tagliaferri, organizes annual Yoga conferences and, in particular, promotes artistic and Olympic Yoga sports. It also publishes *Yoga Sports Journal.*

> San Luis 3369, (7660) Mar del Plata, Pcia de Buenas Aires, Argentina; phone 5423-923303; fax 5423-756555; e-mail matcomp@statics.com.ar; Web site www.sportscenter.com.ar/

Australia and New Zealand

International Yoga Teachers Association, directed by Susan Kirkham, has a membership of several hundred Yoga teachers in New Zealand and Australia and offers teacher-training courses. The Association publishes a quarterly newsletter for members.

> 35 Ranelagh Street, Karori, Wellington 5, New Zealand; phone 04-476-4337; fax 04-476-0317; e-mail kirkham@actrix.gen.nz

The Meditation Institute, directed by Shanti Gowans, offers spiritually based classes on Hatha Yoga, meditation, and yogic philosophy, as well as retreats.

> P.O. Box 3512, Southport, Queensland, Australia 4215; phone 07-5531-6593; fax 07-5592-0592

India

Bihar School of Yoga, founded in 1963 and today directed by Swami Niranjananda Sarasvati, is today acknowledged for its high standards of teacher training and advanced programs, especially in Kriya Yoga and Kundalini Yoga. It also has a Yoga university.

> Ganga Darshan, Munger 811 201, Bihar, India; phone 06344-22430; fax: 06344-20169

Gitananda Ashram, established by the late Dr. Swami Gitananda Giri and presently headed by Meenakshi Devi, is a very active school with many programs, including a correspondence course, and the monthly magazine *Yoga Life* (see the "Peeking into Periodicals" section, later in this appendix).

16-A Mattu Street, Chinnamudaliarchavady, Kottakuppam (via Pondicherry), Tamil Nadu 605 104, India

Krishnamacharya Yoga Mandiram, founded by T.K.V. Desikachar (the son of Krishnamacharya), preserves the rich heritage of the late Yoga Master Professor Sri T. Krishnamacharya. It offers training programs and Yoga therapy classes, as well as publications.

13,4th Cross Street, Ramakrishnanagar, Madras, India 7998; phone 91-44-493-7998

Ramamani Iyengar Memorial Yoga Institute, founded and directed by B. K. S. Iyengar, is the hub of the world's most widespread style of Hatha Yoga — Iyengar Yoga. The Institute has trained thousands of Yoga teachers.

1107-B/1, Shivajinagar, Pune 411 016, India

Tapping into Yoga Props

We discuss the use of props in Chapter 17. Here are some addresses to help acquaint you with the possibilities. Also, *Yoga Journal* is an excellent source for companies specializing in Yoga props, such as mats, blocks, and straps, as well as outfits, and so on.

Body Slant: Gravity inversion tool invented by Larry Jacobs, founder and director of Age in Reverse Inc., P.O. Box 1667, Newport Beach, CA 92663; phone 800-443-3917.

Eye Bags (Relaxation in a Bag): Founded by Shelly Greenberg, offers relaxation and Yoga props, plus T-shirts. 7603 Granada Drive, Bethesda, MD 20817; phone 888-MRE-YOGA; e-mail info@moreyoga.com; Web site www.moreyoga.com.

Harmony screens: Nonelectronic relaxation devices available from Yoga Research Center. For address, see the "Yoga research organizations" section, earlier in this appendix.

Hugger Mugger: Yoga props and products, including mats, bolsters, blocks, straps, and Yoga clothing. Founded by Sarah Chambers. 31 W. Gregson Ave, Salt Lake City, UT 84115; phone 800-473-4888.

Invertebod: Inversion device invented by Leroy R. Perry D.C, founder and director of International Sports Medicine Institute. Inquiries to Brilhante, 3283 Motor Ave, West Los Angeles, CA 90034; phone 800-Bad-Back or 223-2225.

Checking Out Top-notch Web Sites

Yoga's presence on the Internet is growing rapidly. Here are some excellent sites for you to visit. Most of them contain links to other sites.

Hindu Tantrik Homepage. A fine Tantra site maintained by Michael Magee, translator of several Sanskrit texts. www.hubcom.com/tantric/

Samata Yoga Center. Web site of Larry Payne's User Friendly Yoga Program. Includes color photos of annual retreats, videos, audios, and books. www.samata.com/

Sivananda Om Page. Maintained by the organization of Swami Vishnudevananda, this award-winning site has over 100 pages and 170 graphics. www.sivananda.org/misc/faq/faq.htm

Yoga Research Center. This is a good first site to visit. It contains numerous articles on various (theoretical and practical) aspects of Yoga and has many links to other sites on Yoga, Hinduism, and Buddhism. `www.yogaresearchcenter.org`

Yoga Teacher Directory. A list of names and addresses of participating Yoga teachers in the United States. `www.yogasite.com/teachers.html`

Lingering at the Yoga Library

The following resources are among the better books available today on Yoga and Yoga-related topics. They represent a small selection from a huge body of literature. If you have Internet access, check out the long list of Yoga books available on `amazon.com`.

Reference works

The Shambhala Encyclopedia of Yoga by Georg Feuerstein. Boston, MA: Shambhala Publications, 1997 — This award-winning illustrated work contains over 2,000 entries.

The Yoga Tradition: Its History, Literature, Philosophy, and Practice by Georg Feuerstein, Prescott, AZ: Hohm Press, 1998 — With its 720 pages and numerous illustrations, this is the most comprehensive overview of the Yoga tradition available today.

General introductions (with a traditional orientation)

The Shambhala Guide to Yoga, by Georg Feuerstein, Boston, MA: Shambhala Publications, 1996.

The Tree of Yoga, by B.K.S. Iyengar, Boston, MA: Shambhala Publications, 1989.

Hatha Yoga (beginners and advanced)

The Breathing Book: Good Health and Vitality Through Essential Breath Work by Donna Farhi, New York, NY: Henry Holt, 1996.

Hatha Yoga: The Hidden Language by Swami Sivananda Radha, Porthill, ID: Timeless Books, 1987.

The Heart of Yoga: Developing a Personal Practice by T. K. V Desikachar. Rochester, VT: Inner Traditions, 1995 — The authoritative book on the Viniyoga approach to Hatha Yoga.

Light on Pranayama: The Yogic Art of Breathing by B. K. S. Iyengar, New York, NY: Crossroad, 1985.

Light on Yoga by B. K. S. Iyengar, New York, NY: Schocken Books, 1966.

The New Yoga for People Over 50 by Suza Francina, Deerfield Beach, FL: Health Communications, 1997.

Philosophy of Hatha Yoga by Usharbudh Arya, Honesdale, PA: Himalayan International Institute, 1988.

Power Yoga: The Total Strength and Flexibility Workout by Beryl Bender Birch, New York, NY: Fireside Books, 1995 — A manual for more athletic practitioners.

Relax and Renew: Restful Yoga for Stressful Times by Judith Lasater, Berkeley, CA: Rodmell Press, 1995.

A Systematic Course in the Ancient Tantric Techniques of Yoga and Kriya by Swami Satyananda Saraswati, Monghyr, India, Bihar School of Yoga, 1981 — This voluminous manual is available in the United States through `amazon.com`.

Yoga for Body, Breath, and Mind: A Guide to Personal Reintegration by A. G. Mohan, Portland, OR: Rudra Press,1993.

Yoga: The Spirit and Practice of Moving Into Stillness by Erich Schiffman, New York, NY: Pocket Books, 1996.

Yoga for Your Life: A Practice Manual of Breath and Movement for Every Body by Margaret and Martin Pierce, Portland, OR: Rudra Press, 1996.

Raja Yoga (classical Yoga)

The Essence of Yoga by Bernard Bouanchaud, Portland, OR: Rudra Press, 1997.

Raja-Yoga by Swami Vivekananda, New York, NY: Ramakrishna-Vivekananda Center, 1982.

The Yoga-Sutra of Patanjali: A New Translation and Commentary by Georg Feuerstein, Rochester, VT: Inner Traditions, 1989.

Jnana Yoga

Jnana-Yoga by Swami Vivekananda, New York, NY: Ramakrishna-Vivekananda Center, 1982.

Ramana Maharshi and the Path of Self-Knowledge by Arthur Osborne, York Beach, ME: Samuel Weiser, 1995.

Bhakti Yoga and Karma Yoga

Karma-Yoga and Bhakti-Yoga by Swami Vivekananda, New York, NY: Ramakrishna-Vivekananda Center, 1982.

The Yoga of Spiritual Devotion: A Modern Translation of the Narada Bhakti Sutras by Prem Prakash, Rochester, VT: Inner Traditions International, 1998.

Tantra and Kundalini Yoga

Energies of Transformation: A Guide to the Kundalini Process by Bonnie Greenwell, Saratoga, CA: Shakti River Press, 1995.

The Kundalini Experience: Psychosis or Transcendence? by Lee Sannella, Lower Lake, CA: Integral Publishing, 1992.

Kundalini Yoga for the West by Swami Sivananda Radha, Spokane, WA: Timeless Books, 1978.

Layayoga: An Advanced Method of Concentration by Shyam Sundar Goswami, Rochester, VT: Inner Traditions International, 1999 — The single most comprehensive work on Laya Yoga and Kundalini Yoga, based on and containing numerous quotations from the Hindu scriptures.

Living With Kundalini: The Autobiography of Gopi Krishna ed. Leslie Shepard, Boston, MA: Shambhala Publications, 1993.

The Serpent Power by John Woodroffe (Arthur Avalon), Mandras, India: Ganesh & Co., 1974 — Available in the United States through amazon.com.

Tantra: The Path of Ecstasy by Georg Feuerstein, Boston, MA: Shambhala Publications, 1998.

Meditation, mantras, and prayer

Healing Words by Larry Dossey, San Francisco, CA: HarperSanFrancisco, 1993.

Mantra & Meditation by Usharbudh Arya, Honesdale, PA: Himalayan International Institute, 1981.

Meditation For Dummies by Stephan Bodian, Foster City, CA: IDG Books Worldwide, Inc., 1998.

Somatics and Somatic Yoga

How Yoga Works: An Introduction to Somatic Yoga by Eleanor Criswell, Novato, CA: Freeperson Press, 1989.

Somatics: Reawakening the Mind's Control of Movement, Flexibility, and Health by Thomas Hanna, Reading, MA: Addison-Wesley, 1988.

Yoga therapy

Phoenix Rising Yoga Therapy: A Bridge from Body to Soul by Michael Lee, Deerfield Beach, FL: Health Communications, 1997.

Yoga for Common Ailments by Robin Munro, R. Nagarathna, and H. R. Nagendra, New York, NY: Simon & Schuster, 1990.

Yoga and wellness

Ancient Insights for Modern Healing by Gary Kraftsow, New York, NY: Penguin, forthcoming 1999 — a comprehensive work on Yoga therapy based on the Viniyoga approach of T. K. V. Desikachar.

Diet and health

Eat More, Weigh Less: Dr. Dean Ornish's Life Choice Program for Losing Weight Safely While Eating Abundantly by Dean Ornish, New York, NY: Harper Mass Market Paperbacks, 1997.

Everyday Cooking With Dr. Dean Ornish: 150 Easty, Low-Fat, High-Flavor Recipes by Dean Ornish, New York, NY: HarperCollins, 1997.

Full Catastrophe Living: Using the Wisdom of Your Body and Mind to Face Stress, Pain and Illness by Jon Kabat-Zinn, New York, NY: Delta Books (Dell Publishing), 1990.

McDougall's Medicine: A Challenging Second Opinion by John McDougall, Piscataway, N.J: New Century Publishers, 1985.

The McDougall Program: Twelve Days to Dynamic Health by John McDougall, New York, NY: NAL Books, 1990.

Meaning and Medicine: A Doctor's Tales of Breakthroughs and Healings by Larry Dossey, New York, NY: Bantam Books, 1991.

The Yoga of Nutrition by Omraam Mikhael Aivanhov, Fréjus, France: Prosveta, 1982 — Available in the United States.

Ayurveda and herbs

Ayurveda: A Life of Balance — The Complete Guide to Ayurvedic Nutrition & Body Types with Recipes by Maya Tiwari, Rochester, VT: Healing Arts Press, 1995.

Ayurvedic Healing: A Comprehensive Guide by David Frawley, Salt Lake City, UT: Passage Press, 1989.

Ayurveda and the Mind: The Healing of Consciousness by David Frawley, Twin Lakes, WI: Lotus Press, 1997.

The Yoga of Herbs: An Ayurvedic Guide to Herbal Medicine by David Frawley and Vasant Lad, Santa Fe, NM: Lotus Press, 1988.

Sexuality and spirituality

The Alchemy of Love and Sex by Lee Lozowick, Prescott, AZ: Hohm Press, 1996.

The Little Book for Lovers by Dana Goodwin, Rockport, MA: Element Books, 1995.

Passions of Innocence: Tantric Celibacy and the Mysteries of Eros by Stuart Sovatsky, Rochester, VT: Destiny Books, 1994.

Sacred Sexuality by Georg Feuerstein, Los Angeles, CA: J. P. Tarcher, 1993.

Sex and Yoga by Nancy Phelan and Michael Volin, New York, NY: Harper & Row, 1967.

Sexual Secrets by Nik Douglas and Penny Slinger, New York, NY: Destiny Books, 1979.

Inspirational Yoga literature

Autobiography of a Yogi by Paramahamsa Yogananda, Los Angeles, CA: Self-Realization Fellowship, 1987. Another edition by Crystal Clarity in Nevada City, CA, 1987.

Daughter of Fire by Irina Tweedie, Nevada City, CA: Blue Dolphin Press, 1986.

Masters of Mahamudra by Keith Dowman, Albany, NY: SUNY Press, 1985.

The Notebooks of Paul Brunton by Paul Brunton, Burdett, NY: Larson Publications, 1984-99, 16 volumes.

Play of Consciousness by Swami Muktananda, San Francisco, CA: Harper & Row, 1978.

Sanskrit classics on Yoga

The Bhagavad Gita by Winthrop Sargeant, Albany, NY: SUNY Press, 1984.

The Concise Yoga Vasiṣṭha by Swami Venkatesananda, Albany, NY: SUNY Press, 1984.

God Talks with Arjuna: The Bhagavad Gita by Paramahansa Yogananda, Los Angeles, CA: Self-Realization Fellowship, 1995, 2 volumes.

Teachings of Yoga by Georg Feuerstein, Boston, MA: Shambhala Publications, 1997.

Upaniṣads by Patrick Olivelle, London: Allen & Unwin, 1932.

General Yoga topics

The Art of Positive Feeling by Swami Jyotirmayananda, South Miami, FL: Yoga Research Foundation, 1997.

Dancing with Śiva: Hinduism's Contemporary Catechism by Satguru Sivaya Subramuniyaswami, Concord, CA: Himalayan Academy, 1996 — an excellent starting point for Yoga students who want to explore Hinduism.

The Future of the Body: Explorations Into the Further Evolution of Human Nature by Michael Murphy, Los Angeles, CA: Jeremy Tarcher, 1992 — The author, cofounder of the Esalen Institute, offers a vast amount of information about the extraordinary potential of the human body-mind.

Golden Rules for Everyday Life by Omraam Mikhaël Aïvanhov, Fréjus, France, Prosveta: 1990 — Available in the United States.

Health, Healing and Beyond: Yoga and the Living Tradition of Krishnamacharya. T.K.V. Desikachar (contributor), R.H. Cravens, 1998.

Lucid Dreaming by Stephen LaBerge, New York, NY: Ballentine, 1985.

Lucid Waking: Mindfulness and the Spiritual Potential of Humanity by Georg Feuerstein, Rochester, VT: Inner Traditions International, 1997.

The Mystery of Light: The Life and Teaching of Omraam Mikhaël Aïvanhov by Georg Feuerstein, Lower Lake, CA: Integral Publishing, 1998.

The Nine Stages of Spiritual Apprenticeship: Understanding the Student-Teacher Relationship by Greg Bogart, Berkeley, CA: Dawn Mountain Press, 1997 — An excellent balanced discussion about teachers and disciples from a psychological and spiritual perspective.

The Relaxation Response by Herbert Benson, New York, NY: Avon Books, 1976.

The Tibetan Book of Living and Dying. Sogyal Rinpoche et al, San Francisco, CA: HarperSanFrancisco, 1992 — A beautiful and helpful book on the almost forgotten art of dying with mature awareness.

A Year to Live: How to Live this Year As If It Were Your Last by Stephen Levine, New York, NY: Bell Tower, 1997 — An important practical book for those taking the inevitability of death seriously.

Yoga of the Heart by Alice Christensen, New York, NY: Daybreak Books (Rodale Press), 1998 — One of few books to deal with the moral principles of Yoga.

Peeking into Periodicals

Here are the names and addresses of the better-known periodicals dealing with Yoga from various points of view. Although certainly not exhaustive, the list can give you a start in the right direction.

Hinduism Today: A monthly magazine for students of Yoga and Hinduism.

> Himalayan Academy, 107 Kaholalele Road, Kapaa, HI 96746-9304

*International Journal of Yoga Therapy (*formerly *Journal of the International Association of Yoga Therapists):* An annual journal for professionals interested in the restorative applications of Yoga.

> Yoga Research Center, P.O. Box 1386, Lower Lake, CA 95457

Mountain Path: A monthly magazine by students of Ramana Maharshi's Jnana Yoga.

> Sri Ramanasramam, P.O. [note to readers: no box number], Tiruvannamalai 606 603, India

Yoga & Health: A monthly magazine.

> Yoga & Health, 21 Caburn Crescent, Lewes, East Sussex BN 7 1NR, Great Britain

Yoga and Total Health: A monthly magazine published by the Yoga Institute of Santacruz.

> Santacruz East, Shri Yogendra Marg, Prabhat Colony, Mumbai (Bombay) 400 055, India

Yoga International. A bimonthly magazine.

> Himalayan International Institute, RR1, Box 407, Honesdale, PA 18431

Yoga Journal:. The most widely distributed (bimonthly) magazine on Yoga in the world.

> Yoga Journal, 2054 University Avenue, Berkeley, CA: 94704

Yoga Life: A monthly magazine published by Swami Gitananda's school.

> Yoga Life, c/o ICYER, 16-A Mattu Street, Chinnamudaliarchavady, Kottakuppam (via Pondicherry), Tamil Nadu 605 104, India

Yoga Rahasya. A quarterly magazine dedicated to the teachings of B. K. S. Iyengar.

> IYNAUS, c/o Laura Allard, 1420 Hawthorne Avenue, Boulder, CO 80304; or Yoga Rahasya, c/o Sam N. Motiwala, Palia Mansion, 622 Lady Jehangir Road, Dadar, Mumbai 400 014, India

Yoga World A quarterly newsletter for teachers and students, edited by Georg Feuerstein, Richard Rosen, and Richard Miller.

> Yoga Research Center, P.O. Box 1386, Lower Lake, CA 95457

Hearing All the Latest on Audio- and Videotapes

Many Yoga teachers have produced their own audio- and videotapes, of varying quality. Here we bring you a small selection of those tapes that we have listened to or watched and can recommend (including our own!). For a long list of available tapes, visit amazon.com online.

Audiotapes

Basic Daily Routine by John Schumacher

The Business of Teaching Yoga by Larry Payne

Healthy Back Exercises for High Stress Professionals by Larry Payne

Introducing Yoga: Its Purpose and Approaches by Georg Feuerstein

Meditation: An Invitation to Inner Growth by Swami Chetanananda

Relax with Yoga during Pregnancy by Leslie Goldstein

Rest, Relax, and Sleep by Lilias Folan

Spiritual Growth through Yoga by Georg Feuerstein

User Friendly Yoga, Levels 1 and 2 by Larry Payne

User Friendly Back Yoga by Larry Payne

Yoga in the Land of Oz by Georg Feuerstein; released by Yoga Research Center

Videotapes

Hatha Yoga and meditation

Easy Yoga for Seniors: The Self-Help method to a Healthier Mind and Body by Pat Laster

Forever Flexible: The Easy Stretching Program for a More Vital You by Lilias Folan

Gentle Yoga: For the Physically Challenged by Margot Kitchen

Kathy Smith's New Yoga: A Yoga workout for levels 1 and 2 by Kathy Smith with Rod Stryker

Kripalu Yoga/Dynamic: A full, extended dynamic Yoga experience with Stephen Cope

Kripalu Yoga/Gentle: A distinct approach to gentle Yoga experience with Carolyn Lundeen (Sudha)

Lilias! Alive with Yoga: Beginner by Lilias Folan

Lilias! Alive with Yoga: Intermediate by Lilias Folan

Total Yoga: A flowing workout sequence with beginner and intermediate segments by Ganga White and Tracey Rich

User Friendly Yoga: A safe program for beginners and advanced beginners by Larry Payne

User Friendly Back Yoga: A proven program for preventing back problems by Larry Payne

Yoga Alignment and Form: A presentation of alignment and form for all levels with John Friend

Yoga Breathing and Relaxation by Richard Freeman

Yoga for Meditators: An effective video for meditators and yogins by John Friend

Yoga for the Young at Heart: Gentle Stretching Exercises for Seniors by Susan Winter Ward

A series of Yoga videos produced for beginners by LIVING ARTS in conjunction with the *Yoga Journal:*

Yoga for Beginners by Patricia Walden

Yoga for Energy by Rodney Yee

Yoga for Flexibility by Paticia Walden

Yoga for Kids with Marsha Wenig

Yoga for Meditation by Rodney Yee

Yoga for Relaxation with Patricia Walden

Yoga for Strength by Rodney Yee

Spiritual teachers

For fine videotapes of spiritual teachers like Ramana Maharshi, Ramakrishna, Nisargadatta Maharaj, and Anandamayi Ma, we can heartily recommend the *Inner Directions Catalog* (which also includes books).

> Inner Directions, P.O. Box 231486, Encinitas, CA: 92023; phone 760-599-4075; fax 760-599-4076

Index

Notes

Notes

Notes

Notes

Notes

Notes

Notes

Notes